Dictionary of Cognitive Science

Neuroscience, Psychology, Artificial Intelligence, Linguistics, and Philosophy

Olivier Houdé, Editor
with
Daniel Kayser, Olivier Koenig,
Joëlle Proust, François Rastier

Vivian Waltz, Translator
Christian Cavé, Scientific Advisor

PSYCHOLOGY PRESS
New York and Hove

Published in 2004 by
Psychology Press, LTD.
29 West 35th Street
New York, NY 10001
www.psypress.com

Published in Great Britain by
Psychology Press, LTD.
27 Church Road
Hove, East Sussex
BN3 2FA

Psychology Press, LTD., is an imprint of the Taylor & Francis Group.
Printed in the United States of America on acid-free paper.

Originally published as *Vocabulaire de sciences cognitives: Neuroscience, psychologie, intelligence artificielle, linguistique et philosophie,* edited by Olivier Houdé, Daniel Kayser, Olivier Koenig, Joëlle Proust, François Rastier.
© Presses Universitaires de France, 1998

Published with the participation of the *Ministère français chargé de la Culture – Centre National du Livre* (French Ministry of Culture – National Book Center).

10 9 8 7 6 5 4 3 2 1

Library of Congress Cataloging-in-Publication Data

Vocabulaire de sciences cognitives. English.
  Dictionary of cognitive science : neuroscience, psychology, artificial intelligence, linguistics, and philosophy / Olivier Houdé, editor, with Daniel Kayser ... [et al.] ; Vivian Waltz, translator ; Christian Cavé, scientific advisor.
      p. cm.
Includes bibliographical references and index.
  ISBN 1-57958-251-6
1. Cognitive science—Dictionaries.   I. Houdé, Olivier. II. Title.
  BF311.V56713 2003
  153'.03—dc21
                                            2003011554

Dictionary of
Cognitive Science

Editor

OLIVIER HOUDÉ   Professor, Université Paris 5-René Descartes; member, Institut Universitaire de France, Groupe d'Imagerie Neurofonctionnelle (GIN), Centre National de la Recherche Scientifique (CNRS), Commissariat à l'Énergie Atomique (CEA), Université de Caen, and Université Paris 5. (Psychology)

Section Editors

DANIEL KAYSER   Professor, Université Paris 13, France. (Artificial Intelligence)

OLIVIER KOENIG   Professor, Université Lyon 2; member, Institut Universitaire de France. (Neuroscience)

JOËLLE PROUST   Director of Research, Centre National de la Recherche Scientifique (CNRS), Institut Jean Nicod, Paris, France. (Philosophy)

FRANÇOIS RASTIER   Director of Research, Centre National de la Recherche Scientifique (CNRS), Models, dynamics, corpora, Université Paris 10, France. (Linguistics)

Contributors

ANNE ABEILLÉ   Professor, Université Paris 7; member, Institut Universitaire de France. (Linguistics)

CLAUDE BASTIEN   Professor, Université Aix-Marseille 1, Aix-en-Provence, France. (Psychology)

JANINE BEAUDICHON   Professor Emerita, Université Paris 5, France. (Psychology)

JOSIE BERNICOT   Professor, Université de Poitiers, France. (Psychology)

CLAUDE BONNET   Professor, Université Louis Pasteur, Strasbourg, France. (Psychology)

PAUL BOURGINE   Research Engineer, Centre National de la Recherche Scientifique (CNRS), Centre de Recherche en Épistémologie Appliquée (CREA), Paris, France. (Artificial Intelligence)

JEAN-FRANÇOIS CAMUS   Professor, Université de Reims, France. (Psychology)

ROBERTO CASATI   Director of Research, Centre National de la Recherche Scientifique (CNRS), Institut Jean Nicod, Paris, France. (Philosophy)

MICHEL CHAROLLES   Professor, Université Paris 3, France. (Linguistics)

BERNARD CROISILLE   M.D., Hôpital Neurologique, Lyon, France. (Neuroscience)

PHILIPPE DAGUE   Professor, Université Paris 13, France.

JEAN DECÉTY   Director of Research, Institut National de la Santé et de la Recherche Médicale (INSERM), Unit 280, Lyon, France; Professor, University of Washington. (Neuroscience)

STANISLAS DEHAENE   Director of Research, Institut National de la Santé et de la Recherche Médicale (INSERM), Unit 562, Service Hospitalier Frédéric Joliot, Orsay, France. (Neuroscience)

MICHEL DENIS   Director of Research, Centre National de la Recherche Scientifique (CNRS), Vulnerability, adaptation, and psychopathology, Hôpital Pitié-Salpêtrière, Paris, France. (Psychology)

JÉRÔME DOKIC   Master Lecturer, Université de Rouen, France. (Philosophy)

PASCAL ENGEL   Professor, Université Paris 4; member, Institut Universitaire de France. (Philosophy)

MICHEL FAYOL   Professor, Université de Clermont-Ferrand, France. (Psychology)

JACQUES FERBER   Professor, Université Montpellier 2, France. (Artificial Intelligence)

JEAN-MICHEL FORTIS   Researcher, Centre National de la Recherche Scientifique (CNRS), History of linguistic theory, Université Paris 7, France. (Linguistics)

BERNARD FRADIN   Director of Research, Centre National de la Recherche Scientifique (CNRS), Formal linguistics, Université Paris 7, France. (Linguistics)

JACQUES FRANÇOIS	Professor, Université de Caen, France. (Linguistics)
JEAN-GABRIEL GANASCIA	Professor, Université Paris 6, France. (Artificial Intelligence)
DANIEL GAONAC'H	Professor, Université de Poitiers, France. (Psychology)
MALIK GHALLAB	Director of Research, Centre National de la Recherche Scientifique (CNRS), Laboratoire d'Analyse et architecture des Systèmes (LAAS), Toulouse, France. (Artificial Intelligence)
JEAN-ÉMILE GOMBERT	Professor, Université Rennes 2, France. (Psychology)
LAURENT GOSSELIN	Professor, Université de Rouen, France. (Linguistics)
JEAN-PAUL HATON	Professor, Université Nancy 1; member, Institut Universitaire de France. (Artificial Intelligence)
YVETTE HATWELL	Professor Emerita, Université Grenoble 2, France. (Psychology)
MAYA HICKMANN	Director of Research, Centre National de la Recherche Scientifique (CNRS), Cognition and development, Université Paris 5, France. (Psychology)
OLIVIER HOUDÉ	Professor, Université Paris 5; member, Institut Universitaire de France. (Psychology)
PIERRE JACOB	Director of Research, Centre National de la Recherche Scientifique (CNRS), Institut Jean Nicod, Paris, France. (Philosophy)
DANIEL KAYSER	Professor, Université Paris 13, France. (Artificial Intelligence)
MAX KISTLER	Master Lecturer, Université de Clermont-Ferrand, France. (Philosophy)
OLIVIER KOENIG	Professor, Université Lyon 2; member, Institut Universitaire de France. (Neuroscience)
JACQUES LAUTREY	Professor Emeritus, Université Paris 5, France. (Psychology)
PIERRE LIVET	Professor, Université Aix-Marseille 1, Aix-en-Provence, France. (Philosophy)
TODD LUBART	Master Lecturer, Université Paris 5, France. (Psychology)
ANNE-MARIE MELOT	Researcher, Centre National de la Recherche Scientifique (CNRS), Groupe d'Imagerie Neurofonctionnelle, Université de Caen and Université Paris 5, France. (Psychology)
JACQUES MOESCHLER	Professor, Université de Genève, Switzerland. (Linguistics)
LORENZA MONDADA	Professor, Université de Bâle, Switzerland. (Linguistics)
SYLVAIN MOUTIER	Master Lecturer, Université Paris 5, France. (Psychology)
JACQUELINE NADEL	Director of Research, Centre National de la Recherche Scientifique (CNRS), Vulnerability, adaptation, and psychopathology, Hôpital Pitié-Salpêtrière, Paris, France. (Psychology)
GABRIEL OTMAN	Translator, specialist in terminology, France. (Linguistics)
ÉLISABETH PACHERIE	Researcher, Centre National de la Recherche Scientifique (CNRS), Institut Jean Nicod, Paris, France. (Philosophy)
JACQUES PITRAT	Honorary Director of Research, Centre National de la Recherche Scientifique (CNRS), Paris, France. (Artificial Intelligence)
MARIE-HÉLÈNE PLUMET	Master Lecturer, Université Paris 5, France. (Psychology)
VIVIAN POUTHAS	Director of Research, Centre National de la Recherche Scientifique (CNRS), Cognitive neuroscience and brain imaging, Université Paris 6, France. (Psychology)
JOËLLE PROUST	Director of Research, Centre National de la Recherche Scientifique (CNRS), Institut Jean Nicod, Paris, France. (Philosophy)
FRANÇOIS RASTIER	Director of Research, Centre National de la Recherche Scientifique (CNRS), Models, dynamics, corpora, Université Paris 10, France. (Linguistics)
ANNE REBOUL	Director of Research, Centre National de la Recherche Scientifique (CNRS), Institut des Sciences Cognitives, Lyon, France. (Linguistics)
FRANÇOIS RECANATI	Director of Research, Centre National de la Recherche Scientifique (CNRS), Institut Jean Nicod, Paris, France. (Philosophy)
GEORGES REY	Professor, University of Maryland, College Park. (Philosophy)
MARC RICHELLE	Honorary Professor, Université de Liège, Belgium. (Psychology)
MARIE-CHRISTINE ROUSSET	Professor, Université Paris 11, France. (Artificial Intelligence)
JUAN SEGUI	Director of Research, Centre National de la Recherche Scientifique (CNRS), Experimental psychology, Université Paris 5, France. (Psychology)
ÉRIC SIÉROFF	Professor, Université Paris 5, France. (Neuroscience)
ARLETTE STRERI	Professor, Université Paris 5, France. (Psychology)
JACQUES VAUCLAIR	Professor, Université Aix-Marseille 1, Aix-en-Provence, France. (Psychology)
ANNIE VINTER	Professor, Université de Bourgogne, Dijon, France. (Psychology)
DANIEL WIDLÖCHER	Professor Emeritus, Université Paris 6, France. (Psychology)

Preface: Finding Your Way through the Forest

STEPHEN M. KOSSLYN
DEPARTMENT OF PSYCHOLOGY
HARVARD UNIVERSITY, CAMBRIDGE, MASS.

The advent of neuroimaging has been widely hailed as a turning point in the study of the mind. For the first time, we can obtain pictures of how the brain is activated while people perform specific tasks. This, we are told, is a watershed event; the relation of mind and brain is no longer mysterious and ethereal, but instead is observable and palpably concrete. Many researchers seem to believe that from here on, it's just a mopping up operation; more studies need to be conducted, and after the results are in we will understand not only how the mind works, but also how it arises from the brain.

I wish I could be so sanguine. I worry that much of the dramatic progress in cognitive science never made it to cognitive neuroscience — but am cheered by the prospect that this book might serve to right this situation.

What's bothering me? First, consider the typical neuroimaging study today. I don't want to single out anyone in particular as the guilty party, and it really isn't necessary to do so; the tendency I've noticed is possibly now the norm, and even if not it is very widespread. A typical study goes like this: Show people pictures of faces and other objects while assessing activation in their brains, and find an area that lights up only (or most strongly) to faces. Aha, you've discovered the "Face Area." Or, ask people to watch another person perform an action, and then ask them to perform the action themselves. Areas that are activated similarly when only observing as when performing are "Imitation Centers." Or, ask people to read words that have negative valence and words that have neutral valence. Areas that are more activated by negative words are involved in "Negative Emotions." What do all of these studies have in common? The brain activation is interpreted using common sense and intuitions about the effects of stimuli on the brain. Since faces activate a brain area more than do other stimuli, that area must be involved in representing faces; since there's a correspondence between observing and performing in some brain areas, those areas must connect the two kinds of activities; since words that label negative emotions activate some areas more than do other words, those areas must be involved in emotion.

The theories in much of cognitive neuroscience have rapidly evolved into what used to be known as "functional anatomy." In the present incarnation, theories ascribe certain functions to brain areas based on observations about what activates them. This is in fact a kind of neophrenology; the goal is to characterize what parts of the brain do by making direct connections between a brain area and obvious properties of the stimuli and responses that are associated with its activation.

In my view, this is a step backwards, for two reasons. First, the only way to understand a representation or process is by considering it in the context of an information-processing system (e.g., Fodor, 1975). Thus, instead of simply looking for correlations between stimulus or response properties and activation, one needs to think about the brain as a system and what that system is doing to accomplish specific tasks. Representations are repositories of information; but representations convey information only because the appropriate processes are available. By analogy, to a blind man, chalk marks on a blackboard are meaningless (in fact, they may as well not exist); the marks convey information only because they can be interpreted. Second, as soon as one starts thinking in terms of information-processing systems, one realizes that common sense can't characterize the nature of internal representations nor how they are processed. Information-processing systems, by definition, take some input and produce an output. Depending on the problems that need to be solved by the system, different aspects of the input will be used. And there is no reason why the aspects of the input that are useful to the system in a particular circumstance should be intuitively obvious. It's not even obvious that *Force = Mass × Acceleration*, something we experience many times each day, so why should it be obvious how brain events carry out specific tasks?

How can we describe information-processing systems? The heart of cognitive science focuses on just this question. Cognitive science, in effect, has developed a language for describing information processing. This language hinges on the notion of computation. According to this idea, processing systems typically are composed of sets of subsystems that work in concert to perform a task (Kosslyn and Koenig, 1992; Simon, 1981). Each subsystem is defined by the input it receives, the output it produces, and the operation that transforms the input to output.

Moreover, these subsystems can be described at multiple levels of analysis. Marr (1982), for example, famously proposed an initial distinction between delineating *what* a subsystem does versus *how* it accomplishes that process. In the first case, the theorist analyzes a problem confronted by a system as a whole in terms of the input that's available and the output that must be produced. This analysis hinges on the concept of division of labor, and the goal is to specify a set of computations that divides the large problem. For example, the large problem might be recognizing an object one sees, and the individual computations would include those that detect edges and organize the input into shapes that are likely to correspond to an object or parts thereof, those that compare such organized shapes to shapes previously stored in memory, and so on. Each of these computations is specified in terms of what it accomplishes. The analysis becomes increasingly concrete when the theorist considers how each computation is actually accomplished. For each computation, one can characterize an algorithm, a step-by-step procedure that actually carries out the operation of transforming input to output. In fact, it's typically relatively easy to propose several possible algorithms—and sorting among them becomes a major focus of subsequent research. In addition, algorithms can be mapped into the brain itself, charting the specific neural tissue and operations that carry out each step of the processing. Again, there is usually more than one way, in principle, that the brain could carry out an algorithm—and (decidedly nonphrenological) brain research is necessary to sort among them.

Cognitive science is an inherently interdisciplinary enterprise. Different disciplines lend different insights into how to characterize the problems to be solved, how to characterize the decomposition of processing into sets of subsystems, and how to characterize the algorithms and their implementation in the brain. Linguistics, for example, plays a crucial role in characterizing what problems need to be solved during language and how to characterize representations and accompanying processes, anthropology can help characterize problems (such as those involved in mate selection) that are posed by evolutionary imperatives, computer science can characterize types of algorithms that will in principle produce specific outputs on the basis of specific inputs, and so on.

From this perspective, instead of concluding that one has found a "face area" when faces are the optimal stimulus, one might ask whether the area registers biologically important stimuli. And in fact, Ganis et al. (unpublished) found that pictures of genitalia activate the "face area" as strongly or stronger than faces. Or, instead of thinking of "imitation" as a basic process, one would be led to try to think through how input images could be converted, step-by-step, into output instructions. Or, instead of assuming that certain words activate "negative emotions" one might ask whether such words ready the brain to execute specific types of actions (such as approaching or withdrawing; Davidson, 2002). The computational approach leads one to look beneath the surface, to think about what one would need to do if one were actually *building* a system that performed the requisite task. And it is within this framework that one interprets results from empirical studies.

All of this is daunting. At first glance, it might appear that to do cognitive science well one needs to know too much. One needs to know about computational systems and about various fields of inquiry. And the problem is even worse if one wants to use cognitive science approaches to characterize what the brain does. That's where this book comes in. I am reminded of a parable (which I was told is Indian in origin). Let me risk recounting it, in hopes that it will be illuminating: A bunch of animals in the forest were concerned because their children were up to no good. They were loitering in the clearings, hanging around the trail corners. The adult animals got together one evening to discuss this sorry start of affairs, and quickly converged on the time-worn, tried-and-true solution: school. Put the kids in classrooms, keep them off the streets. And then the issue of curriculum raised its head. The squirrels said, "tree climbing; we've got to include tree climbing." And the bears said "Digging; it's critical to become good at digging." And the birds said "Don't forget about flying!" So, they gathered up all the young animals and put them in school. And soon, you know what they had? Little baby birds with broken wingtips from trying to dig, and little baby bears with broken backs from trying to fly, and so on. Now, you might think that the moral of the story is that we should find out who's a bird and who's a bear, and if you are bear you dig and if you are a bird you fly. But I don't think that's the point. Instead, in my view we should find out who's a bird and who's a bear, and if you are a bird you should know that you are terrific at flying, but should dig in an archeological dig where you can use your claws to make precise and delicate excavations. And if you are a bear, you should know that you are good at digging deep holes, and if you want to fly—get in an airplane!

The point is, to do cognitive science well we each must specialize in one of the parent disciplines, but should also know enough to collaborate with those in other disciplines. The present book is just what the doctor ordered for this tack. The key concepts in virtually all of cognitive science are described clearly and concisely, in enough detail that the reader can know where to begin in collaborating with colleagues in other disciplines. As such, this book may play a major role in introducing the conceptual sophistication developed over decades to new generations, allowing them to build on what's come before instead of trying to start from scratch. Such accumulation of knowledge is the heart of what commonly is regarded as progress in science.

Olivier Houdé and authors have done a major service in compiling the material in this volume, and all of us birds and bears owe them a debt of gratitude.

BIBLIOGRAPHY

Davidson, R. J. (2002). Anxiety and affective style: Role of prefrontal cortex and amygdala. *Biological Psychiatry, 51*, 68–80.

Fodor, J. A. (1975). *The language of thought*. Sussex: Harvester Press.

Kosslyn, S. M., & Koenig, O. (1992/1995). *Wet mind: The new cognitive neuroscience*. New York: Free Press.

Marr, D. (1982). *Vision. A computational investigation into the human representation and processing of visual information*. San Francisco: W.H. Freeman.

Simon, H. A. (1981). *Sciences of the artificial*. Cambridge, MA: MIT Press.

Foreword

The Transcontinental Development of Cognitive Science

OLIVIER HOUDÉ
LA SORBONNE, PARIS
MARCH 2003

The first cognitive science research center, the Center for Cognitive Studies, was founded at Harvard University in 1960 by the psychologists Jerome Bruner and George Miller (Miller, 2003). Since then, great American thinkers like the linguist Noam Chomsky and the philosopher Jerry Fodor have created—and still are nourishing—important new lines of research in this field, namely regarding language (Chomsky) and "language of thought" (Fodor). Another example is the close connection established in the 1990s between cognitive psychology and neuroscience (notably, with brain-imaging techniques), through the pioneering work of two other Americans, Michael Posner and Stephen Kosslyn, on visuospatial attention and mental imagery, respectively. For the most part, then, cognitive science is American. But digging a little deeper, we can see that it is also fundamentally European (Houdé and Mazoyer, 2003). Two examples of its European roots concern the formalization and automatization of thought and the cerebral bases of thought, both founding themes of cognitive science.

The seeds of the formalization of thought were initially sown by the French philosopher René Descartes in the seventeenth century. Descartes argued that thinking is reasoning, and that reason is a chain of simple ideas linked together by applying strict rules of logic. Descartes, with his *cogito ergo sum*, was the very first precursor of cognitive science (even if he was wrong about the dualism of mind and brain). Then, in the nineteenth century, it was an English mathematician, George Boole, who invented symbolic calculus, where such logical operations as *or*, *and*, and *if-then* are expressed as simple mathematical computations on 0 and 1. Boole's dream was to translate all operations of the human mind into an elementary mathematics. Part of this dream was realized in the twentieth century by the

Swiss psychologist Jean Piaget (Bruner's professor), who showed how elementary psychological mechanisms (mental actions and operations) gradually construct logical and mathematical thinking between infancy and adulthood. This was also shown by the French neurobiologist Jean-Pierre Changeux in his neural Darwinism, which describes the tight links between logic, mathematics, and the brain, links we can now observe directly by means of functional brain imaging (Houdé and Tzourio-Mazoyer, 2003).

It was another French philosopher, Julien Offray de La Mettrie, who planted the seeds of the automatization of thought in the eighteenth century. La Mettrie dared claim that human beings were machines (according to Descartes, only animals were so). Based on this premise, La Mettrie began his mechanistic attempt to naturalize the human mind. This was in fact one of the most original ideas that came out of the Age of Enlightenment in France. The idea took on a more modern form in the twentieth century, when the English mathematician Alan Turing imagined a virtual device (the Turing machine) that could translate any humanly computable mathematical problem into a sequence of simple operations, thereby inventing the algorithm, the basis of what was to become computer science and the germ from which artificial intelligence was born.

The second European root of cognitive science, the cerebral bases of thought, dates back to the early nineteenth century, when the Austrian neurologist, Franz Josef Gall, ventured the idea that the human mind is divided into multiple mental functions, and that each of these functions corresponds to a part of the cerebral cortex. Gall is cited by Fodor in the introduction of his seminal book, *The Modularity of Mind*, which has made an indelible mark on computational research in cognitive science. Gall's localization method, or "phrenology" (interpretation of bumps on the skull), was quite fanciful, however, and it was not until the 1860s that the French neurologist Paul Broca achieved the first scientific localization of a mental function (language) in the human brain. Cognitive brain mapping was thus launched. The project was pursued in the twentieth century, first in cognitive neuropsychology on brain-damaged patients (as Broca had done) and later (in the 1990s) via functional brain imaging of healthy subjects.

As this brief history shows, the growth of what is now called cognitive science—although first instituted as an academic discipline in the United States—has taken place on both sides of the Atlantic. Clearly, cognitive science is an international, collective enterprise. Today, whether it be in cognitive neuroscience, cognitive psychology, artificial intelligence, cognitive linguistics, or philosophy of mind, we find major research centers across North America, Europe, and Japan.

Psychology Press now offers this English translation of the *Vocabulaire de Sciences Cognitives*, the first reference work of its kind published in France. It is perhaps also because of France's long-standing encyclopedic tradition, initiated by Denis Diderot and Jean Le Rond d'Alembert in the eighteenth century and maintained today in many domains of knowledge (including history, philosophy, science, law, political science, and literature) by the Presses Universitaires de France. The present dictionary was updated and adapted for the American edition (particularly the examples used in cognitive linguistics) and meticulously translated by Vivian Waltz, to whom, as Editor-in-Chief, I would like to express my deepest gratitude for her truly exceptional work. My thanks are also extended to the Section Editors—Daniel Kayser (artificial intelligence), Olivier Koenig (cognitive neuroscience), Joëlle Proust (philosophy of mind), and François Rastier (cognitive linguistics)—for their assistance in resolving the many intractable problems that inevitably arose in translating a technical book of so broad a scope. I hope this dictionary will be useful to the English-speaking public, and that it will reinforce the transcontinental development of cognitive science.

BIBLIOGRAPHY

Boole, G. (1854). *An Investigation of the Laws of Thought, on Which Are Founded the Mathematical Theories of Logic and Probabilities*. London: Macmillan.

Changeux, J.-P., & Connes, A. (1998). *Conversations on Mind, Matter, and Mathematics*. Princeton, NJ: Princeton University Press.

Edelman, G., & Changeux, J.-P. (2000). *The Brain*. New Brunswick, NJ: Transaction Books.

Encyclopedia of Diderot and d'Alembert Collaborative Translation Project at www.hti.umich.edu/d/did/

Fodor, J. (1983). *The Modularity of Mind*. Cambridge, MA: MIT Press.

Fodor, J. (2000). *The Mind Doesn't Work That Way: The Scope and Limits of Computational Psychology*. Cambridge, MA: MIT Press.

Hauser, M., Chomsky, N., & Fitch, W. (2002). The faculty of language: What is it, who has it, and how did it evolve? *Science, 298*, 1569–1579.

Houdé, O., & Mazoyer, B. (2003). The roots of cognitive science: American, yes, but european too. *Trends in Cognitive Sciences, 7*, 283–284.

Houdé, O., & Tzourio-Mazoyer, N. (2003). Neural foundations of logical and mathematical cognition. *Nature Reviews Neuroscience, 4*, 507–514.

Julien Offray de La Mettrie. (1996). *Julien Offray de La Mettrie: Machine Man and Other Writings* (A. Thomson, Trans. and Ed.). Cambridge, England; New York: Cambridge University Press.

Kosslyn, S. (1994). *Image and Brain*. Cambridge, MA: MIT Press.

Miller, G. A. (2003). The cognitive revolution: A historical perspective. *Trends in Cognitive Sciences, 7*, 141–144.

Posner, M. (1993). Seeing the mind. *Science, 262*, 673–674.

Posner, M., & Raichle, M. (1994). *Images of mind*. New York: Freeman.

Introduction: A New Puzzle of the Mind

Abduction, action, aging, animal cognition, artificial life, attention, autism, belief, categorization, cognitive development, cognitive psychiatry, cognitivism, communication, computational analysis, connectionism, consciousness, constructivism, context, control, creativity, desire, differentiation, discourse, dynamic system, emergence, emotion, epistemic, functional neuroimaging, functionalism, infant cognition, information, intentionality, knowledge base, language, language of thought, learning, localization of function, logic, memory, mental imagery, metacognition, mind, modularity, naturalization, neural Darwinism, neuropsychology, number, object, perception, pragmatics, propositional attitude, psychophysics, rationality, reading, reasoning, representation, robotics, schizophrenia, semantics, semiotics, space, symbol, syntax, theory of mind, time, will, writing . . . and more.

All of these entries figure in this *Dictionary of Cognitive Science*, which brings together the essential contributions of cognitive neuroscience, cognitive psychology, artificial intelligence (AI), cognitive linguistics, and the philosophy of mind. Cognitive science stands out today as a new field of knowledge in which experimentation, modeling, and state-of-the-art technology are combined in an attempt to uncover the mystery of the mind and how it is embodied in matter: the brain, the body, and the computer.

To compile this dictionary, we began by setting up a five-member editorial board that included a specialist from each of the core disciplines of cognitive science: cognitive neuroscience, cognitive psychology, AI, cognitive linguistics, and the philosophy of mind. After drawing up a list of the key terms that would become the dictionary entries, the editors asked various authors to write the definitions applicable to their particular discipline. In an attempt to best render the complexity of the terms, the definitions are usually encyclopedic, in the sense that the notion is defined by presenting multiple approaches and models and referring to important related notions. Although the dictionary has a single overarching theoretical and epistemological orientation, the authors sometimes set forth different or even opposing points of view on a given issue. This approach makes the book an interdisciplinary composite of selected entries, with variable contributions from each discipline. The term *cognitive science*, in the singular form, was chosen for the dictionary's title to clearly reflect the unity that is emerging from this new interdisciplinary framework, but that form and the plural *cognitive sciences* are found throughout the book.

Before going into how the dictionary might best be used as a reference tool (see *Guidelines for Dictionary Users* at the end of this introduction), let us describe the overall scientific background of each of the concerned disciplines. Below, the five editors present their individual disciplines, taking the unifying approach that drives the cognitive sciences today.

COGNITIVE NEUROSCIENCE

The 1990s were the decade of the brain. These years enabled us to better understand how the human brain functions and how our thinking is able to emerge from it. To conduct research in this field, psychologists (from cognitive psychology), artificial intelligence specialists, and neuroscientists must work closely together. It was out of this cross-disciplinary collaboration that cognitive neuroscience was born.

The aim of cognitive neuroscience is to understand the nature and structure of our mental operations. The approach is computational, in that mental activities are described in terms of the processing subsystems needed to perform each of the elementary tasks involved in carrying out a particular mental activity, such as reading a word or a sentence, recognizing an object perceived visually, solving an arithmetic problem, and so forth. The processing subsystems are identified on the basis of functional and anatomical brain data, and the cognitive processing models proposed are tested using computer simulation experiments. In short, a model of mental functioning in cognitive neuroscience must be both plausible at the neural level and compatible with the results of simulation experiments.

Computational analysis and computer simulation models should not be confused, however. A computational analysis is a logical thought process aimed at determining what properties a given system must have in order to execute a given behavior. It generally leads to postulates about what processing subsystems must be included in the system for it to produce a specific behavior in response to a particular input signal. By contrast, a computer simulation model is a computer program that simulates the operations of one or more of the subsystems whose existence was postulated in the computational analysis. The analysis thus serves to build a particular simulation model, which in turn can be used to test its validity.

Processing subsystems are considered to be individual neural networks or groups of networks operating interactively with each other. Such *neuralnets* can be described at various levels of detail, either as subsystems of variable coarseness, or as smaller assemblies permitting a finer-grained description of our mental activities. A subsystem is characterized in terms of input, operations on that input, and output.

Cognitive psychologists and cognitive neuroscientists pursue the same goal: to understand how the cognitive system functions. But psychologists have traditionally studied mental events independently of the brain, in the same way as the information-processing operations executed by a computer can be studied without considering the physical characteristics of the machine. The cognitive neuroscience approach differs from psychology in this respect. It rests on the idea that cognitive activities are what the brain does, so describing mental processes requires data about the brain. This does not mean that a description of cognitive processes can be replaced by a description of brain mechanisms; rather, it is postulated that thought does not come forth from just any substrate, and that that substrate, the brain, conditions the possible forms that thinking can assume.

Researchers in AI have developed computer models of information processing. In the same manner as one can test the behavior of a Formula-One racing car by building a model and observing its behavior in an aerodynamic tunnel, one can test a theory of information processing by programming a computer to simulate a cognitive process. But the goal of computer modeling in cognitive neuroscience is not simply to devise any model capable of producing the behavior in question. The idea is rather to determine how a model that possesses the structure and properties of the brain can generate that behavior. Hence, such a model must be based on knowledge of the brain.

An impressive amount of work in psychophysiology and psychobiology has revealed that studies on the brain-behavior relationship can lead to important discoveries without bringing information-processing hypotheses to bear. The cognitive neuroscience approach tends to show that even greater progress can be made by taking information-processing data into account, by way of a computational type of approach.

Cognitive neuroscience came to be in the 1990s. These years were stamped by the first cognitive neuroscience summer school at Harvard University and the creation of the *Journal of Cognitive Neuroscience* at MIT Press. The boom in this new discipline has two origins. The first is related to advances in computer science, where increasingly powerful machines are offered at ever more attractive prices. The implications of this progress are enormous. Large numbers of researchers now have computers sophisticated enough to simulate cognitive activities in artificial neural networks (connectionist models). Further, the availability of these high-performance computers has supported the development of extremely powerful functional brain-imaging techniques such as positron emission tomography (PET), functional magnetic resonance imaging (fMRI), and magnetoencephalography (MEG). These techniques enable investigators to observe the activity of the intact brain of humans or animals, and to determine what regions are involved in a given cognitive process. Computers are indispensable here, as much for driving the imaging devices as for recording and analyzing the output data. Indirectly, then, the development of computer science is what allowed cognitive neuroscience to take a tremendous leap forward, through the use of techniques that have contributed significantly to furthering our knowledge of the mechanisms of the brain.

The possibility of observing the intact brain in this direct way as it performs various cognitive tasks initiated a genuine revolution in the entire field of cognitive science. The brain-imaging data gathered for certain cognitive tasks has been related to behavioral observations of brain-damaged patients, or to the results of mental chronometry experiments in cognitive psychology. While each approach has its limitations and its specific potential sources of error, the findings obtained using different techniques are matched, and their respective contributions are combined, to gain an overall understanding of mental mechanisms. This is the second origin of the success of cognitive neuroscience.

Because it is interdisciplinary in nature, cognitive neuroscience overlaps with other fields, particularly cognitive psychology and AI. However, in order to clearly mark the boundaries (albeit artificial ones) between the disciplines in this dictionary, the cognitive neuroscience definitions given here focus on the "sciences of the brain."

COGNITIVE PSYCHOLOGY

While cognitive neuroscience, as it is presented above, is a recent discipline, this is far from true of scientific psychology, which originated more than a hundred years ago. Except for the behaviorist period in the early twentieth century, when certain psychologists striving for rigor surrendered in the face of the unobservable (what happens between the stimulus and the response), the issues raised today in cognitive science are the ones that have always been posed by psychologists, namely, understanding the operations of the mind, their development, and their dysfunction. In addition, from the outset, relations with biology, on the one hand, and with philosophy (from which psychology descended) on the other, were close knit. As Marc Jeannerod humorously wrote about the birth of psychology in the nineteenth century: "Two fairies, Biology and Philosophy, were hovering over the cradle. Both were trying to win the newcomer's favor: 'She looks just like me,' said Biology; 'She's the spitting image of me,' replied Philosophy. The newborn quickly proved rebellious and ungrateful, ready to disown her ancestors." Psychology then set out to establish itself as an independent discipline for studying the operations of the human mind (or for some, human behavior only), using the experimental method and the principles of psychophysics. Little by little, as the twentieth century progressed, psychology achieved recognition as an academic discipline in its own right.

In the light of its roots in philosophy and biology, it is not surprising that today's psychology is often regarded as the central, unifying discipline of the cognitive sciences. Having become a full-grown, healthy adult, the child is no longer rebellious or ungrateful toward her ancestors, who—now called *cognitive neuroscience* (anchored in biology) and the *philosophy of mind*—are still taking an interest in her. In the meantime, with the arrival of the computer, a younger sister named Artificial Intelligence was born, and then it was Psychology's turn to exclaim, "She looks like me!" A few cousins, such as Linguistics and Logic, were right there on the new scene.

At the time of the "cognitive revolution" (to borrow Howard Gardner's expression) that marked the second half of the twentieth century, "cognitive" psychology was confounded with cognitivism. In this respect, psychology, being the science of mental life, is a special science; it is the science of the language of thought, a concept proposed by Jerry Fodor (a student of the linguist Noam Chomsky) to refer to a formal inner language consisting of syntactic rules and symbols. In reference to the mind-computer analogy, radical cognitivists such as Philip Johnson-Laird argued that the physical nature of the brain (neural hardware) imposes no constraints on thought per se (mental software); thought, being made up of rules and symbols, could in principle be implemented on a computer as well (electronic hardware). This view, initially formulated by the logician and philosopher Hilary Putnam, is the functionalist doctrine, according to which the only things that count are the cognitive functions under study (the software) and their interactions; the cerebral or electronic structures underlying those functions matter little. With the arrival of the 1990s, hailed as "the decade of the brain" (see *cognitive neuroscience* above), this radical cognitivism was denounced. A testimony to the change in orientation that ensued was the appearance of connectionism, a branch of AI aimed at developing artificial neural networks to simulate cognitive functions. Even more markedly, functional brain-imaging techniques were introduced and rapidly led cognitive psychologists to begin directly exploring the brain-mind relationship, whether in the study of perception, motricity, attention, language, memory, mental imagery, or reasoning. In a 1993 article entitled "Seeing the Mind," the psychologist Michael Posner wrote, "The microscope and telescope opened vast domains of unexpected scientific discovery. Now that new imaging methods can visualize the brain systems used for normal and pathological thoughts, a similar opportunity may be available for human cognition" (*Science, 262,* 673–674).

Before the introduction of functional brain imaging, the two methods generally used in psychology and neuropsychology to study the functioning of the mind and its relationship to the brain were mental chronometry and the lesion paradigm (also, but less often, electroencephalography or EEG, the study of evoked potentials). Mental chronometry, the most widespread method in experimental psychology, attempts to infer the mental algorithms of human beings by measuring their processing time and the errors they make. The lesion paradigm is used to investigate cognitive dysfunction in brain-damaged patients, in view of determining what structures are involved in normal brain functions. Considerable progress has been made using these methods and they are still being effectively applied today. However, they suffer from a number of serious limitations, one of which is difficulty interpreting the results, owing to their indirect nature. Compared to these classical methods, neurofunctional imaging offers a possibility never experienced in the history of psychology: the ability to directly visualize brain activity in normal human beings, while they are carrying out cognitive tasks as varied as preparing for a movement, reading a word, imagining a scene, or solving a problem. Today's psychologists must master the basic principles of the various neuroimaging techniques (PET, fMRI, and MEG) in order to design suitable experimental protocols for interdisciplinary research that merges disciplines like cognitive neuroscience and psychology, and even AI and the philosophy of mind.

Without knowing whether the history of science will dub functional brain imaging "the microscope of psychology," it has become evident that it is no longer possible for any major research laboratory to practice experimental psychology without relying on these techniques. The question now raised is: What new ways of testing cognitive models have been introduced by functional brain imaging? For neuroscientists, psychologists, and philosophers, this question is historically related to René Descartes's postulation of dualism between the mental world (cognitive functions) and the physical world (brain and body). What indeed is left (or will be left) of Cartesian dualism? The most radical materialists would answer, "Nothing!" But as the philosopher John Searle so rightly pointed out, the new materialists unknowingly accept the categories and the vocabulary of dualism. They are in some sense doomed to acknowledge the dichotomy of the physical and the mental by their very own claim that one of the terms of the dichotomy contains everything while the other is empty. Paradoxically, then, they do not deny Descartes's way of framing the debate.

In fact, the point of view that truly overthrows the Cartesian framework and the disciplinary breakdown that follows from it (neuroscience/psychology) consists in arguing that neurofunctional imaging techniques are able to delineate a radically new scientific object that falls outside the categories of dualism. Everything seems to suggest indeed that images of the brain in action—that is, as the subject executes an experimental task requiring a specific cognitive function—are pictures of an "object" that is neither matter alone (materialism) nor mind alone (classical cognitivism). Nor is it their union, in the Cartesian sense of a mysterious interaction between two components, one that can be subjected to mechanistic analysis and one that cannot.

But exactly what scientific object is at issue? Even if today we have a feeling of what it might be, coming up with a precise definition will remain a challenge in the years to come, an ambitious and fascinating challenge. A convincing example of this is found in the brain images obtained by Stephen Kosslyn, which bring out the interrelationships between mental-image generating (mind) and topographic representations of the primary visual cortex (matter). It has even been demonstrated that this brain region changes topographically in accordance with whether the mental images generated by the subject correspond to small, medium-sized, or large objects.

However, this enterprise has only just begun, and many points remain obscure. As contemporary philosophers of the mind have stressed, the unanimous antidualism that reigns in the cognitive sciences is more a reflection of agreement on the epistemologically hopeless nature of Cartesian dualism than it is a shared view of the paths that should be explored in order to relate psychological functions clearly and accurately to physical mechanisms. In cognitive psychology as in other disciplines, a model is defined by a syntax and a semantics. With neurofunctional imaging, the syntax, derived from the mind-computer analogy during the 1970s and 1980s, is now defined in cerebral terms: the physicochemical and neuroanatomical properties of the brain. The semantics correspond to the spatial and temporal projection of that syntax onto a psychologically meaningful reality (with resolution constraints that depend upon the imaging technique used). New theoretical and methodological debates are already tackling the issue of the various possible ways of achieving this projection and the validity of each one. It should nevertheless be stressed that symbolic or connectionist computer simulations of cognitive functions remain useful, as do classical paradigms such as mental chronometry and lesion studies, but as direct complements of imaging techniques. The idea is to tightly articulate these approaches when designing experimental procedures and validating models (in particular, by referring to a computational analysis of the mind).

With these new cards in its hand, cognitive psychology has changed considerably at the theoretical level. One example illustrating this impact is how recent brain-imaging data have led to the revision of the classical—and above all theoretical—separation of psychological functions (perception, attention, memory, language, mental imagery, reasoning, executive control, etc.), in such a way that from now on, multiple complex brain networks are brought to bear in accounting for a given task (even if earlier neuropsychological findings on the structural localization of brain functions have been largely confirmed). Along with this reconfiguration, key concepts such as the modularity of the mind and the executive-control center have been challenged, and in some cases redefined (in terms of weak modularity for the former, and large-scale synchronization of neuron assemblies or cognitive modules for the latter). Another example of a theoretical—and even paradigmatic—innovation is the new approach to mental illness, which has traditionally been studied in clinical psychopathology (said to be noncognitive, nonexperimental) and, more specifically, in psychoanalysis. Here also, the impetus provided by the discovery of new connections between cognitive psychology, brain-imaging techniques, genetic research, and clinical psychopathology has reframed the problem in disorders like autism, schizophrenia, and others. The Cognitive Psychiatry entry in this dictionary brings this out by reminding us that Sigmund Freud's very first psychoanalytic research was already a model for neurocognitive psychopathology. Why not strive once again for a new unity in psychology?

But isn't cognitive psychology too often mistaken in describing a "cold mind," a rational mind devoid of emotion, one with no body? Clearly, this criticism holds for the "computer mind" of early cognitivism. Today, however, neurocognitive psychology has begun to sketch the portrait of a "mind-brain-body" where emotions play an essential role. This new picture is illustrated by Antonio Damasio's work and his somatic marker theory. Damasio describes the mind and its most complex operations as being "rooted in the flesh" and deems the absence of bodily emotions to be what prevents us from being "truly rational" (*see* Emotion in this dictionary).

Although cognitive psychology has surely evolved in the recent past, psychologists have not "lost their souls" because of it—on the contrary. Take the case of functional brain imaging, where brain specialists obviously play an essential role—there is nothing "functional" about brain imaging other than its use of the experimental procedures (cognitive tasks, mental chronometry, etc.) and theoretical concepts of psychology. More than ever, then, the skills and competencies of psychologists are a necessity. In cognitive science, the specificity of psychologists lies precisely in their ability to design experimental procedures, and to utilize both sophisticated techniques and very simple situations (consider, for example, the simplicity and ingeniousness of some of the tasks devised in child psychology). Over and above their role in designing procedures, the specificity of psychologists also lies in their direct experimentation, not only on human subjects from infancy to adulthood, but also on other animals.

Cognitive psychology can thus look forward to a favorable climate in the future, and to new and challenging problems that it can solve by pooling its resources with those of neuroscience, AI, linguistics, and philosophy. In addition, it must continue to play its unifying role in the cognitive sciences. It was in this spirit of combining disciplinary knowledge with an interdisciplinary approach that the psychology definitions in this dictionary were written.

ARTIFICIAL INTELLIGENCE

Artificial intelligence made its debut in the 1950s with the appearance of the first computers and cybernetics. An unprecedented, highly ambitious project started to take shape: using computers to simulate processes attributed to human intelligence. In fact, "artificial intelligence" is an ancient myth that has been passed down and reshaped through the centuries, particularly during the Age of Enlightenment with its upsurge of the mechanical arts (which gave us Julien Offroy de La Mettrie's "machine man," after Descartes's "animal machines"). AI took its first steps in the second half of the twentieth century, in the areas of game theory and theorem proofs. In this founding context, it was Alan Turing who forcefully proposed the idea of an intelligent, nonhuman creature. Very rapidly, AI began to fascinate specialists in other disciplines, notably psychologists, linguists, and philosophers. Nascent cognitivism then took an interest in the computer as a symbol manipulator (a feature common to the computer and the human mind).

This sudden interest in their discipline sometimes led AI researchers to overestimate their chances of success on problems whose difficulty they could not assess. Their lack of caution in a domain where so much was ideologically and epistemologically at stake was a severe discredit to AI's reputation and punctuated its history with alternating periods of infatuation—with its expert systems around 1980, and then connectionism and "artificial life" following the growth of cognitive neuroscience—and periods of disenchantment, although these vicissitudes did not prevent the discipline from constituting a core doctrine over the years.

The place of AI in cognitive science ranges from the most boastful to the most humble, depending on how it is perceived. The boastful view would proclaim, for one thing, that AI's expansion is at the heart of the movement that triggered or at least strongly stimulated the upsurge of interest in cognition exhibited by the neighboring disciplines, and second, that the paradigms introduced by AI do much of the work for the other disciplines, leaving no other task for cognitive psychology than observing how human intelligence instantiates the paradigms, for neuroscience, than showing how neuronal substrates embody them, and for philosophy, than agreeing to be supplanted. The humble view, by contrast, would hold that AI must be confined to putting the models devised in psychology, neuroscience, linguistics, and so forth into computerized format, and that doing so would at best demonstrate that the simulated behavior is a good approximation—for the part deemed significant—of the observed behavior. In this case, it would be the task of philosophers to assess the epistemological significance of this partial validation. Most AI researchers, particularly those who contributed to this dictionary, have views somewhere between these two extremes.

One can hypothesize that intelligence is an abstract quality of which, to date, only human performance has afforded a glimpse. The role of AI within the cognitive sciences is primarily to try to differentiate between what pertains intrinsically to that quality and what depends on its biological realization, and, more specifically, on the particularities of the human species.

AI's most important epistemological contribution to the question of cognition is its in-depth study of how to find a happy medium between the expressive power of the models of reality built and used by the intelligence and the ability to make timely decisions. Under certain hypotheses, it is indeed impossible to reconcile a rich representation and an effective decision-making mechanism, no matter what mode (biological, computer-based, or other) is used to build the mechanism. This is why anything that enters into our understanding of this AI-specific task is essential here: complexity, control, expressiveness, logic, metacognition, reasoning, representation, and semantic networks. Other subjects, such as logic and algorithmic complexity, are far from being specific to AI, but are part of what has given the discipline its role in solving the problem of cognition. The expressiveness-efficiency tradeoff mentioned above is only highly critical for certain decision-making hypotheses. Over the past fifteen years or so, a number of very different hypotheses on this issue have been stated, or rather reinstated, putting AI in a key position in the current debate between the various approaches, centered on the notions of symbol, connectionism, artificial life, learning, and so on.

Notwithstanding the cognitive orientation of this dictionary, a view of AI that conforms to the place it occupies within computer science must be given here. This implies presenting certain basic concepts such as function, information, and language, and especially certain computer-related notions either originating in AI (for example, inheritance, object-oriented programming, and distributed artificial intelligence) or formulated elsewhere but currently affecting AI (for example, constraint-based programming). Although these tools have generally been developed with a resolutely technical outlook, their impact on cognitive science can prove to be great.

AI also has its "old standbys": robotics, pattern recognition, problem solving, communication, language understanding, representation of uncertainty (fuzzy logic), and so forth. For quite some time now, theoretical and practical developments in robotics have enabled AI to tackle problems of philosophical interest, such as how to represent action (and its consequence, the so-called frame problem). AI has earned its standing in cognitive science because of its many applications now implemented in computer programs. The expert systems of the late 1970s and early 1980s gave way to such research topics as knowledge bases, knowledge acquisition, and knowledge validation. New functionalities were then added, including explanation and diagnosis (where abduction plays an important role), particularly diagnosis of physical systems, which led to the development of some useful models of qualitative physics.

All these facets of the discipline show how the idea of an intelligent nonhuman creature gradually took shape alongside—and sometimes in close connection with—the psychological study of human intelligence, thereby defining a specific branch of cognitive science. The approach taken to define the AI entries in this dictionary involved bringing to bear three aspects of AI: certain theoretical results whose epistemological contribution is of interest to cognitive science, developments likely to supply it with useful tools, and the traditional topics studied in AI. This should provide full coverage of the state of the art in this domain.

COGNITIVE LINGUISTICS

In the Western philosophical tradition, language has always been regarded as a means of access to knowledge. Cognitive linguistics is reestablishing its ties with this tradition, which existed well before linguistics was instituted as an academic and scientific discipline in the early nineteenth century, but it is obviously doing so under new conditions.

The history of cognitive linguistics dates back to the mid-twentieth century. Cybernetics was responsible for paving the way for the cognitive approach. In the early 1950s, information theory began influencing linguistic theories, and the first language-processing systems were developed (automatic translation, speech analysis and synthesis). As early as 1955, Chomsky proposed his generative grammar based on formal language theory.

Formal language theory posits a strict kinship between grammar theory and automaton theory. The theoretical grounding of linguistics in formal language theory could then be associated with experimental validation: a computerized grammar should be able to automatically generate all correct sentences of a language.

Psycholinguistics, instituted in the early 1960s under the impetus of George Miller, appropriated the correlated task of validating Chomsky's proposals. The interrelationships established between formal linguistics, cognitive psychology, and computer science provided the bases for the so-called symbolic paradigm of classical cognitivism: thought is conceived of as a rule-based sequence of operations on symbols, in the manner of computer algorithms. The language of thought, borrowed from the philosophical tradition by Fodor in the 1970s, plays the same role for the brain as machine language plays for the computer. It structures mental representations as logical propositions, which natural languages are designed to express. This means that linguistics no longer has a privileged rapport with the social sciences. According to Chomsky, linguistics must first be reduced to psychology and then become part of biology; and the universal grammar is regarded as a (hypothetical) component of our genetic makeup.

After the 1970s, these research aims and themes—characterized by the primacy of syntax and a formal approach to cognition—were contested by proponents of generative semantics such as George Lakoff and Charles Fillmore. The result was a shift of interest from syntax to semantics (particularly lexical semantics) and a questioning of the logical representation format; prototype theory, borrowed from anthropology and cognitive psychology (Brent Berlin, Eleanor Rosch), was thought to demonstrate the non-Aristotelian nature of lexical structures. In the cognitive grammars that appeared in the 1980s with Lakoff and Ronald Langacker, linguistic operations, seen as paths in an abstract space, were a testimony to a generalized neolocalism. The localistic hypothesis, which stipulates in particular that case relations have a spatial character, was extended to all fundamental linguistic relations. Cognitive grammars place the computation paradigm in opposition to the perception paradigm, borrowing from transcendental philosophy (Immanuel Kant) concepts such as schematism, and using the idea of frames or forms of the imagination to account for language understanding in terms of mental scenes. The reshaping of phenomenological topics by Terry Winograd and Mark Johnson stressed the role of bodily experience in the exploration of semantic space.

This research trend found support in the connectionist approach to artificial intelligence (the offspring of cybernetics, which tried to simulate brain activity on the computer by means of formal neural networks). Connectionist systems produce the best results for automatic speech-perception, particularly when it comes to recognizing incomplete or noisy patterns. Within this neoassociationist paradigm, linguistic operations are fashioned after perceptual processes. Connectionism counters classical cognitivism's favored symbolic level with a subsymbolic level (using Paul Smolensky's term), formed by the constituents of the symbols.

While these two paradigms disagree as to the nature of the postulated mental operations, they nevertheless adopt the same mentalistic conception of language, which explains linguistic facts in terms of the mental or cerebral states they are thought to reflect. The two paradigms also share the objective of developing computer simulations of mental processes. Cognitive linguistics has had a considerable impact on the entire discipline, not only through its relationships with neighboring disciplines, but also in the very definition and conceptualization of the object under study, the goals to pursue, and potential technical applications.

At the epistemological level, linguistics has been the primary social science included in the cognitive-science group since the mid-1970s. This explains the development of new exchanges with AI as well as renewed exchanges with the sciences of the brain. General linguistics, a descriptive and nonpredictive discipline, has been contested by universal grammars, with their claimed capability of generating all possible languages. These grammars stand out from others by the methodology they use (including various logics such as organon), the nature of their theories (aimed at formalization), and the scientific status of linguistics, which, rather than being a social science, could become a branch of mathematics, according to Richard Montague, or of the life sciences, according to Chomsky. The nonformal cognitive grammars developed over the past fifteen years or so are no less universalistic. They strive to describe the basic mental operations assumed to be at work in all languages.

General linguistics, which has been under constant development since the nineteenth century, studies three major types of diversity: the synchronic diversity of natural languages (of which there are at least three thousand), their diachronic diversity (constants and variables over time), and their internal diversity (dialects, sociolects, etc.). By contrast, cognitive linguistics deals more with language in general than with particular natural languages; at most, it studies only the standard usage of a small number of natural languages from the synchronic viewpoint. Beyond their role in constituting a cognitive linguistics, cognitive theories have influenced all branches of linguistics, and the concepts proposed therein have spread throughout the discipline; for example, the concept of typicality is now commonly used in lexicology. Finally, new areas of applied linguistics are currently being connected to cognitive research through their inclusion in the field of AI. This is true, for instance, of human-machine dialogue, automatic speech analysis and synthesis, automatic text generation and understanding, and knowledge representation. Whether or not it is aimed at simulating mental processes, this research has proven highly useful from a heuristic standpoint. However, the computerizability criterion is subject to question: what is operational in practice is not necessarily so in theory.

As the principal social science among the core disciplines of cognitive science, linguistics may be assigned a specific task in the future: that of articulating the social and cognitive sciences by bringing cultural factors to bear in cognition. The linguistics definitions in this dictionary were written from the cognitive angle described above, with a view of the discipline as it evolved through fifty years of enhancements and contrasts.

PHILOSOPHY OF MIND

Philosophy's contribution to cognitive science, especially the philosophy of mind, does not reside solely in the role it has traditionally played in the history of science (in mathematics, physics, biology, psychology, and so on), that is, doing the groundwork for scientific analyses and then stepping back in the face of the science now standing on its own. Three reasons account for the fact that philosophy has made a deeper and more lasting contribution to the development of the cognitive sciences than it has to the other sciences. First of all, philosophy is the only discipline able, in its official capacity, to address the question of the foundations of cognitive science. Yet this question is crucial for validating the object of study shared by a group of disciplines that otherwise possesses a subject matter and a methodology of their own. Second, philosophy supplies some of the conceptual instruments that enable the various branches of cognition to coordinate their research. Finally, philosophy does not settle for merely proposing a synthetic and critical point of view—permitting a finer analysis of the methods used and argumentation about the merits of the results obtained—as it does for other sciences; it also offers the cognitive disciplines some new theoretical hypotheses, and it can even participate in testing them.

When a science is being created or is going through a critical period, it behooves us to wonder about the exact rationale that intrinsically and objectively justifies the definition of the subject matter studied by that science. This type of inquiry into the legitimacy conditions of the corresponding quest for knowledge is called *foundational research*. Typically, foundational research examines the nature of the object under study, the adequacy of the methods used relative to that object, and finally, the validity of those methods. In the case of cognitive science, the disciplines involved each possesses its own subject matter and methods. The role of philosophy is therefore not to ground each of these sciences, but to justify the focusing of their joint efforts on a new domain named *cognition*, that is, any kind of information processing that enables an organism (or, more generally, a system) to build representations of its environment, store them, and combine them for planning its actions.

This objective, shared by the various cognitive sciences, does not result solely from the development of computer technology. One of its oldest roots lies in the work of philosophers and logicians in the seventeenth century. We know that Gottfried Leibniz attempted to elaborate a characteristic language that could replace natural thinking with a calculus (rightly called a *calculus ratiocinator*). His aim was to enhance creativity and reduce error by fully describing the symbolic and calculatory aspects of thought. What Leibniz could not achieve owing to the incomplete state of logic at the time became possible when logic reached its full developmental peak. At the turn of the twentieth century, Gottlob Frege devised a logical ideography that included quantification theory and provided a means for formally representing any domain of knowledge. In the 1930s and the years that followed, two other logicians (logico-mathematicians), Alan Turing and Alonzo Church, took another decisive step in the foundation of cognitive science by positing that any form of calculation can be mechanized: in principle, all computational processes can be represented formally, and all representations of this type can be translated into the formal system of the universal Turing machine. The last step involved supporting the hypothesis that all forms of thought presuppose the utilization of a calculus. Here again, philosophers, such as Putnam and Fodor, played a key role at the foundational level by devising the analogy between an individual's mental states and the logical states of a Turing machine. This analogy underlies the idea that mental states, although always realized by physical states, can be characterized not in terms of their realization, but in terms of the systematic relationships they have with other states and with the perceptual input and behavioral output of the cognitive system to which they belong.

Initially, the prevailing position involved seeing cognitive processes as constituted by computational processes that operate on sequences of symbols representing properties or states of affairs. However, connectionist models cast doubt on the privileged rank given to the symbolic approach. Note, though, that while rejecting the idea of rules applied to symbol sequences and adopting models based on spreading activation in a network of formal neurons, connectionist models nevertheless remain tied to the computational nature of cognition in a modified sense of the term. This raises new foundational questions concerning the relationship between the physical level and the representational level, often regarded as emergent.

The above analysis of the foundations of cognitive science—to which philosophers and logicians have been contributing extensively—gives an account of its major stages and orientations. Analogous developments are described here in this introduction in relation to cognitive neuroscience, cognitive psychology, artificial intelligence, and cognitive linguistics.

When it comes to conceptual instruments, cognitive science is still drawing on philosophy for conceptual tools and interdisciplinary materials. Both the supporters and the opponents of functionalism, for example, can appreciate the clarification afforded by the distinction between the different ways of identifying mental states with physical states, depending on whether one is dealing with type physicalism, as were the first functionalists (David Armstrong, David Lewis), or token physicalism (Fodor, Putnam). Functionalism has sparked many philosophical debates about the limits of this theory. Ned Block pointed out the shortcomings of the postulated "multirealizability" of mental states and raised the issue of qualitative states, or *qualia*, which cannot be adequately explained in functionalist terms. Other philosophers, such as Searle, attracted the attention of cognitive scientists to how little hope there is of solving the problem of the semantic content of cognitive states in purely computational terms.

The philosophy of language initially emerged as one of the domains where substantial conceptual exchange took place between philosophy and the other cognitive disciplines. Paul Grice's work on the concept of meaning inspired many cognitive linguists, psychologists, and anthropologists, as did work by John Austin and Searle on speech act theory. Saul Kripke's work on reference has also spread widely across the fields of linguistics and AI.

It is obviously the philosophy of mind that has furnished the greatest number of topics for reflection to this interdisciplinary community. Philosophy's plan to naturalize intentionality, understood to be a representational capacity, has captured the interest of all of the cognition-related disciplines. Contemporary thinking about the various levels of consciousness has opened up new areas for joint study, where neuroscientists are establishing privileged ties with philosophers, psychologists, and psychiatrists. Another compelling question posed in the cognitive community concerns naive theories of mind: How do subjects understand or "theorize" their own mental states and those of others? The various existing views (for example, "theory" theories and simulation-based theories) draw their substance as much from work in philosophy as from developmental or psychiatric arguments.

The traditional task of philosophy is not to explore natural reality or the experience one has of it, but rather to understand how the explanatory concepts, theories, or strategies used either in common sense or by the sciences are organized. Such philosophers as John Haugeland and Robert Cummins were instrumental in popularizing the problems that have arisen in cognitive psychology or AI, and the solutions that have been proposed.

However, philosophers have not confined themselves to the role of providing conceptual descriptions and clarifications of cognitive theories. They have not only criticized work done in other disciplines, particularly psychology and linguistics, but have proposed modifications or new avenues of research. Fodor, Donald Davidson, and Daniel Dennett, for example, have made a deep imprint on research in cognitive psychology, both through their criticism (e.g., Davidson's objection to the a priori character of an interpretation scheme that does not allow one to infer the independent reality of the mental state being interpreted) and through their own proposals (e.g., Fodor's hypothesized modularity of the mind).

In a reciprocal way, philosophy has largely benefited from the contributions of other cognitive disciplines: in the 1960s, Chomsky showed philosophers how linguistics has updated the debate between empiricists and rationalists; since the 1980s, psychologists of reasoning have questioned the classical view of the rational subject, and so on. Examples of how philosophy has been enriched are abundant and clearly suggest that pursuing interdisciplinary research will prove to be fruitful on all sides.

The philosophy definitions in this dictionary cover the three facets presented above: the foundations of cognitive science, the conceptual instruments provided by philosophy, and the dynamics of interdisciplinarity.

DICTIONARY OF COGNITIVE SCIENCE

All of these approaches, from cognitive neuroscience to the philosophy of mind, through cognitive psychology, artificial intelligence, and cognitive linguistics, forcefully assert themselves today as bodies of knowledge whose pieces form a new jigsaw puzzle of the mind. But putting such a puzzle together takes time and patience. Moreover, it requires solid interdisciplinary knowledge. In this respect, the *Dictionary of Cognitive Science* is a tool that provides a wealth of information and a firm basis for reflection, or even debate, not only for students, professors, and researchers in each of the disciplines involved, but also for a large cultivated readership.

Here, then, is a new dictionary to add to the library of contemporary science. In science as in life, there are special times when forces combine and rare phenomena arise. Cognitive science today seems to be benefiting from this kind of synergy. The present dictionary hopes to be its echo.

Olivier Houdé (cognitive psychology)
Daniel Kayser (artificial intelligence)
Olivier Koenig (cognitive neuroscience)
Joëlle Proust (philosophy of mind)
François Rastier (cognitive linguistics)

GUIDELINES FOR DICTIONARY USERS

Each entry is broken down into as many as five sections, depending on the number of disciplines to which it is applicable. For example, *Action* has a definition in cognitive neuroscience, cognitive psychology, AI, and the philosophy of mind. Other entries are relevant to a single discipline. For example, *Localization of Function* is defined solely in cognitive neuroscience.

To avoid redundancy, entries shared by several domains but employed in the same sense in each are defined only once (for example, *Logic* has a definition in AI alone).

Many cross-references are given to refer readers to other relevant entries in the dictionary or to another definition within the same entry.

SELECTED BIBLIOGRAPHY

Austin, J. (1962). *How to do things with words.* Cambridge, MA: Harvard University Press.

Block, N., Flanagan, O., & Güzeldere, G. (Eds.). (1997). *The nature of consciousness: Philosophical debates.* Cambridge, MA: MIT Press.

Chalmers, D. (2002). *Philosophy of mind: Classical and contemporary readings.* New York: Oxford University Press.

Chomsky, N. (1955/1975). *The logical structure of linguistic theory.* New York: Plenum.

Chomsky, N. (1969). *Aspects of the theory of syntax.* Cambridge, MA: Harvard University Press.

Chomsky, N. (1995). *The minimalist program.* Cambridge, MA: MIT Press.

Crumley, J. (1999). *Problems in mind: Readings in contemporary philosophy of mind.* New York: McGraw-Hill.

Damasio, A. (1994). *Descartes' error: Emotion, reason, and the human brain.* New York: Putnam.

Damasio, A. (1999). *The feeling of what happens: Body and emotion in the making of consciousness.* New York: Harcourt Brace.

Davidson, D. (1980). *Essays on actions and events.* Oxford, England: Clarendon Press.

Davidson, D. (1984). *Inquiries into truth and interpretation.* Oxford, England: Clarendon Press.

Davis, M. (2000). *The universal computer: The road from Leibniz to Turing.* New York: Norton.

Debenham, J. (1998). *Knowledge engineering: Unifying knowledge base and database design.* Berlin, Germany; New York: Springer-Verlag.

Dennett, D. (1987). *The intentional stance.* Cambridge, MA: MIT Press.

Dennett, D. (1991). *Consciousness explained.* Boston: Little Brown.

Dreyfus, H. (1979). *What computers can't do: The limits of artificial intelligence.* New York: Harper Collins.

Dreyfus, H. (1992). *What computers still can't do: A critique of artificial reason.* Cambridge, MA: MIT Press.

Farah, M., & Feinberg, T. (Eds.). (2000). *Patient-based approaches to cognitive neuroscience.* Cambridge, MA: MIT Press.

Fodor, J. (1975). *The language of thought.* New York: Crowell.

Fodor, J. (1983). *The modularity of mind.* Cambridge, MA: MIT Press.

Fodor, J. (2000). *The mind doesn't work that way: The scope and limits of computational psychology.* Cambridge, MA: MIT Press.

Frackowiak, R., Friston, K., Dolan, R., Mazziotta, J., & Frith, C. (Eds.). (1997). *Human brain function.* San Diego, CA: Academic Press.

Gardner, H. (1987). *The mind's new science: A history of the cognitive revolution; with a new epilogue by the author: Cognitive Science after 1984.* New York: Basic Books.

Gazzaniga, M. (Ed.). (2000). *The new cognitive neurosciences* (2nd ed.). Cambridge, MA: MIT Press.

Gregory, R., & Zangwill, O. (Eds.). (1998). *The Oxford companion to the mind.* New York: Oxford University Press.

Grice, H. P. (1989). *Studies in the way of words.* Cambridge, MA: Harvard University Press.

Halligan, P., & David, A. (2001). Cognitive neuropsychiatry: Towards a scientific psychopathology. *Nature Reviews Neuroscience, 2,* 209–215.

Haugeland, J. (Ed.). (1997). *Mind design II: Philosophy, psychology, and artificial intelligence* (Rev. ed.). Cambridge, MA: MIT Press.

Hauser, M., Chomsky, N., & Fitch, W. (2002). The faculty of language: What is it, who has it, and how did it evolve? *Science, 298*, 1569–1579.

Holland, J. (1975). *Adaptation in natural and artificial systems: An introductory analysis with applications to biology, control, and artificial intelligence.* Ann Arbor, MI: University of Michigan Press.

Jackendoff, R. (2002). *Foundations of language: Brain, meaning, grammar, evolution.* Oxford, England; New York: Oxford University Press.

Jeannerod, M. (1996). *De la physiologie mentale* [Mental physiology]. Paris: Odile Jacob.

Johnson-Laird, P. (1988). *The computer and the mind: An introduction to cognitive science.* Cambridge, MA: Harvard University Press.

Kitamura, T. (Ed.). (2001). *What should be computed to understand and model brain function? From robotics, soft computing, biology and neuroscience to cognitive philosophy.* River Edge, NJ: World Scientific.

Kitcher, P. (1992). *Freud's dream: A complete interdisciplinary science of mind.* Cambridge, MA: MIT Press.

Kosslyn, S. (1994). *Image and brain: The resolution of the image debate.* Cambridge, MA: MIT Press.

Kosslyn, S., et al. (1995). Topographical representations of mental images in primary visual cortex. *Nature, 378*, 496–498.

Kosslyn, S., & Koenig, O. (1992/1995). *Wet mind: The new cognitive neuroscience.* New York: Free Press.

Kosslyn, S., & Rosenberg, R. (2001). *Psychology: The brain, the person, the world.* Boston: Allyn & Bacon.

Kripke, S. (1972). *Naming and necessity.* Oxford, England: Blackwell.

Langacker, R. (1987–1991). *Foundations of cognitive grammar* (Vols. 1–2). Stanford, CA: Stanford University Press.

Levesque, H., & Lakemeyer, G. (2001). *The logic of knowledge bases.* Cambridge, MA: MIT Press.

Murphy, R. (2000). *An introduction to AI robotics.* Cambridge: The MIT Press.

Posner, M. (1993). Seeing the mind. *Science, 262*, 673–674.

Posner, M., & Raichle, M. (1994/1997). *Images of mind.* New York: Freeman.

Putnam, H. (1979). *Philosophical papers* (2nd ed.). Cambridge, England; New York: Cambridge University Press.

Putnam, H. (1988). *Representation and reality.* Cambridge, MA: MIT Press.

Pylyshyn, Z. (1986). *Computation and cognition: Toward a foundation for cognitive science.* Cambridge, MA: MIT Press.

Roland, P. (1993). *Brain activation.* New York: Wiley-Liss.

Searle, J. (1983). *Intentionality: An essay in the philosophy of mind.* New York: Cambridge University Press.

Searle, J. (1992). *The rediscovery of the mind.* Cambridge, MA: MIT Press.

Sharma, T. (2003). *Brain imaging in schizophrenia: Insights and applications.* London: Remedica.

Standish, R., Abbass, H., & Bedau, M. (2003). *Artificial life VIII: Proceedings of the Eighth International Conference on Artificial Life.* Cambridge, MA: MIT Press.

Turing, A. M. (1992). *Collected works of A. M. Turing: Mechanical intelligence* (D. C. Ince, Ed.). Amsterdam; New York: North-Holland.

Winograd, T. (1983). *Language as a cognitive process.* Reading, MA: Addison-Wesley.

Winograd, T., & Flores, F. (1986). *Understanding computers and cognition: A new foundation for design.* Norwood, NJ: Ablex.

A

ABDUCTION

Artificial intelligence. — According to the philosopher and logician Charles Peirce, *abduction* is the reasoning process by which we initially limit the number of hypotheses likely to explain a given phenomenon (→ EXPLANATION, REASONING AND RATIONALITY). For the logical implication $A \supset B$, deduction given A consists in inferring B (→ LOGIC). Abduction given B consists in considering A as the cause of B (→ CAUSALITY AND MENTAL CAUSATION). While the former assertion is logically correct, the latter cannot be declared so unless additional information is obtained. Say we know that A is the only possible cause of B; then it is legal to infer A from B. More generally, if we assume, given a set of causes A_i of B such that $A_i \supset B$, that there are no other causes (which, from the logical standpoint, amounts to *completing* the theory with $\vee A_i \equiv B$), then inferring by abduction the disjunction $\vee A_i$ based on B is logically correct because it is a simple deduction in the completed theory.

Peirce insisted on the difference between abduction and *induction*. Induction consists in generalizing an idea based on observations already made, and it is widely used in symbolic learning (→ LEARNING, SYMBOL). For Peirce, induction has no inherent originality because it merely verifies preexisting suggestions. Abduction is much more powerful; it requires assuming something of a different nature than what has already been observed, often something that would be impossible to discern directly (for example, B is observable, but not its primary causes A_i).

Artificial intelligence (AI) frequently uses abductive reasoning as a method for generating hypotheses about a series of events, given a theory of the domain (→ DOMAIN SPECIFICITY). The privileged area of application is diagnosis. *Abductive diagnosis* originated in the medical field, where causal models of diseases (primary causes) and the symptoms that ensue (observed effects to be explained) provide a natural theory for the domain. This approach was later extended to the assessment of *artifacts* (man-made devices), where theory T (a description of the to-be-diagnosed system) contains the axioms that describe abnormal outcomes, and the axioms act as the hypotheses. David Poole offers us the following definition of abductive diagnosis: Given theory T and a set of observations *OBS*, abductive diagnosis is a minimal set E of hypotheses (parsimony principle) such that $T \cup E$ is coherent and logically implies *OBS*, a minimal explanation of the observations. Abductive diagnosis has been generalized as well to handle cases where the theory also contains axioms describing correct behaviors, and as such, it combines hypotheses about normality with hypotheses about abnormality.

Alongside abductive diagnosis, but from the opposite viewpoint, *coherence-based diagnosis* was developed. Coherence-based diagnosis looks solely at correct behaviors (easier to obtain in the case of artifacts) and does not presuppose knowledge of the nature of any abnormalities or their effects. It is based on the refutation of any hypothesis about correct behavior that contradicts the theory and the observations; a coherence-based diagnosis is thus a minimal set E of nonnormality hypotheses such that $T \cup OBS \cup E$ is coherent. This type of diagnosis is much less restrictive, since it merely restores coherence to the observations rather than trying to explain them. It too has been generalized by incorporating knowledge of flaws.

Given that each theory "trespasses" on the other's domain, it seems natural to try to find a unifying framework that might bring them together. This can be done by separating the observations one wants to explain from those one need not refute and still be satisfied. By letting the observations one wants to explain vary between the null set and the set of all observations, one obtains a series of logical definitions of the diagnosis, ranging from a purely coherence-based one to a purely abductive one.

Note that abduction is a form of *nonmonotonic reasoning*, one of whose prototypes is precisely diagnosis since its explanations are subject to revision. It should also be noted that abduction plays an important role in many other problem-solving tasks ($\rightarrow$ PROBLEM SOLVING) including planning, natural language comprehension ($\rightarrow$ LANGUAGE), automatic learning ($\rightarrow$ AUTOMATISM), and so on. In psychology, it is studied from the standpoint of two fundamental processes: hypothesis formulation based on knowledge stored in memory ($\rightarrow$ MEMORY), and hypothesis testing, where one of the questions that arises concerns the nature of the rule that stops the new-hypothesis generation process.

PHILIPPE DAGUE

SELECTED BIBLIOGRAPHY

Fodor, J. (2000). *The mind doesn't work that way: The scope and limits of computational psychology*. Cambridge, MA: MIT Press.

Gabbay, D., Kruse, R., & Smets, P. (Eds.). (2000). *Handbook of defeasible reasoning and uncertainty management systems: Vol. 4. Abductive reasoning and learning*. Dordrecht, The Netherlands: Kluwer.

Josephson, J., & Josephson, S. (Eds.). (1994). *Abductive inference: Computation, philosophy, technology*. Cambridge, England; New York: Cambridge University Press.

Peirce, C. (1998). *The essential Pierce: Selected philosophical writings, 1893–1913* (N. Houser & C. Kloesel, Eds.). Bloomington, IN: Indiana University Press

Peng, Y., & Reggia, J. (1990). *Abductive inference models for diagnostic problem-solving*. Berlin, Germany; New York: Springer-Verlag.

Poole, D. (1989). Explanation and prediction: An architecture for default and abductive reasoning. *Computational Intelligence, 5*, 97–110.

Poole, D. (1989). Normality and faults in logic-based diagnosis. *AJCAI–1889: Proceedings of the 11th International Joint Conference on Artificial Intelligence,* 1304–1310.

ACTION

Psychology. — *Motor action* is understood to mean the occurrence of a movement made up of three stages: planning, programming, and motor execution. Only the last stage is directly observable and brings about a change in the environment. The first two stages, elaborated mentally before the onset of the action, determine the goal and the strategy to adopt (planning), and the sequence of movements to make (programming). Proper execution of a motor action requires the subject to process two types of sensory information (→ INFORMATION, PERCEPTION): (1) *exteroceptive information* drawn from "external space" (outside the body), which can be auditory, visual, olfactory, or somesthetic, and which acts both as a trigger and a guide for the motor action as it occurs in the environment; and (2) *proprioceptive information* drawn from "internal space" (inside the body). For an action to be performed efficiently, subjects must know their position relative to external space (→ SPACE) and sense the position of their body segments, both before beginning to move (*statesthesia*) and during motion (*kinesthesia*). Motor actions can be distinguished from *movement reflexes*, which are elementary, rapid responses to external demands integrated at the bone marrow level, as well as from *automatic responses* (→ AUTOMATISM), executed essentially in the brainstem and basal ganglia. A motor action is a voluntary movement (→ CONTROL, WILL) to the extent that it is an expression of the individual's *intentions*. It originates in a neural command generated in the cortex (see *neuroscience* below), either consecutive to or simultaneously with the integration of exteroceptive and proprioceptive sensory information.

It might seem absurd to grant a predominant role to the brain in the programming and control of all actions, from finger flexing to locomotion, given that the human body is known to be capable of mobilizing as many as 792 distinct muscle groups, each containing a thousand or so fibers. The number of possible ways of acting upon the world is virtually infinite. However, within this wide range, there are movements with a recognizable form (walking, grasping an object, eating, etc.). Certain constraints thus impose limitations on the range of possibilities, although not in a rigid way, so that the motor system is still able to generate new forms of action (dancing, skiing, playing a musical instrument). How does the organism go about controlling this potential? Nicolas Bernstein showed us a way to understand how complex activity is controlled: let the muscles and joints that receive the commands do some of the work. It suffices to group the muscles and joints into larger systems, or *synergies*, and then to have these larger units control part of the movement. This type of organization has been demonstrated for locomotion, bimanual coordination, and facial expressions: the brain delegates tasks to the periphery. Alain Berthoz supplemented this idea of a motor synergy, viewed as a genuine movement unit, with that of a strategy, and together, these two ideas can account not only for the richness of our most complex behaviors but also for how they are executed. If each synergy constitutes a clearly localized movement unit, then by means of neural network flexibility ($\rightarrow$ NEURAL NETWORK), a set of local synergies becomes organized into behavioral strategies guided by more general mechanisms. In humans, such strategies can be anticipated, chosen, and mentally simulated before execution.

To produce an efficient movement, certain conditions of tonicity and posture must be met. Newborns and young infants fall far short of satisfying these requirements ($\rightarrow$ INFANT COGNITION). Among the many infant gesticulations, researchers distinguish several categories of movements and then define their significance and function ($\rightarrow$ FUNCTION).

1. Independently of all external stimulation, the organism has its own motricity, called *motility*, which is part of our fetal ($\rightarrow$ FETAL COGNITION) and neonatal endowment. Motility is a kind of "background noise" in which behaviors with a coherent spatiotemporal structure can be detected. Spontaneous fetal motility, observed using ultrasound testing, can be clearly differentiated by the second month and prefigures certain movements in the newborn. Some researchers consider fetal motility to be a precursor of newborn behavior, while others see it as an epiphenomenon caused by nerve maturation and devoid of any adaptive function. According to Heinz Pretchl, fetal changes in position facilitate blood circulation, prevent tissue adhesion, and fashion the body's architecture, and as such, they have an immediate functional role. In contrast, eye movements or pseudorespiration movements occur idly and prepare the organism for extrauterine life.

2. *Rhythmies* are original, stereotyped behaviors. They are observed by the second day after birth and are executed repeatedly at a pace of about one per second. More than forty forms have been distinguished, and such movements are known to take up as much as forty percent of the infant's life in the first year. The opening-closing of a hand, extension-flexion of an arm or leg, kicking, head turning, and trunk swaying are the most noticeable forms. Some movements, in particular neonatal ones, are not triggered randomly but follow the beat of the body's intrinsic rhythm, a veritable "internal clock" in the nervous system ($\rightarrow$ TIME AND TENSE) thought to control motor output for durations of a few minutes or so. Certain rhythmies may also have an interactive social function, that of inhibiting or triggering adult behaviors ($\rightarrow$ COMMUNICATION, INTERACTION, SOCIAL COGNITION).

3. *Reflexes* exist before birth and can be seen in the fetus and the premature infant. Today, 73 reflexes have been inventoried in infants, and their presence at the infant clinical examination is a testimony to the proper functioning of the organism. Postural reflexes appear later. Both archaic and postural reflexes disappear in normal children within two or three months after birth, while other reflexes turn into voluntary behaviors. Jean Piaget referred to the latter as *reflex schemes*. These initially awkward, inefficient structures are consolidated by exercise and later transformed into *action schemes*, the "preludes" to intelligence ($\rightarrow$ COGNITIVE DEVELOPMENT).

4. *Aimed motor acts* of an intentional nature are assumed to be absent in the newborn. However, certain mature, organized behaviors of late onset exhibit a morphology similar to that of reflex movements. For example, walking and object grasping are observable behaviors in newborns; after briefly disappearing, these behaviors reemerge and mark off the main stages of motor development in the child. An ongoing problem is understanding the structural and functional similarities of these two types of behavior so as to establish a link between them.

If in the infant these various forms of motricity mainly reveal maturational processes, action in the child may be a more or less effective means of obtaining information about the world and detecting its regularities. This type of "learning through action" ($\rightarrow$ LEARNING) can be achieved by acting upon material objects, upon one's own body or that of others, or even upon one's thoughts and symbolic expressions. Two ways of learning through action have been proposed, one by Burrhus Skinner and the other by Piaget.

Instrumental or *operant conditioning*, which we owe to Skinner, is a form of conditioning (although not the same as Ivan Pavlov's classical conditioning) based on an association between the organism's *response* and the *reinforcement* of that response. The reinforcement may be *positive*, either because it causes an appetitive stimulus or reward to appear (approval, food, etc.) or because it eliminates an aversive stimulus (punishment, electric shock, etc.). In contrast, a reinforcement is *negative* when it is followed by the withdrawal of an appetitive stimulus or when the behavior triggers the appearance of an aversive stimulus. Instrumental conditioning is thus both a source of learning and a means of restricting, selecting, or even modulating the actions that allow the child to adjust to the environment. A perfect example of a teaching application of instrumental conditioning is *programmed learning*, where the learner, whether a child or an adult, acquires schoolbook knowledge and know-how at his/her own pace through the provision of ongoing feedback to responses or actions in the form of immediate consequences or outcomes.

Although the relationship between an organism's responses and reinforcements can be quantified in instrumental conditioning, where both are directly observable, Piaget's cognitivist approach is more structuralistic and qualitative. It grants action an essential role as a source of knowledge and as an organizing principle of thought. By manipulating, searching for, and operating in various ways upon objects, and, more generally, by carrying out activities in and on the world, children organize and structure both the external world and their internal world of thought. Children's actions and the effects of those actions not only enable them to detect physical regularities in the environment (*empirical abstraction*), but also lay the foundation for question asking and hypothesis making, for reasoning about the world (*reflective abstraction*) (→ REASONING AND RATIONALITY). Logical operations in the child and adolescent (→ LOGIC), as genuine actions that are internalized and coordinated, enable them to manipulate symbolically represented knowledge and know-how, acquired through practical actions carried out at a younger age (→ SYMBOL).

The study of motricity in adults suffered for quite some time from methodological and technical constraints. It was not until the 1980s that an interest was taken in the most abstract level of action, approached mainly through the analysis of the execution of fine movements such as pointing, reaching for a spatial target, grasping or manipulating objects, and eye saccades during reading (→ READING). Studies in these areas have provided insight into the relationships between central commands and peripheral adjustments. One study on the kinematic analysis of the hand approaching an object showed that the trajectory speed can be described by a slightly asymmetrical bell curve, a form of invariance that accounts for an infinite number of analogous movements. The speed of the hand increases rapidly until it reaches a peak and then decreases as it approaches the target. This analysis led to the general hypothesis that *goal-oriented movements* are made up of two parts, an initial movement triggered by a central motor command and a final adjustment made under the continuous control of vision (Marc Jeannerod). Going beyond this general scheme, each particular movement that transports the hand is specified in terms of its direction, amplitude, speed (duration), and effector (right or left hand). A chronometric analysis of the motor program is then conducted based on reaction time.

The now classic concept of *motor program* is grounded in the observation that individuals organize, prepare, and plan their movements. In the computer metaphor first proposed in the cognitive psychology of information processing (→ COGNITIVISM), biological movements are seen as taking place sequentially within hierarchies that define the different levels of execution. More recently, in the *nonlinear dynamic approach* initiated by Bernstein, which opposes the traditional theory, biological movement is defined instead as a system of elements interacting in parallel (→ DYNAMIC SYSTEM). Moving away from the computer metaphor, one can rethink the problem of motor control in terms of energy flow. Instead of a motor program, this synergistic view proposes the idea of a control parameter whose variations cause *movement discontinuities* of varying abruptness (for example, a change of regime in the continuous stream of animal locomotion, as in walking, trotting, or galloping), with an *order parameter* that restabilizes the system. One advantage of this theory is that it accounts for and analyzes the transitions between changes of any form.

ARLETTE STRERI

Neuroscience. — Living beings have the capacity to act upon their environment and even modify it according to their own internal plan. An action thus involves a plan that aims for a goal. More generally, actions are approached in cognitive neuroscience in terms of voluntary motricity (→ WILL). To be accomplished, an action necessarily brings into play various neural structures involved in the different stages of motor control (→ CONTROL): intention, planning, programming, and execution.

Representation is a key concept in models of how actions are controlled (→ REPRESENTATION). It is used by such authors as Jeannerod to refer to mental information about the goal and consequences of an action, and the neural processes assumed to take place before execution.

For a long time, knowledge in neurophysiology was acquired through animal studies and through observation in neurological clinics. Such studies pointed out the respective roles of hierarchically organized parts of the nervous system: the bone marrow, the brainstem, the basal ganglia, the cerebellum, and the cortex. Today, brain imaging techniques (→ FUNCTIONAL NEUROIMAGING) offer dynamic insight into this organization, not only in neurological patients but also, and especially, in normal subjects. In addition, these techniques can furnish information about the initial stages in the organization of an action by permitting the exploration of the neuronal substrate of motor representations (see studies by Jeannerod and Jean Decéty, for example). These techniques have brought to light the various nerve structures involved in the initial organizational stages of an action (motor preparation, motor imagery; → MENTAL IMAGERY), namely, the premotor cortex, the lateral cerebellum, the inferior parietal lobe, and the anterior cingulate cortex. In studies by Muriel Roth, Decéty, and their collaborators, functional nuclear magnetic resonance imaging (fMRI) has revealed the implication of the primary motor cortex in action-related representations.

JEAN DECÉTY

Artificial intelligence. — In artificial intelligence, investigators *formalize* action by devising operational models of the conditions and the effects of changes in the world (→ model). The idea is to be able to utilize such models to predict, plan, or even act rationally in the real world via robots (→ ROBOTICS) or in a virtual world via software-driven agents. Specific formalizations have been proposed for different types of actions (e.g., movements) each based on its own theories (e.g., geometry and dynamics). Formal models are necessary but they are too limited. For instance, when an agent moves, the movement has nongeometric effects, both on the objects it carries and on its environment. Logical formalizations of action strive for a broad expressive scope (→ EXPRESSIVENESS, LOGIC). They require restrictive hypotheses such as discrete time, or more often, changes in the state of the world (→ TIME AND TENSE). Accordingly, an action whose effects are continuous cannot be accounted for unless it is broken down into a sequence of discrete changes. The world is thus described as a series of *states*, and states remain stable until an action is triggered. A state has several possible pasts and futures: a partial order of states is a reflection of incomplete knowledge.

How does state E, represented by a set of logic formulas, describe an action that transforms E, and how does one calculate the resulting state E'? Solutions to this problem have been sought in extensions of classical logic (which is monotonic and does not handle change) or outside logic altogether.

Situation calculus falls into the first category. Only a few additions to first-order logic need be introduced, namely, a predicate *hold* (p, E) (property p holds in state E) and a function *result* (A, E), which denotes state E' resulting from action A triggered in E. An action is described by its *preconditions* (the set of necessary and sufficient properties for its occurrence) and its *effects* (the set of properties that are always true in the state resulting from its execution). A basic axiom says that in any state E where the preconditions of A are satisfied, the effects of A are true in resulting state

E'. But this does not suffice: we do not know how to deduce the status in E' of other properties of the world untouched by the effects of A ($\rightarrow$ FRAME PROBLEM).

A representation system using operators of state changes, called *strips* ($\rightarrow$ REPRESENTATION), solves this problem using set theory, without relying on logic. The state, the preconditions, and the effects are described explicitly by sets of properties (rather than by formulas). These descriptions are assumed to be complete, and the world is assumed to be closed (whatever is not stated as true, is false). A is applicable in E if its preconditions are included in E. E' is calculated by taking the algebraic sum in E of the effects of A. Any property not modified by this operation subsists between E and E'. This offers a very simple solution to the problem encountered in the above approach, but poses some new problems. It is indeed very difficult to exhaustively describe all effects and all preconditions of a given action in all situations. Opening a door, for instance, can induce effects such as a draft or better lighting in the hallway. The problem of determining the ramifications of an action entails coming up with a synthesis of all induced effects based, for example, on the axioms of that domain ($\rightarrow$ DOMAIN SPECIFICITY). An analogous problem is encountered for the preconditions (the door must not be locked, blocked by an obstacle, barred, etc.). Various approaches have been used in trying to solve these problems. In most cases, the resulting state is determined both by an *inference mechanism* (changes deduced from stated information; $\rightarrow$ REASONING AND RATIONALITY) and by an *extralogic mechanism of minimal change* (whatever subsists implicitly). The idea here is that the action transforms the world locally. Globally it is invariant, unless information allows one to deduce otherwise. Thus, among the possible E' states compatible with the axioms describing the action and the domain, the one chosen will be the closest one to state E. Criteria for defining proximity, which must not depend on the syntactic form of the representation, are difficult to define and implement, and rarely lead to the selection of a single resulting state.

Alongside these studies, others attempt to extend the computational capabilities of representing action plans by change-of-state operators. This type of representation has been extended, for instance, to entities such as actions with conditional effects, certain induced effects (for example, moving a box moves its content), the resources used up or required by an action, the duration of an action and how its effects are spread across time, and the timing of an action with respect to contingent events. Planning is very much a combinatory problem. With the help of heuristics, it is possible to synthesize relatively complex plans involving parallel actions, multiple goals, and an evolving environment.

However, the hypothesis that there exist complete reliable models, as required in the approaches outlined above, is hardly acceptable in practice.

This fact has provided the incentive in many studies, particularly in decision theory, to look for a way to handle the incompleteness and uncertainty of the models, the nondeterminism of actions (including perception and communication; → COMMUNICATION, PERCEPTION), changes in the world, and the to-be-optimized utility functions expressing the state of the world.

MALIK GHALLAB

Philosophy. — An action differs from a simple movement by the fact that it was caused in a fitting way by the agent's intentions, desires, and beliefs (→ BELIEF, CAUSALITY AND MENTAL CAUSATION, DESIRE, WILL). Deliberately shoving someone is an action, but incidentally shoving that person while tripping over something is not. However, there are several ways of describing one and the same act. For example, pulling the trigger, putting a bullet through someone's heart, killing someone, taking the law into one's own hands: How many actions are accomplished here?

The initial task for a theory of action is to define a criterion for identifying or *individuating* an action. First, the *type* of act should be distinguished from an occurrence or *token* of that type (→ TYPE/TOKEN). Killing someone is a type of act, defined as something any agent does that causes the death of another person, and it can be realized by many possible singular events (*a* poisons *b,* *c* stabs *d,* etc.).

Three types of theories have been proposed to describe the individuation of actions. At one extreme, represented by Alvin Goldman, an action is individuated by the properties used to describe it. For example, pulling the trigger is a different action from putting a bullet through someone's heart insofar as the two descriptions are potentially independent of each other. Situated at the other extreme, Donald Davidson contends that the action in this example is individuated by the movement of the finger on the trigger, but also includes every consequence of that (intentional) movement. All of these descriptions of this particular act of killing characterize the same action. An intermediate position holds that an action can have constituents that are themselves actions or events caused by those actions.

Philosophers have noted that an event that is the product of an action can satisfy the agent's intention only if it happens in the desired way. Davidson illustrates this with the example of a mountain climber who, troubled by his desire to no longer risk his own life in order to ensure the safety of his fellow climber, involuntarily lets go. His intention is realized, but the realization was not intentional. John Searle resolves this difficulty by making distinctions among *prior intention, intention in action,* and *physical event.* The mountain climber may have formed a prior intention to perform the action of letting go, without yet forming the intention in action that causes the physical movement of letting go. It is the intention in action that, by virtue of its content, sets the conditions of satisfaction of the intentional action.

An action can be physical or mental. If it is physical, the *intentional content* consists of an outside event whose occurrence depends on the execution of a movement by the agent (or, for speech acts, the production of an utterance; → PRAGMATICS). If it is mental, the intentional content consists of a mental event (or disposition) that the agent decides to have occur within him/herself.

JOËLLE PROUST

SELECTED BIBLIOGRAPHY

Austin, J. (1962). *How to do things with words*. Cambridge, MA: Harvard University Press.

Bernstein, N. A. (1967). *The coordination and regulation of movement*. New York: Pergamon Press.

Berthoz, A. (2002). *The brain's sense of movement* (G. Weiss, Trans.). Cambridge, MA: Harvard University Press. (Original work published 1997.)

Catania, C., & Harnad, S. (Eds.). (1988). *The selection of behavior: The operant behaviorism of B. F. Skinner*. Cambridge, England; New York: Cambridge University Press.

Collins, H., & Kusch, M. (1998). *The shape of actions: What humans and machines can do*. Cambridge, MA: MIT Press.

Davidson, D. (1980). *Essays on actions and events*. Oxford, England: Clarendon Press.

Decéty, J. (1998). *Perception and action: Recent advances in cognitive neuropsychology*. Hove, England; Philadelphia: Psychology Press.

Dokic, J., & Proust, J. (Eds.). (2002). *Simulation and knowledge of action*. Philadelphia: J. Benjamins.

Gazzaniga, M. (Ed.). (2000). *The new cognitive neurosciences* (Section IV, *Motor systems*) (2nd ed.). Cambridge, MA: MIT Press.

Jeannerod, M. (1997). *The cognitive neuroscience of action*. Oxford, England; Cambridge, MA: Blackwell.

Kortenkamp, D., Bonasso, R., & Murphy, R. (Eds.). (1998). *Artificial intelligence and mobile robots: Case studies of successful robot systems*. Menlo Park, CA: AAAI Press.

Morik, K., Kaiser, M., & Klingspor, V. (Eds.). (1999). *Making robots smarter: Combining sensing and action through robot learning*. Boston: Kluwer.

Piaget, J. (1952). *The origins of intelligence in children* (M. Cook, Trans.). New York: International Universities Press. (Original work published 1936.)

Piaget, J. (1976). *The grasp of consciousness: Action and concept in the young child* (S. Wedgwood, Trans.). Cambridge, MA: Harvard University Press. (Original work published 1974.)

Roth, M., et al. (1996). Possible involvement of primary motor cortex in mentally simulated movement: A functional magnetic resonance imaging study. *NeuroReport, 7*, 1280–1284.

Searle, J. (1983). *Intentionality: An essay in the philosophy of mind*. New York: Cambridge University Press.

Thelen, E., & Smith, L. (Eds.). (1994). *A dynamic systems approach to the development of cognition and action*. Cambridge, MA: MIT Press.

ACTIVATION/INHIBITION

Neuroscience. — *Activation* refers to a rapid increase in the excitability of the nervous system; *inhibition* refers to a decrease or slowing down of the system's spontaneous activity. At the neural level, inhibition can be presynaptic or postsynaptic.

The term *activation* is frequently used in brain-imaging studies ($\rightarrow$ FUNC-TIONAL NEUROIMAGING) to mean that a brain region increases its metabolic rate in conjunction with a given task.

It is widely agreed that under normal perfusion conditions, the regional cerebral blood flow (rCBF) is a reflection of local synaptic activity. Energy is consumed at the synaptic level, mainly by the excitatory postsynaptic potentials. Membrane repolarization is a highly energy-consuming process. Restoring concentration levels in the intracellular and extracellular fluids is directly linked to the functioning of the ATP-dependent Na^+-K^+ pump. Inversely, postsynaptic inhibition induced by THIP (4,5,6,7-tetrahydroisoxazolo(5,4)-pyridine-3-ol) injection, an agonist of γ-aminobutyric acid (GABA) decreases rCBF. A coupling has been shown to exist between rCBF and the metabolic consumption of oxygen. Although the mechanism by which rCBF and brain metabolism are coupled is still unknown, it has been established that the rCBF is modified by metabolism, probably in response to the energy needs of metabolic substrates and metabolite clearance.

In studies on activation, a brain region is said to be activated by a task only if it increases its metabolism over that of a reference task. This *subtraction method* is based on the assumption that activation conditions are additive. Ideally, the target condition includes every kind of processing required in the reference condition, plus that of the function under study ($\rightarrow$ FUNCTION). The validity of this assumption cannot be guaranteed, particularly in the study of cognition, where the reference condition is difficult to define. The problem is less critical in sensory studies, where the activation conditions are defined by measurable physical parameters (such as color, contrast, and luminance in the case of vision, for example) ($\rightarrow$ PERCEPTION, PSYCHOPHYSICS).

In addition to the fact that the activation levels common to the two tasks are disregarded, they are difficult to interpret. The problem is that an increase in activity may be a sign of greater inhibition of a structure situated downstream; inversely, a decrease in activity may reflect the downstream inhibition of some structures and the disinhibition of others, with the net result being activation of the latter.

The fact that the rCBF reflects local synaptic activity has a significant impact on how brain activation images are interpreted. When an rCBF increase is observed in one cerebral region, it must be interpreted in terms of its known afferents. Moreover, like excitatory processes, inhibitory processes can cause local rCBF increases. As for the deactivations observed by means of the subtraction method, they tell us which brain regions are more active in the reference condition than in the target condition.

JEAN DECÉTY

Psychology. — In psychology, the mechanisms of activation and inhibition must be studied jointly in order to understand how the cognitive system selects information during task execution (→ INFORMATION). Traditionally, *selective attention* has been seen as a function of activation (→ ATTENTION). In this view, after initial automatic processing (→ AUTOMATISM), relevant information is selected (earlier or later, depending on the locus of the "selective filter") by means of an activation mechanism (*facilitation*). At that point, any irrelevant information, which must be ignored, dissipates passively over time, and because it is not activated or facilitated, it is not processed cognitively. An alternative conception, the *attention-inhibition view*, has gradually gained ground on the classical attention-activation theory. In this new approach, the essential mechanism of selective attention is inhibition, that is, the active blocking of irrelevant information in working memory (→ MEMORY). Here, the cognitive processing of relevant information, after selection, is not seen as being due to specific activation-facilitation, but to the fact that there is no longer any interference from inhibited irrelevant information.

For psychologists, the question becomes how can these two possible modes of cognitive selection be distinguished experimentally. The paradigm designed to do this is *negative priming*. Let *a* be a situation where the subject has to respond to S1 (the relevant stimulus) while ignoring S2 (the irrelevant stimulus). Let *b* be the next situation where the subject unexpectedly has to respond to S2, or in another condition, to S3 (a new stimulus). The attention-activation view says that, during the first phase (*a*), S2 dissipates passively over time. If, when the second phase (*b*) begins, the effect of S2 has not yet completely disappeared from memory, then S2 (now the relevant stimulus) is facilitated with respect to S3. This is the *positive priming effect*, which is usually assessed by measuring reaction time. Still in the activation view, if the initial effect of S2 has completely faded when the second phase begins, then S2 processing will not differ from S3 processing. The alternate view, attention-inhibition, predicts exactly the opposite. In this case, since S2 was initially inhibited—actively blocked—its effect no longer exists in memory due to passive dissipation in memory, so S2 is more difficult to process than S3 due to its earlier inhibition. This is negative priming.

Under the impetus of Steven Tipper, who introduced the concept of negative priming into cognitive psychology, a large number of experimental studies have confirmed the existence of this phenomenon in a wide variety of tasks, including identification (picture naming, word naming, letter identification), categorization (semantic categorization, lexical decision; → CATEGORIZATION, LEXICON, SEMANTICS), matching (letter matching, shape matching), counting (→ NUMBER), and localization (→ SPACE). All of these studies have brought the inhibitory control of cognition into the foreground within the past decade (→ CONTROL), and negative priming is now taken to be an indicator of the existence and efficiency of the inhibition mechanism. But new and more precise questions have arisen. For example, exactly what is it that is inhibited: the response, the perception, the representation (→ PERCEPTION, REPRESENTATION)? Does inhibition depend on task requirements? Is there a single inhibition mechanism or are there many? What parameters affect negative priming, given that in certain cases the expected effect is not observed? How is episodic memory involved in negative priming?

In addition to its role in research on selective attention and negative priming, the concept of inhibition, with its long and diverse history (Charles Sherrington, Ivan Pavlov, Sigmund Freud, and other investigators), is benefiting today from a new surge of interest in cognitive psychology. Also contributing to the reemergence of inhibition are the study of developmental and interindividual differences (→ COGNITIVE DEVELOPMENT, DIFFERENTIATION), the growing impact of cognitive neuroscience (recent shift of the computer metaphor of activation to the neuronal metaphor of both activation and inhibition; see *neuroscience* above), connectionist models (role of inhibition in network robustness; → CONNECTIONISM, NEURAL NETWORK), and new connections between psychopathology and the cognitive sciences (cognitive models of mental disorders based on executive dysfunction and inefficient inhibition; → COGNITIVE PSYCHIATRY).

Accordingly, one of the current criticisms of neostructuralist or neo-Piagetian models of developmental psychology is that, like Jean Piaget's theory, they all model the coordination-activation of structural units, not selection-inhibition. Yet many authors, including Adele Diamond, Frank Dempster, Katherine Harnishfeger, and Olivier Houdé, have shown that in a variety of domains, such as object construction, number, categorization, and reasoning (→ OBJECT, REASONING AND RATIONALITY), cognitive development must be regarded not only as the gradual acquisition of knowledge (or of increasingly complex structures), but also as hinging on the ability to inhibit reactions that hinder the expression of knowledge already in place. New psychological and neurocognitive models of development have been proposed from this perspective (→ NEUROPSYCHOLOGY); most of these models rely on the concepts of executive function, efficient/inefficient inhibition, and resistance to interference. Comparative studies have also been conducted on specific cognitive tasks in order to compare the performance of children to that of adult patients who, following damage to the prefrontal cortex, exhibit executive dysfunction of inhibitory control (difficulty inhibiting routine cognitive systems, according to Tim Shallice's model).

However, inhibitory control is not limited to the executive functions of the prefrontal cortex in complex cognitive tasks (categorization, reasoning, etc.). Inhibition in fact takes on many forms in the neural and cognitive system (see the generality of the negative priming effect above). One example is found in work by the physiologist Alain Berthoz, who stresses the essential role of inhibitory control in visual exploration behavior. The challenge for future research will be to join the new functional neuroimaging techniques (→ FUNCTIONAL NEUROIMAGING) with the behavioral study of cognitive function using a symbolic and/or connectionist approach, while clearly specifying what relies on the mechanisms of activation and inhibition, and at what processing level those mechanisms operate.

OLIVIER HOUDÉ

SELECTED BIBLIOGRAPHY

Bechtel, W., & Abrahamsen, A. (2002). *Connectionism and the mind: Parallel processing dynamics and evolution* (2nd ed.). Oxford, England: Blackwell.

Berthoz, A. (2002). *The brain's sense of movement* (G. Weiss, Trans.). Cambridge, MA: Harvard University Press. (Original work published 1997.)

Dagenbach, D., & Carr, T. (Eds.). (1994). *Inhibitory processes in attention, memory, and language.* San Diego, CA: Academic Press.

Dempster, F., & Brainerd, C. (Eds.). (1995). *Interference and inhibition in cognition.* San Diego, CA: Academic Press.

Diamond, A. (1991). Neuropsychological insights into the meaning of object concept development. In S. Carey & R. Gelman (Eds.), *The epigenesis of mind: Essays on biology and cognition.* Hillsdale, New Jersey: Erlbaum.

Ghatan, P., Hsieh, J., Petersson, K., Stone-Elander, S., & Ingvar, M. (1998). Coexistence of attention-based facilitation and inhibition in the human cortex. *NeuroImage, 7*, 23–29.

Houdé, O. (2000). Inhibition and cognitive development: Object, number, categorization, and reasoning. *Cognitive Development, 15*, 63–73.

Houdé, O. (2001). Interference and inhibition (Psychology of -). In J. Smelser & P. Baltes (Eds.), *International encyclopedia of the social and behavioral sciences* (pp. 7718–7722). Amsterdam; New York: Elsevier.

Konishi, S., Nakajima, K., Uchida, I., Kikyo, H., Kameyama, M., & Miyashita, Y. (1999). Common inhibitory mechanism in human inferior prefrontal cortex revealed by event-related functional MRI. *Brain, 122*, 981–991.

Roland, P. (1993). *Brain activation.* New York: Wiley-Liss.

Shepherd, G. (1974). *The synaptic organization of the brain.* New York: Oxford University Press.

Smith, R. (1992). *Inhibition: History and meaning in the sciences of mind and brain.* Berkeley, CA: University of California Press.

Tipper, S. P. (1995). The negative priming effect: Inhibitory priming by ignored objects. *Quarterly Journal of Experimental Psychology, 37A*, 571–590.

AGING

Psychology. — Aging is a process that leads not only to physical and physiological weakening (see *neuroscience* below), but also to the slow deterioration of mental functions. Cognition in the elderly is characterized by a decline in the *information-processing systems* (→ INFORMATION) that results in slower processing, generally manifested as an increase in reaction time. The decline is not uniform: it is greater for some cognitive functions such as memory than it is for others like language (→ LANGUAGE, MEMORY). And even within one and the same function, some processes may be less adversely affected than others. This fact has made it possible to dissociate the different components of memory: when tested specifically, working memory and episodic memory appear to be altered the most. In addition, the data very often bring out substantial interindividual variability (→ DIFFERENTIATION). Increasing heterogeneity of cognitive performance with age and across individuals is a basic indicator of aging, and therefore should be explored as such.

There are two main ways of approaching age-related effects on cognitive functions. One approach looks at specific factors and tries to determine what processing components are altered by age. The other considers general factors (John Cerella, Timothy Salthouse) and interprets aging in terms of a reduction in the availability of processing resources rather than in terms of alterations of specific cognitive mechanisms. The latter approach is based on the finding that age-linked deficits are found only for tasks with a heavy cognitive load, that is, complex or difficult tasks that involve processing at deep levels and require simultaneously controlling the storage and manipulation of information (*dual tasks*) (→ ATTENTION, CONTROL). However, some findings do not support the hypothesis of a single general factor that accounts for the slowing of cognitive operations. Studies on response time, for example, have shown that the relative processing-time increase in elderly subjects compared to young adults depends on what cognitive function is called upon. Accordingly, the slowing coefficient is not as great on verbal tasks (lexical decision making, semantic categorization, etc.) as on other tasks (→ CATEGORIZATION, LEXICON, SEMANTICS). In current models, many of the age-related differences observed in a variety of situations depend on a combination of parameters that correspond to a small number of general factors (smaller resource pool, but also alteration of control and planning processes, lack of flexibility) and several specific factors.

This multifactor approach leads us to reject the earlier view that cognitive aging consists of a generalized and systematic decline. Age effects can vary as a function of the particular constraints of each task and the characteristics of each subject. In this light, it becomes important to search for factors that optimize behavior (favorable contextual conditions; → CONTEXT AND SITUATION) and to identify the adaptive strategies by means of which the elderly make the most of their capacities in their normal activities, and in doing so, reduce or even eliminate the differences brought about by their age.

An important problem in aging studies is being able to determine whether pathological aging involves qualitative changes or simply magnifications of what is observed in normal aging.

VIVIANE POUTHAS

Neuroscience. — The deterioration of intellectual performance with age is accompanied by morphological and metabolic alterations, presumably physiological, whose link to degenerative dementias such as *Alzheimer's disease* still poses many problems. Not only in aging, but also throughout development and in most pathological states of the brain (→ NEURO-PSYCHOLOGY), *neural network plasticity* is achieved through an ongoing renewal process brought about by an equilibrium between cell proliferation and cell death (of glial cells only, since neurons are postmitotic and can therefore only decrease in number) and by the remodeling of the dendritic arborization. Plasticity lessens with age, however, especially in the crucial memorization regions of the hippocampus (→ MEMORY). From a macroscopic standpoint, physiological aging is characterized by a decrease in the weight and volume of the brain (two percent per decade after age fifty). This *cerebral atrophy* varies across individuals and may even taper off in very old subjects. Scanning and magnetic resonance imaging (MRI) can be used to assess atrophy by looking at sulcus and ventricle widening (→ FUNCTIONAL NEUROIMAGING). Contrary to earlier observations, morphometric methods have revealed that neocortical neuron density is not considerably reduced, suggesting that age-related atrophy is related instead to neuron cell-body shrinking and impoverished dendritic arborization. An intracellular accumulation of lipofuscin is also observed, along with senile plaque lesions and neurofibrillary and granulovacuolar degeneration (the last three types of damage are not as great, though, and do not occur outside the hippocampus as often as in Alzheimer's disease). Alteration of the neurotransmitter systems (dopamine, acetylcholine, GABA) is particularly pronounced in the hippocampus. Metabolism tests yield an overall decrease in cerebral blood flow (xenon-133, HMPAO) and lower cortical uptake of oxygen and glucose (positron emission tomography).

Despite their respective methodological biases, cross-sectional and longitudinal studies alike have shown that physiological cognitive aging does exist. It is thus important to understand it in order to be able to say when a given cognitive behavior is still normal and when it has crossed the boundary and should be considered pathological (see *psychology* above). The decline is characterized by a twofold heterogeneity between and within individuals. Here again, this heterogeneity must be recognized, since a demential process that sets in can only inflate the differences observed in the normal population (→ DIFFERENTIATION). In the case of attentional processes, *divided attention* (selection of the most relevant message among several candidates) is thought to be more age sensitive than attention focused on one information source (→ ACTIVATION/INHIBITION, ATTENTION, INFORMATION). Age also has differential effects on memory, depending on the type of process at stake. Roughly, active working memory, recent memory, episodic memory, serial memory, free retrieval, and explicit memory are more adversely affected by aging than are immediate passive memory, remote memory, semantic memory, logical memory, retrieval by recognition, and implicit memory. A distinction is traditionally made between *fluid intelligence* (rapidity of mental processes and the ability to abstract, generalize, make inferences, and simultaneously process several pieces of information; → CONTROL, REASONING AND RATIONALITY) and *crystallized intelligence* (lexicosemantic knowledge, culturally acquired concepts; → CONCEPT, LEXICON, SEMANTICS), the latter being less sensitive to aging than the former. This sharp distinction has now been qualified for verbal performance, which declines moderately after the age of seventy but not to the same extent or manner for each component of language (→ LANGUAGE). For example, lexical retrieval, an active lexical search process, declines more than naming, which appears to be more affected by a decrease in the accessibility of the lexicon than by its own specific alteration. Oral comprehension may deteriorate due to limitations in working memory capacity. In narrations by elderly subjects, syntactic structures are simplified and more grammatical mistakes are made, whereas lexical diversity, number of words, and utterance length are not altered (→ GRAMMAR, SYNTAX, TEXT). Spontaneous speech turns out to be more elaborate, with longer and more complex sentences (→ DISCOURSE). Automatic processes, where conscious attention is not necessary, appear to remain intact, while controlled processes, which are effortful and require conscious analysis, decline (→ AUTOMATISM, CONTROL). In short, aging seems to slow down the processing speed of mental operations and decrease the ability to simultaneously carry out complex cognitive operations.

The incidence of *neurodegenerative diseases* (Alzheimer's and Parkinson's diseases, etc.) is correlated with age, but much is still unknown about the links between these diseases and biological aging. The assumed mechanisms are genetic, trophic, or cytotoxic. As a possible final route for different neurodegenerative mechanisms, an intracellular excess of calcium is promoted by the formation of free radicals, an excess of excitatory amino acids (glutamate, aspartate), alterations of mitochondrial energy metabolism, and the overactivation of cellular enzymes. Another important process is *apoptosis* (genetically programmed cell death), which is different from pathological cell death brought about by necrosis. As the result of an equilibrium between proapoptotic genes ("suicide" genes) and antiapoptotic genes (survival genes), apoptosis occurs both in physiological (embryonic and fetal development of nerve circuits) and pathological conditions. Its involvement is certain, but to different degrees as yet unspecified in many diseases, some of which are degenerative (Alzheimer's disease, amyotrophic lateral sclerosis, Parkinson's disease, HIV encephalopathies, stroke, prion-linked diseases, Huntington's disease, and spinal muscular atrophy).

Alzheimer's disease (AD) is a degenerative dementia that leads to death within seven or eight years. It is characterized by the progressive alteration of memory, behavior, personality, speech, and gestural and visuospatial functions. Along with the presence of an apoe4 allele, age is the main risk factor of late sporadic forms of AD, but recent studies seem to show that its prevalence reaches a plateau after age ninety-five. Mutations on chromosomes 21, 14, and 1 are the cause of early familial dominant-autosomic forms. Cortical atrophy, which is more pronounced in the internal temporal regions, is secondary to a neurofibrillary degeneration-linked neuron loss. Although also present in normal aging, senile plaques and neurofibrillary and granulovacuolar degeneration are nevertheless denser and more diffuse in AD. Three regions are damaged: the limbic system first (hippocampus-amygdala complex and entorhinal, para-hippocampal, and cingulate cortices), parietal, temporal, and prefrontal associative neocortical areas, and certain nuclei of the diencephalomesencephalic regions (nucleus basilis) and the brainstem. Senile plaque density is correlated with cognitive deterioration in Alzheimer patients. There are two opposing paradigms for explaining the links between aging and AD: a physiological one in which cognitive aging is the inevitable consequence of advancing age, and a nosological one according to which one or more diseases (degenerative dementias) of unknown cause set in.

BERNARD CROISILE

SELECTED BIBLIOGRAPHY

Binstock, R., & George, L. (Eds.). (2001). *Handbook of aging and the social sciences* (5th ed.). San Diego, CA: Academic Press.

Birren, J. (Ed.). (1996). *Encyclopedia of gerontology: Age, aging, and the aged.* San Diego, CA: Academic Press.

Birren, J., & Schaie, W. (Eds.). (1996). *Handbook of the psychology of aging* (4th ed.). San Diego, CA: Academic Press.

Graf, P., & Ohta, N. (Eds.). (2002). *Lifespan development of human memory.* Cambridge, MA: MIT Press.

Masoro, E., & Austad, S. (Eds.). (2001). *Handbook of the biology of aging.* San Diego, CA: Academic Press.

Perfect, T., & Maylor, E. (Eds.). (2000). *Models of cognitive aging.* Oxford, England; New York: Oxford University Press.

Troster, A. (Ed.). (1998). *Memory in neurodegenerative disease: Biological, cognitive, and clinical perspectives.* Cambridge, England; New York: Cambridge University Press.

ANIMAL COGNITION

Psychology. — Although animal intelligence was already a theme of ancient writings (in Western tradition, at least since Plato and Aristotle), René Descartes's doctrine of *dualism* (→ DUALISM/MONISM) has played a major role in modern scientific thinking about animal cognition. According to Descartes, animals are like automata and as such, are devoid of reason. By separating the mind ($\rightarrow$ MIND) from the mechanical characteristics of bodies, which are common to all organisms, Descartes's dualism and "animal-machine" theory nevertheless paved the way to modern physiology and later to *comparative psychology*. The latter field grew, in particular, out of Darwinism and its hypotheses on kinships among animal species. According to Charles Darwin, all animal species are situated along a continuum that encompasses not only anatomy but also mental faculties. This evolutionary theory provided the groundwork for the comparative study of intelligence across species, and in particular, between animals and humans. Human psychology added a number of unifying concepts applicable to all "intelligent" behaviors, such as problem solving and attention. These concepts, in conjunction with representation and memory supplied by information theory ($\rightarrow$ ATTENTION, INFORMATION, MEMORY, REPRESENTATION), laid a solid foundation for the upsurge of a cognitive psychology, both animal and human, that could stand up against behaviorism's innate learning models ($\rightarrow$ LEARNING). Another contribution of human psychology was to devise methods (such as mental chronometry) for the experimental study of cognition, which both complemented and extended methods borrowed from conditioning procedures.

Entertaining the idea that there is an animal cognition underlying learned behaviors is justified insofar as explanations in terms of conditioning cannot account for the complexity of learning. But this initial definition, adopted merely by a process of elimination, must be supplemented with positive elements such as reliance on central *information processing systems* in the form of, say, internal representations of objects or situations, possessed by animals and man.

From this angle, the organism (animal or human) is seen as an information extractor and processor and an inference generator, whether at the lower levels of sensorimotor integration or at the higher levels of problem solving and reasoning ($\rightarrow$ REASONING AND RATIONALITY). The contemporary study of animal cognition thus deliberately makes use of metaphors in which animals cognize as they transform information and make decisions. The main characteristic of this approach, then, is that it considers every animal to be an actor in the adaptive process, an actor that selects and processes information in order to adapt. Any area of activity can be analyzed accordingly through this "cognitivist filter": memory, problem solving, reasoning, self-recognition, knowledge attribution ($\rightarrow$ THEORY OF MIND), and so on.

The study of animal cognition has two major branches: comparative psychology and ethology. Starting from these two main disciplines, three distinct perspectives can be discerned in investigations of animal cognition: the *synthetic approach*, the *psychology of cognition*, and *cognitive ethology*.

1. The synthetic approach, sometimes called *ecological*, is used by researchers such as Allan Kamil and Paul Rozin, whose orientation is biological. They stress adaptation factors in animals and their ability to solve problems in their natural environment. Some of the most preferred topics of these ethologists are the organization of memory and behavior during foraging activities, perception and learning of communication signals (such as bird calls) (→ COMMUNICATION, PERCEPTION), and recognition of conspecifics.

2. In the psychology of cognition, researchers such as Herbert Roitblat, Herbert Terrace, and Jacques Vauclair take a more psychological approach. They conduct cross-species comparisons in the laboratory to detect the general, common cognitive mechanisms responsible for the intake and processing of information from the environment. All types of cognitive processing are likely to be addressed in this research trend, including perception, attention, and problem solving (as the animal processes inert objects in the environment), as well as cognitive mechanisms that take effect during communication and social relations (for example, intentionality and theories of mind; → INTENTIONALITY).

3. Finally, cognitive ethology encompasses researchers who, under the impetus of Donald Griffin, take a comparative viewpoint in order to study thought, consciousness (→ CONSCIOUSNESS), beliefs (→ BELIEF), and, in a broader way, the "mental experiences of animals."

Each of the three approaches has its strong points and shortcomings. Briefly, the synthetic approach, whose main goal is to specify the biological context in which cognitive processes have evolved, is limited to comparisons between animal species with a phylogenetic kinship but different cognitive problems, or between unrelated species with the same cognitive problems (for example, species that inhabit the same ecological niche). The results of this type of research should provide greater insight into the impact of evolutionary mechanisms on cognition, and show how cognitive processes are in fact specialized adaptations to the demands of the environment. The psychology of animal cognition takes a general approach, since its aim is to detect identical cognitive traits across species, sometimes species that are phylogenetically far removed from each other. One of its contributions should be to narrow the range of plausible explanations of cognition, particularly those related to the possession and use of articulated language (→ LANGUAGE). Finally, cognitive ethology also postulates the existence of complex cognitive mechanisms in all animals, regardless of their phylogenetic position, and one of the future tasks in its ambitious plan to study animal consciousness is to devise a suitable methodology for this object of study.

JACQUES VAUCLAIR

Philosophy. — From a philosophical point of view, posing the problem of animal cognition means questioning the validity limits of the concepts of cognition and the mind (→ MIND) and distinguishing between cognitive species with and without language (→ LANGUAGE). Davidson regards this question as merely a colorful (and sometimes emotional) way of posing the problem of the nature of thought. Note, however, that the answer given to this question nevertheless defines the conditions for the ethics of human-animal interaction.

One of the more common objections to the hypothesized existence of animal thought is the argument that animals are incapable of speech. In fact, it was for the same kind of reason, but in reverse—that is, that animals seemed to possess linguistic capabilities—that philosophers of ancient times and the classical age endowed the animal kingdom with the ability to think and reason (→ REASONING AND RATIONALITY) and adopted a *continuum-based position* in matters of animal cognition, deemed to differ only in degree from human cognition. The early philosophers advanced three types of arguments: (1) external language, which seems to be what enables animals to profitably cooperate in joint actions, presupposes an internal representation of cooperative situations (→ ACTION, REPRESENTATION, SOCIAL COGNITION); (2) imitation of human language by animals (magpies, parrots, etc.) presupposes the capacity to represent the imitated utterances; and (3) the problem-solving capabilities of certain animals presuppose the ability to reason. Against this continuationist doctrine, Descartes raised the following three objections: (1) if animals are capable of thinking, they should be capable of making themselves understood by us, given that "they have several organs equivalent to ours"; (2) the essence of language does not inhere in the ability to emit signals, but in the ability to compose signs in order to be understood (→ COMMUNICATION, SIGN), or, stated in another way, the use of language implies an *intention* to signify and a structured capacity to employ a linguistic system, both of which are beyond the scope of animals; and (3) mastery of language goes hand in hand with mastery of rational thinking, and consequently, it is because animals are devoid of reason that they cannot speak.

But Descartes's arguments can be questioned: (1) even though animals do not have external language, they may have internal means of representation; (2) an animal might be capable of utilizing representations without being in a position to employ them to communicate with other individuals, be they conspecifics or otherwise (but Descartes was right on one point: what is improperly called "animal communication" is often nothing more than the transmission and utilization of information, without the intention of having other individuals recognize an intent to communicate a message); and (3) it is not the mechanical or more generally material nature of a device that renders it unsuited to rationality; what makes the difference is the type of machine it instantiates. Any mind, by the sheer fact that it computes, must go through states formally equivalent to those of a Turing machine, and must be realized physically (→ TURING MACHINE).

Reflection about intentionality has pointed out the conditions in which the internal states of an animal can afford it cognizance of the world, that is, support the construction of a representation of the world that is geared to its needs (→ GOAL, INTENTIONALITY). Animal cognition requires the animal to be able to store in memory and later utilize information extracted from certain invariants and certain dynamics of the environment (→ IN-FORMATION, MEMORY), and to represent those invariants in a self-removed or "detached" manner. One can assume that the capacity to integrate perceptions cross-modally plays a crucial role in the extraction of the spatiotemporal invariants that constitute representations of objects and events (→ PERCEPTION). From a philosophical standpoint, the capacity to correct one's perceptual input in a systematic manner (*perceptual recalibration*)—which governs the extraction of invariants—plays a crucial role in building a veridical representation of the world. This capacity, present in birds, reptiles, and mammals, but probably absent in insects, could serve as the criterion for drawing the line between animals with and without cognition.

JOËLLE PROUST

SELECTED BIBLIOGRAPHY

Davidson, D. (1985). Rational animals. In E. Lepore & B. McLaughlin (Eds.), *Actions, events: Perspectives on the philosophy of Donald Davidson.* Oxford, England: Blackwell.

Descartes, R. (1999). *Discourse on method* (D. M. Clarke, Trans.). London: Penguin Books. (Original work published 1637.)

Gallistel, C. (Ed.). (1992). *Animal cognition.* Cambridge, MA: MIT Press.

Griffin, D. (2001). *Animal minds: Beyond cognition to consciousness.* Chicago: University of Chicago Press.

Hauser, M. (2000). *Wild minds: What animals really think.* New York: Henry Holt.

Hauser, M., Chomsky, N., & Fitch, W. (2002). The faculty of language: What is it, who has it, and how did it evolve? *Science, 298,* 1569–1579.

Panksepp, J. (1998). *Affective neuroscience: The foundations of human and animal emotions.* New York: Oxford University Press.

Ristau, C. (Ed.). (1991). *Cognitive ethology: The minds of other animals. Essays in Honor of Donald R. Griffin.* Hillsdale, NJ: Erlbaum.

Tomasello, M., & Call, J. (1997). *Primate cognition.* Oxford, England; New York: Oxford University Press.

Vauclair, J. (1996). *Animal cognition: An introduction to modern comparative psychology.* Cambridge, MA: Harvard University Press.

ARTIFICIAL LIFE

Artificial intelligence. — The recent interest in *artificial life* is part of a tradition initiated by cybernetics, which offers a common conceptual framework for studying both natural and artificial objects. Artificial life represents an important conceptual advancement in modern science, and attempts to bridge the gap between the mind, life, and matter (→ MIND).

In postulating that life is a property not of matter, but of a way of organizing matter, the study of artificial life attempts to gain insight into what differentiates the sciences of matter from the sciences of life. In postulating that at the heart of all cognitive faculties is the faculty to be alive, it attempts to bring the cognitive sciences and the life sciences closer together. Because it takes an interest in the *emergent properties* of life as an organized form of matter, artificial life can be regarded as a synthetic biology (→ EMERGENCE). And because in doing so, it takes an interest in a class of systems endowed with cognitive faculties greater than those of living systems, it can be viewed as a theory of *autonomous systems*.

Artificial life, like biology, is a scientific field devoted to understanding whatever is alive. Unlike biology, however, it is less concerned with the analytic properties of living organisms than with their emerging synthetic properties. It focuses accordingly on abstracting the fundamental life processes, in order to study the dynamic principles that manifest those emerging properties, and then strives to test those principles on appropriate physical media. John von Neumann's self-reproducing automata, Aristid Lindenmayer's systems for morphogenesis, and John Holland's genetic algorithms for evolutionary phenomena are all examples of the abstraction of the fundamental processes of living things.

How did the metabolites responsible for the cycles and hypercycles of cellular metabolism get selected? How does a vast number of cells get organized into types of cells in order to form a multicellular being capable of self-repair? How do immense collections of lymphocytes manage to make the vital distinction between the self and the nonself? How can a large number of species coevolve within the ecosphere? How can we grasp all these phenomena of emergence, in which systems maintain their organization in an autopoietic manner? At every level, life is the seat of self-organization processes, between order and chaos. A major heuristic of artificial life is the hypothesis that life is situated at the transition point between order and disorder, on the brink of chaos, where the large interactive systems are at their peak of complexity.

In postulating that life is a property not of matter but of a way of organizing matter, artificial life provides a route for experimentation on physical media other than the carbon chains found in living organisms. In particular, the study of the large *interactive systems* that make up living beings, viewed as complex evolutive cosystems, is approached by means of modeling and simulation. Although some simulations are performed on analogical physical media, the computer is usually the privileged instrument: in this sense, artificial life also encompasses a computational biology.

As a discipline at the crossroads of biology, artificial intelligence (AI), and the cognitive and physical sciences, artificial life is based on the premise that the core cognitive faculty is in the capacity to live, that is, to maintain one's viability and autonomy in diverse and ever-changing environments (→ CONSTRUCTIVISM). This capacity to live is rooted in a sensorimotor apparatus (→ ACTION, PERCEPTION). The mind ceases to be separate from the body as it is in Cartesian dualism (→ DUALISM/MONISM), and cognition is no longer solely the work of a pure mind that manipulates symbols (→ COGNITIVISM, SYMBOL). It is the emergence of a world of meanings for a given mind existing within a body. Finally, an autonomous system cannot be conceived of in isolation: its viability depends on symbiotic interactions with an environment composed of other autonomous systems. This dependence becomes crucial during social interactions between individuals of the same species, a perfect example being insect societies (→ ANIMAL COGNITION, COMMUNICATION, INTERACTION, SOCIAL COGNITION). *Collective intelligence* is regarded as the ability of a society of autonomous systems to be better at solving their viability problem collectively rather than individually (→ DISTRIBUTED INTELLIGENCE).

To understand autonomous systems, artificial life strives to discover their fundamental dynamic principles. Research in this area benefits from knowledge acquired in AI, from connectionist approaches for its cognitive aspects (→ CONNECTIONISM), and from game theory for studying social interaction. In designing and experimenting with autonomous agents, the study of artificial life sheds new light on traditional engineering fields such as robotics and control theory (→ CONTROL, ROBOTICS), while introducing concepts derived from biology such as viability, autonomy, adaptation, and collective intelligence.

PAUL BOURGINE

SELECTED BIBLIOGRAPHY

Adami, C. (1998). *Introduction to artificial life*. New York: Springer.

Boden, M. (Ed.). (1996). *The philosophy of artificial life*. Oxford, England; New York: Oxford University Press.

Bonabeau, E., Dorigo, M., & Theraulaz, G. (1999). *Swarm intelligence: From natural to artificial systems*. New York: Oxford University Press.

Dasgupta, D. (Ed.). (1999). *Artificial immune systems and their applications*. Berlin, Germany; New York: Springer-Verlag.

Fogel, G., & Corne, D. (2003). *Evolutionary computation in bioinformatics*. San Francisco, CA: Morgan Kaufmann.

Holland, J. (1975). *Adaptation in natural and artificial systems: An introductory analysis with applications to biology, control, and artificial intelligence*. Cambridge, MA: MIT Press.

Koza, J., Bennett, F., André, D., & Keane, M. (Eds.). (1999). *Genetic programming III: Darwinian invention and problem solving*. San Francisco, CA: Morgan Kaufmann.

Mitchell, M. (1990). *An introduction to genetic algorithms*. Cambridge, MA: MIT Press.

Standish, R., Abbass, H., & Bedau, M. (Eds.). (2003). *Artificial life VIII: Proceedings of the Eighth International Conference on Artificial Life*. Cambridge, MA: MIT Press.

ASPECT

Linguistics. — The concept of *aspect*, which appeared in Russian grammars of the nineteenth century and rapidly spread to all Slavic languages, took a very long time to find its way into the grammars of languages like French and English, which do not have a system of morphological markers devoted to its expression (→ GRAMMAR, MORPHOLOGY). French owes the first real efforts to theorize aspect-related phenomena to Gustave Guillaume. Guillaume distinguished two kinds of time. One serves as a framework for locating occurrences (states or events) in time; the other is internal to the occurrence (the time it takes to unfold), which, strictly speaking, is the aspect of the occurrence (→ TIME AND TENSE). Another distinction that gradually became vital was between two main types of aspect. *Lexical aspect*, which is marked by the verbal lexeme and its semantic-case environment (→ LEXICON, THEMATIC RELATION), defines the type of occurrence. *Grammatical aspect*, essentially expressed by the verb tense and certain adverbs of aspect, is the presentation mode of the occurrence (the way it is perceived or taken into account).

In linguistic studies on lexical aspect, the traditional opposition between verbs of action and verbs of state or being has gradually been replaced by much finer classifications that break down processes into different types. All parts of predication are considered rather than the verb alone as in the past (for example, *to come out* does not express the same type of process in *Pierre is coming out of the kitchen* as it does in *Black smoke is coming out of the chimney*). The classifications proposed are based on (or go against) the now well-known one proposed by Zeno Vendler, who distinguishes states, activities, accomplishments, and achievements. The distinction between these classes is made on the basis of three main features: dynamic, bounded, and punctual. Accordingly, states are [−dynamic], [−bounded], [−punctual]; activities are [+dynamic], [bounded], [−punctual]; accomplishments are [+dynamic], [+bounded], [−punctual]; and achievements are [+dynamic], [+bounded], [+punctual].

The values of these features are attributed by applying tests. For English, (1) if the predicate is compatible with the phrase [*be* Ving] (Ving = present participle of verb), the process is [+dynamic]; for example, *He is walking; *He is liking chocolate* (an asterisk indicates an ungrammatical sequence). (2) If the predicate is compatible with [*for/during* + duration] and incompatible with [*in/within* + duration], the process is [−bounded]; for example, *He walked for two hours; ?*He walked in two hours* (an asterisk preceded by a question mark indicates questionable grammaticality; the sequence could be accepted only in a highly specific context). In other words, the linguistic meaning of the predicate, here *to walk*, does not imply that the process has an end. Different authors also call such processes *imperfective, atelic, inconclusive*, or *extrinsically bounded*. (3) If the predicate is compatible with [*in/within* + duration] and incompatible with [*for/during* + duration], the process is [+bounded]; for example, *?*He drank a lemonade for five minutes; He drank a lemonade in five minutes*. In this case, the linguistic meaning of the predicate (complements included) implies that the process has an end. Other terms used to express boundedness are *perfective, telic, conclusive*, and *intrinsically bounded*. (4) A process is considered [+punctual] if, when the phrase [*took a certain amount of time* Vinf] (where Vinf = verb in the infinitive) is introduced into the utterance, it is interpreted as expressing the duration not of the process itself (which, by definition, is punctual) but of the preparatory phase; for example, *He took two hours to reach the peak* (≅ *before reaching the peak*; punctual process); *He took two hours to read his novel* (≠ *before reading his novel*).

However, applying compatibility tests 1, 2, and 3 above poses some problems, since the process may get "deformed" under the effects of the test. This often happens in cases of contextual polysemy, a common phenomenon (→ CONTEXT AND SITUATION), where detection is unsuccessful without additional tests using paraphrases (as in test 3). For example, I could very well say of a child *He slept within ten minutes*, but it would be incorrect to thereby assume that *to sleep* expresses an accomplishment or an achievement, since in this example, it is the preparatory phase of the process that is at stake. This becomes apparent if we paraphrase the utterance as *Ten minutes went by before he slept*. Similarly, in *He stopped for an hour*, it is the duration of the resulting state that is assessed (being in a stopped state), not the duration of the stopping process itself, which is intrinsically punctual.

By contrast, grammatical aspect is easy to analyze and represent if we make use of the idea of a *reference time frame*, defined as the time span referred to or taken into account (and potentially stated) in the utterance. The various possible relationships between the reference time frame and the time taken by the process define the different types of grammatical aspect: (1) perfective aspect (this term is also confusingly employed by some authors to refer to lexical aspect) or *aoristic aspect*, where the two time frames coincide and the process is thus seen in its entirety, for example, *He slept for two hours;* (2) imperfective or *unaccomplished aspect*, where the reference time frame is included in that of the process, of which neither the beginning nor the end is considered, for example, *At midnight, he was sleeping;* (3) *accomplished aspect*, where the reference time frame succeeds that of the process, of which only the resulting state is declared, for example, *His work had been finished for ten minutes;* (4) *prospective aspect*, where the reference time frame precedes that of the process, of which only the preparatory phase is taken into account, for example, *(I see that) he is going to get sick;* (5) *inchoative aspect*, where the reference time frame (infinitely small) corresponds to the beginning of the process, for example, *He slept at eight o'clock (≅ fell asleep);* (6) *terminative aspect*, where the reference time frame (infinitely small) coincides with the end of the process, for example, *He came home at eight o'clock (≅ arrived);* and (7) *iterative aspect*, where the process is reiterated to form a series, with each occurrence in the series being seen as perfective, but the series itself being presented as unaccomplished, for example, *He had been eating in fifteen minutes for a month.*

Attempts to determine aspect come up against the same obstacles as those encountered in determining temporal relations: the markers are generally polysemous and they interact with each other in a holistic way (→ HOLISM). For instance, in the statement *(At that time) Pierre was sleeping within five minutes*—which could legitimately be followed by something like *but now, he has to read for two hours before he can fall asleep*—the imperfect has an iterative value, *to sleep* means *to fall asleep*, and *within five minutes* does not refer to the duration of the process itself, but to that of its preparatory phase (the time between when Pierre used to go to bed and when he would fell asleep). These meanings are interdependent: it is because the process is interpreted as punctual and inchoative that the circumstantial element expressing duration applies to the preparatory phase, but it is also because of this circumstantial clause that the phase of the process considered is construed to be the initial one.

LAURENT GOSSELIN

SELECTED BIBLIOGRAPHY

Bybee, J., Perkins, R., & Pagliuca, W. (1994). *The evolution of grammar: Tense, aspect, and modality in the languages of the world.* Chicago: University of Chicago Press.
Guillaume, G. (1929/1984). *Temps et verbe: Théorie des aspects, des modes et des temps* [Time and verb: A theory aspects, moods, and tenses]. Paris: Champion.
Vendler, Z. (1967). *Linguistics in philosophy.* Ithaca, NY: Cornell University Press.

ATTENTION

Psychology. — *Attention* encompasses various cognitive activities that are carried out on representations (→ REPRESENTATION) and involve amplification (enhancement) and attenuation (*inhibition*) mechanisms (→ ACTIVA-

TION/INHIBITION); such mechanisms temporarily change the efficiency of our mental processes and have behavioral consequences manifested in the form of benefits.

Attention is related to the way the cognitive system processes information (→ INFORMATION). A *two-stage processing* view, in which an initial parallel-processing stage is followed by a second, sequential stage was first proposed by Donald Broadbent in 1958. Later, in the 1970s, under the impetus of researchers such as Michael Posner, Richard Shiffrin, and Walter Schneider, this view gave way to a new one based on the distinction between two types of processes: *automatic processes*, which are rapid parallel processes that do not require attention (→ AUTOMATISM), and *controlled processes*, which are slow, serial, and strategically determined (→ CONTROL). Anne Treisman's model of feature integration exemplifies this approach. *Target detection* is said to be automatic when it is defined by a single elementary property, on a single dimension such as color, brightness, size, or shape that can be analyzed by prewired, specialized detectors functioning in parallel (the target "pops out" no matter how many distractors are simultaneously present). In contrast, when the target is defined by a combination of two elementary properties belonging to two different dimensions and for which there is no dedicated analyzer, detection is controlled. Acting as a sort of "glue," attention temporarily holds the combination of expected properties together in a coherent representation of the object.

An important dimension of attention is its *selectiveness*. In visuospatial processing (→ SPACE), Posner pointed out the impact of preparatory directing of attention on the efficiency of target detection. He considers attention to correspond to a *focus* on a specific location in the visual scene (→ PERCEPTION). This focusing enhances the processing of information at that location (benefits) and inhibits information located elsewhere (costs). The direction of the focus may be predetermined involuntarily by the unexpected arrival of external peripheral stimulation (*exogenous attention*) or determined voluntarily by a prior strategic decision (*endogenous attention*). David LaBerge suggested that when targets and distractors are located in the same space, sustained attention helps render the target more perceptually salient.

Information to which we do not attend is generally poorly recalled (→ MEMORY). As Fergus Craik and Robert Lockhart showed, memory performance seems to depend on the depth of the cognitive processing carried out during encoding, with encoding depending in turn on the availability of attentional resources.

Various theoretical proposals have been advanced to account for the allocation of attentional resources. Daniel Kahneman suggested the existence of a *central administrator* that prioritizes the different operations.

Alan Baddeley defined a *central executive* that coordinates and integrates representations useful for the current activity. Don Norman and Tim Shallice proposed a *supervisory attentional system* whose function is to ensure some degree of cognitive flexibility; this system is thought to be impaired in cases of frontal brain damage (see *neuroscience* below). The privileged tool of these cognitive "managers" seems to be a set of inhibitory processes capable not only of resisting distraction, but also of avoiding the irruption of routine behavior schemas that turn out to be ineffective, particularly in unfamiliar situations or when new problems must be solved.

JEAN-FRANÇOIS CAMUS

Neuroscience. — Attention is a key concept in understanding how the brain works. It is linked to mental capacity limitations and seems to be the principal factor in controlling cerebral functions and behavior (→ CONTROL). Analysis of the neural characteristics of attention brings out the predominant role played by certain structures. These structures are organized into a complex circuit or *network* (→ NEURAL NETWORK) that is responsible for the fundamental features of attentional processes already noted by William James, namely, selecting what information to process and maintaining (or varying) the processing level (→ INFORMATION). Evidence of such a network involving different encephalic regions has been provided both by neuropsychological research on humans (brain-damage studies, recordings of brain metabolism) and by neurophysiological research on animals (lesions, single-cell recording) (→ FUNCTIONAL NEUROIMAGING, NEUROPSYCHOLOGY).

The selective component of attention chooses what information to process. Clearly, it is not possible to do in-depth processing of all simultaneously incoming information. The necessary choice of what information to process depends on the joint operation of several brain areas or regions. Selective attention thus plays an essential role in visual information intake by selecting information located at a given spot in space (→ PERCEPTION, SPACE). The superior colliculi (mesencephalon), phylogenetically the oldest structures involved in selective attention, seem to be what enable ocular movements to adjust rapidly to a peripheral target. In the brain, certain thalamic nuclei (like the pulvinar) filter information coming into the cortex, and this is what allows attention to be directed at a given source of information. Pulvinar function has been shown to be associated with the allocation of attention, whether *passive* (attention attracted selectively to a sudden change of information) or *active* (attention controlled by central processes). The posterior cortical regions, especially the parietal regions, are involved in the selection of spatial information. Parietal lesions in humans cause *hemineglect*, where the part of the world contralateral to the lesion is ignored: patients with this syndrome have trouble looking at that hemifield and pay no attention to it.

Since the early studies by David Ferrier in the nineteenth century, the prefrontal cortex has been regarded as an associative "supercortex" that is particularly well developed in humans and acts as a veritable controller of behavior. Today's research has shown that this cortical area makes the final decisions about our behavior, such as deciding to inhibit an immediate response (a routine) that is currently irrelevant (→ ACTIVATION/INHIBITION), initiating a processing strategy when a choice has to be made, and planning a behavior sequence. This cortex can thus be considered to act as an attentional system supervisor in selective attention, to borrow Norman and Shallice's terminology. However, unlike the posterior cortex, it is less involved in selecting what information to process than in choosing a processing strategy for complex tasks. In the view of certain researchers like Posner, it is especially the left frontal lobe that plays this role in humans.

Finally, the most general aspect of attention, that is, the overall, undifferentiated level of arousal underlying our mental abilities, depends on the implication of the midbrain reticular formation, whose function was first demonstrated in 1949 by Giuseppe Moruzzi and Horace Magoun. The locus coeruleus is thought to be responsible for variations in the level of vigilance or alertness. This noradrenergic system sends efferences to the greater part of the nervous system, operating in connection with the reticular nuclei of the thalamus and certain frontal regions, especially right frontal ones in humans.

The neural complex just described constitutes the privileged circuit in the nervous system for fulfilling the various functions of attention. Of course, the attentional system is tightly connected to other systems, such as the temporal areas that ensure memory retrieval of already learned information and storage of new information (→ MEMORY). It also works in close connection with the limbic circuit, particularly the cingulate gyrus, which forms the individual's motivation system (→ EMOTION). Finally, the attentional system surely also plays a role in the mechanisms of consciousness (→ CONSCIOUSNESS), for it is in charge of selecting the "object of the consciousness."

ÉRIC SIÉROFF

SELECTED BIBLIOGRAPHY

Baddeley, A., and L. Weiskrantz. (1993). *Attention: Selection, awareness and control.* Oxford, England: Clarendon Press.

Braun, J., Koch, C., & Davis, J. (Eds.). (2001). *Visual attention and cortical circuits.* Cambridge, MA: MIT Press.

Broadbent, D. E. (1958). *Attention and communication.* New York: Pergamon Press.

Cowan, N. (1995). *Attention and memory: An integrated framework.* Oxford, England: Clarendon Press; New York: Oxford University Press.

Dagenbach, D., & Carr, T. (Eds.). (1994). *Inhibitory processes in attention, memory, and language*. San Diego, CA: Academic Press.

Gazzaniga, M. (Ed.). (2000). *The new cognitive neurosciences* (Section V, *Attention*) (2nd ed.). Cambridge, MA: MIT Press.

Ghatan, P., Hsieh, J., Petersson, K., Stone-Elander, S., & Ingvar, M. (1998). Coexistence of attention-based facilitation and inhibition in the human cortex. *NeuroImage, 7*, 23–29.

Humphreys, G., Duncan, J., & Treisman, A. (Eds.). (1999). *Attention, space and action: Studies in cognitive neuroscience*. Oxford, England; New York: Oxford University Press.

LaBerge, D. (1995). *Attentional processing: The brain's art of mindfulness*. Cambridge, MA: Harvard University Press.

Pashler, H. (1998). *The psychology of attention*. Cambridge, MA: MIT Press.

Posner, M., & Raichle, M. (1994/1997). *Images of mind*. New York: Freeman.

Scholl, B. (Ed.). (2002). *Objects and attention*. Cambridge, MA: MIT Press.

AUTISM

Psychology. — In his pioneering work published in 1943, Leo Kanner isolated *autism* as a syndrome characterized by (1) the inability to establish socioaffective relations with others (→ SOCIAL COGNITION), (2) mutism or the incapacity to use language for communicative purposes (→ COMMUNICATION, LANGUAGE), and (3) abnormal responses to the environment (stereotypies, immutability)—all standing out against a normal physical appearance and isolated areas of competency. The symptomatology was later supplemented with another criterion: (4) the appearance of these signs before the age of thirty months. Despite general agreement on these four criteria, it is always difficult to establish an irrefutable diagnosis of autism. Mental deficiencies and other associated impairments, frequent but not necessarily present, are one of the reasons for this uncertainty, which is made worse by the fact that the criteria remained rather subjective for quite some time. *Asperger's syndrome*, another form of autism isolated by Hans Asperger, involves socioaffective impairment associated with normal language development.

Added to the problem of difficulty diagnosing autism is the opposition between two major etiological perspectives: the psychoanalytically oriented approach, which considers the causes to be environmental, and the neurocognitive approach (→ COGNITIVE PSYCHIATRY), which acknowledges a biological etiology of a neurological type. It should be noted, however, that a neurological etiology does not rule out the hypothesis of a primary social or emotional disorder (→ EMOTION).

The diagnosis of autism became more reliable when behavioral criteria were adopted by the *International Classification of Child Psychopathological Diseases* (ICD10) established by the World Health Organization, and in the various versions of the *Diagnostic and Statistical Manual* published by the American Psychiatric Association (current version: *DSM-IV*).

The hypothesis of the biological etiology of autism, along with recognition of the developmental character of the syndrome, led to the recent implementation of simulations of its development based on the assumed primary deficits. The postulates are grounded in ontogenetic models. The many studies revolve around three main models of autism: Peter Hobson's *emotional theory*, in which the initial impairments concern the innate capacity to decode emotions as "transparent mental states"; Sally Rogers and Bruce Pennington's *intersubjective model*, where the neonatal capacity for intermodal transfer linked to imitation is deficient (→ INFANT COGNITION); and Simon Baron-Cohen, Alan Leslie, and Uta Frith's *metarepresentational theory*, according to which the primary deficit concerns the development of a *theory of mind* (→ THEORY OF MIND). While the alleged imitative impairment remains a controversial issue, a consensus has been reached on the emotional and metarepresentational deficits. However, no conclusion can be drawn at present concerning the order of precedence of the deficits.

JACQUELINE NADEL

SELECTED BIBLIOGRAPHY

Baron-Cohen, S., Tager-Flusberg, H., & Cohen, D. (Eds.). (2000). *Understanding other minds: Perspectives from developmental cognitive neurosc*ience. Oxford, England; New York: Oxford University Press.

Frith, U. (1992). *Autism: Explaining the enigma*. Oxford, England; Cambridge, MA: Blackwell.

Hobson, P. (1993). *Autism and the development of mind*. Hillsdale, NJ: Erlbaum.

Mitchell, P. (1996). *Introduction to theory of mind: Children, autism and apes*. London: Arnold.

Nelson, C., & Luciana, M. (Eds.). (2001). *Developmental cognitive neuroscience* (Section VII, *Neurodevelopmental aspects of clinical disorders*). Cambridge, MA: MIT Press.

Rogers, S., & Pennington, B. (1991). A theoretical approach to the deficits in infantile autism. *Development and Psychopathology, 3*, 137–162.

AUTOMATISM

Psychology. — In cognitive psychology, *automatic information processing* is generally qualified as having no attentional load , no controlled processes, a lack of consciousness, parallel operations, and fast execution (→ ATTENTION, CONSCIOUSNESS, CONTROL, INFORMATION).

Richard Schiffrin and Walter Schneider operationalized the opposition between automatic processing and *controlled processing* in an experimental paradigm that became very influential in research on cognitive automatisms. In the task they devised, subjects had to detect previously memorized targets (→ MEMORY) among distractors seen on a sequence of screens. In the first series of trials, the processing time of each screen was a function of the number of items memorized and the number of items presented on the screen. With practice, processing time became considerably shorter and no longer depended on the number of items memorized and presented, as if the items were being processed in parallel. However, the change from controlled processing (dependent on the number of items) to automatic processing (independent of the quantity of information processed) took place only when the targets on consecutive trials were coherent (that is, when the target of one trial was not a distractor of the next).

To show that automatic processing has no attentional load, the most common experimental paradigm used is the *dual-task paradigm*, in which two different tasks are performed at the same time. In one of its variants, subjects are asked to place priority on the task whose degree of automatization is being assessed, in such a way that the second task is executed with residual attentional resources. The amount of attention allocated to the primary task is then assessed indirectly by looking at the performance decline on the secondary task compared to when it was executed alone.

To demonstrate the absence of control in automatic processing, the *Stroop effect* is often used. John Stroop showed that it was particularly difficult to name the color of the ink used to print a word when the word happens to be the name of another color (for example, saying *blue* when the word printed in blue is the word *red*). The difficulty is thought to stem from the fact that word reading is a highly automatized and thus "mandatory" activity that has to be inhibited in order to name the word's color (→ ACTIVATION/INHIBITION, READING). The degree of automaticity in reading (but also difficulty inhibiting this automatism) is measured as the difference between the time taken to name colors in a simple situation and in the Stroop situation. The principle behind the Stroop effect has been generalized to a variety of tasks.

Problems encountered in classifying various processes into the automatic versus controlled dichotomy led to the acknowledgment that the distinction is not so clear cut and that there probably are not any processes that use no attentional resources at all. Instead, there seems to be a continuum along which the amount of allocated attention varies. The nature of automatic processing has also been subject to debate. A theory worth mentioning is Gordon Logan's theory positing that automatization does not consist in executing the same operations faster and thereby disengaging attention, but in directly retrieving from memory-specific solutions to each particular problem already encountered.

JACQUES LAUTREY

Neuroscience. — In the 1880s, the English physician John Hughlings Jackson pointed out the automatic-voluntary opposition in behavior (→ CONTROL, WILL). He also hypothesized the existence of brain mechanisms for automatic processes. In Jackson's view, automatisms call upon processes that are well organized in the nervous system and are thus less fragile in cases of partial neurological lesions (→ NEUROPSYCHOLOGY). In contrast, highly voluntary processes (phylogenetically more recent) are more complex and not very organized; they are less well established in the nervous system and thus more fragile.

An illustration of the robustness of automatic processes can be found in the performance of patients who have lost control over some of their behavior. Take the case of the anomic patient who was asked by Théophile Alajouanine to state the first name of her daughter seated next to her. After failing to name the girl, the woman apologized and turned to her daughter and said, "See, my poor Jeannine, I can't even remember your first name anymore." The daughter's name was thus not lost, but it was available only in ordinary situations. There are many examples of automatisms that subsist after focal brain damage, including uncontrolled processing routines in cases of frontal brain damage, implicit learning abilities in amnesic patients with hippocampal lesions ($\rightarrow$ LEARNING, MEMORY), automatic processing of spatial information in hemineglect patients who are no longer able to direct their attention to the side opposite their lesion ($\rightarrow$ ATTENTION, SPACE), and so on.

The findings suggest that "learned" automatisms, that is, cognitive ones, involve networks that are highly distributed throughout the nervous system. Only attentional processes appear to implicate a set of anatomically and functionally distinct areas ($\rightarrow$ LOCALIZATION OF FUNCTION). However, automatisms of peripheral information processing (for example, the innate faculty to detect elementary features in the visual world such as color, tilt of contrasting lines, etc.) are known to rely on the functioning of specialized cells in the primary cortical areas and specific secondary cortical areas ($\rightarrow$ PERCEPTION). In fact, the question of the neural substrate of cognitive automatisms is certainly one of the least well-understood issues in neuroscience.

ÉRIC SIÉROFF

SELECTED BIBLIOGRAPHY

Dulany, D., & Logan, G. (Eds.). (1992). Views and varieties of automaticity. *American Journal of Psychology, 105* (2).

Logan, G. D. (1988). Toward an instance theory of automatization. *Psychological Review, 95*, 492–527.

Schiffrin, R. M., & Schneider, W. (1977). Controlled and automatic human processing: II. Perceptual learning, automatic attention and a general theory. *Psychological Review, 84*, 127–190.

Uleman, J., & Bargh, J. (Eds.). (1989). *Unintended thought*. New York: Guilford Press.

B

BELIEF

Philosophy. — In everyday usage, a *belief* is a certain psychological state that leads the subject to assent to a given representation whose epistemic status is unsure or doubtful (→ EPISTEMIC, REPRESENTATION). In this sense, a belief is not a piece of knowledge: if X knows that p, then p is true, whereas if X believes that p, p is not necessarily true. Since Bertrand Russell, contemporary philosophers have treated beliefs as *propositional attitudes* endowed with an *intentional* or *semantic content*, that is, capable of being true or false and of representing the world in some fashion (→ INTENTIONALITY, PROPOSITIONAL ATTITUDE, SEMANTICS). A distinction is generally made between the psychological problem, which concerns the nature of the mental state (the belief), and the semantic or logical problem (→ LOGIC), which consists in determining the logical form of belief attributions (X believes that p). But the next problem—that of knowing whether the attributions are about a relationship between the subject and some entity (A proposition? A sentence?)—is closely tied to the first, since one cannot determine whether an attribution is true or false without knowing the psychological nature of the state in question.

The simplest psychological view of beliefs is the *behaviorist* one: beliefs are behavioral dispositions (verbal or nonverbal). But two problems arise: first, one cannot specify the class of behavioral dispositions that corresponds to a belief; second, the dispositions exist only if other mental states exist in return, such as desires (→ DESIRE). A more complex, *disposition-based* conception makes use of this circularity and defines a belief as a propensity to act, provided other mental states exist (→ ACTION). But beliefs and desires are more than just propensities to act; they are also the causes of actions (→ CAUSALITY AND MENTAL CAUSATION). The *functionalist* view defines beliefs as causal or functional roles that take effect (in connection with other mental states) between sensory input and behavioral output (→ FUNCTIONALISM). In certain materialistic versions, functionalism likens these causal structures to types of physical states (David Armstrong) (→ PHYSICALISM). In other versions (Jerry Fodor), beliefs, as causal roles, are realized in multiple ways via various physical tokens that differ across individuals (→ TYPE/TOKEN). In still other versions (Ruth Millikan), beliefs are akin to biological functions determined by natural selection.

There are two main conceptions in the semantics of beliefs as propositional attitudes. In one, beliefs are seen as being about abstract propositions or entities (functions of universes of possibles about truth values) and in the other, beliefs are about sentences expressed in a public language or in a *language of thought* (→ LANGUAGE, LANGUAGE OF THOUGHT). Both views come up against the problem of the individuation of the concerned entities, in addition to the problem of the referential obscurity of the content of propositional attitudes (if X believes that a is F, and if $a = b$, it does not follow that X believes that b is F). According to Fodor, beliefs are computational states mapped to representations (taken to be sentences in the language of thought), which receive part of their content from their causal relations to the outside world. According to Fred Dretske, these representations are functional information structures (physically defined) that covary causally with the environment (→ INFORMATION).

Each of these conceptions treats beliefs (and other intentional mental states) as real states of organisms, and as internal representations (→ EXTERNALISM/INTERNALISM, REALISM). But other philosophers consider beliefs to be general properties of individuals that are inseparable from the mental state attributions they might make, in the third person, within a given physical, social, and communicational environment (→ COMMUNICATION). These philosophers are led to doubt the reality of such states outside of attribution schemas, and construe beliefs as interpretive schemas that allow individuals to explain and predict behavior by virtue of an intentional stance (Daniel Dennett) (→ INTERPRETATION) whose content is necessarily undetermined.

Whether one understands beliefs in this antirealist mode or in a realist mode, two problems remain unsolved. The first is the asymmetry between belief attribution in the third-person or "objective" mode, and belief attribution in the first-person or "subjective" mode (in general, subjects have access to their own beliefs but not to those of another organism). The second problem concerns the nature of the attitude toward a belief, that is, approval of the representation, which presupposes that subjects not only have beliefs but also have beliefs about their own beliefs. In developmental psychology research on beliefs as metarepresentations, and on the formation of a *theory of mind* in the child ($\rightarrow$ METACOGNITION, THEORY OF MIND) may help further our knowledge of the nature of these conditions.

PASCAL ENGEL

SELECTED BIBLIOGRAPHY

Armstrong, D. M. (1968). *A materialist theory of the mind*. London: Routledge.

Dennett, D. (1987). *The intentional stance*. Cambridge, MA: MIT Press.

Dretske, F. (1988). *Explaining behavior: Reasons in a world of causes*. Cambridge, MA: MIT Press.

Dretske, F. (2000). *Perception, knowledge and belief: Selected essays*. Cambridge, England; New York: Cambridge University Press.

Fodor, J. (1987). *Psychosemantics: The problem of meaning in the philosophy of mind*. Cambridge, MA: MIT Press.

Millikan, R. (1984). *Language, thought, and other biological categories*. Cambridge, MA: MIT Press.

C

CATEGORIZATION

Psychology. — *Categorization* is the fundamental adaptive behavior by which we "break down" physical and social reality (→ SOCIAL COGNITION). Its cognitive function is to create the various categories (of objects, individuals, etc.) needed to transform the continuous into the discrete. The traditional, "Aristotelian" view of categorization assumes the logical equivalence of elements in the same category (→ LOGIC), in the sense that they all share the set of necessary and sufficient features that defines the category. This conception left its mark on early work in cognitive psychology, like that of Jerome Bruner, which focused on the formation of well-defined categories. In the first experimental categorization paradigm, objects are constructed by combining a number of dimensions (for example, shape, color, and size) and the subject has to discover the categorization rule arbitrarily chosen by the experimenter. A series of objects is presented, and for each one, the experimenter states whether it belongs to the category, in such a way that after a certain number of objects, it is logically possible to discover the rule with certainty. This paradigm thus examines the subject's ability to analyze and logically process examples and counterexamples by means of hypothesis testing.

This logical view of categorization is also found in developmental psychology in Jean Piaget's work on the emergence of *class logic* (→ COGNITIVE DEVELOPMENT), where categorization is studied in terms of the ability to coordinate the *comprehension* (or *intension*) and *extension* of well-defined categories (the comprehension of a class corresponds to the set of necessary and sufficient features that defines it). In Piagetian theory, this logical capacity does not appear in children until the age of seven or eight, when they begin succeeding at the *quantification of inclusion task* (*Are there more As or more Bs?* in a set of materials where $A > A'$, $A \subset B$, and $A' \subset B$). Success on this task means that the child has acquired a logicomathematical structure capable of analytically processing well-defined hierarchical categories in an inclusive system (additive grouping of classes: composition of the direct operation $A + A' = B$ and the inverse operation $B - A' = A$).

A strictly logical and analytic understanding of categorization thus presupposes treating all categories in fundamentally the same way (except for the fact that some categories are subclasses of others) and also treating all exemplars of the same category in an identical fashion. This view was questioned in Eleanor Rosch's work on "natural" categories, which showed that (1) among the categorization levels in a class-inclusion hierarchy (or *taxonomy*), one level called the *basic level* is psychologically more salient than the others, and (2) exemplars of the same category are not all equally representative or typical of the category. Some exemplars are not very representative of a category and are called *atypical* or *peripheral;* others are highly representative and are called *typical*. The most typical member of a category is the *prototype*, which serves as a reference point, a psychological "landmark" for categorizing new instances. Research conducted under Rosch's impetus has shown that estimates of prototypicality are highly correlated with measures of information processing ($\rightarrow$ INFORMATION). Accordingly, people categorize typical exemplars faster and more accurately than atypical ones. Both children and adults perform better on reasoning tasks if typical exemplars are used (for example, in Piaget's quantification of inclusion task) ($\rightarrow$ REASONING AND RATIONALITY).

The abstraction of a prototype from a set of exemplars produces an *average prototype* or a *modal prototype*. The average prototype is the exemplar that has the mean values of the dimensions that define the structure of the categorized material. The modal prototype is the exemplar that possesses the most frequent features. According to *exemplar models* (as opposed to *prototype abstraction models*), it is not necessary to assume that subjects build statistical summaries (mean or modal prototypes) to represent categories. Categorization can in fact correspond to the clustering of exemplars according to a "family resemblance" (concept taken from Ludwig Wittgenstein) or overall similarity, with each exemplar retaining its own identity. In this case, categorizing a new object involves searching in memory ($\rightarrow$ MEMORY) on the basis of a similarity metric for the exemplars that most closely resemble the object.

Research on this topic attempts to account for the plurality of categorization processes in symbolic or connectionist terms (subsymbolic networks of prototype extraction or exemplar integration) ($\rightarrow$ CONNECTIONISM, SYMBOL) and to specify how these processes are dependent upon the structure of the material and the task demands. Categorization processes can be logical and analytical, or based on the principles of prototypicality and family resemblance (or other criteria such as schemas or scripts, explanatory theories, etc.).

OLIVIER HOUDÉ

Linguistics. — Émile Benveniste defined *linguistic categories* as classes of forms with distinctive features and capable of fulfilling grammatical functions (→ FUNCTION, GRAMMAR), in such a way that the members of the same linguistic category can occur in the same syntactic contexts (→ SYNTAX). These forms (the words of the language) convey both grammatical and semantic information (→ SEMANTICS). Linguistic categories are characterized by elements that are marked or unmarked (for example, *man/woman* in the *human being* category) or elements that exhibit graduality. In the same way as *sparrow, hen,* and *ostrich* occupy distinct positions on the typicality scale of the bird category (see *psychology* above), *icy, cold, cool, warm, hot*, and *boiling* are gradations on the increasing temperature scale of the category of adjectives expressing temperature. The question that arises here is whether psychological approaches to categorization are suited to describing languages. Although George Lakoff contends that studies on linguistic categories provide some of the first evidence of the nature of categorical structures in general, a Rosch-like category is not a lexical class (→ LEXICON), but rather a class of objects or concepts (→ CONCEPT, OBJECT). It is usually called by a name, in which case the names of the language are merely symbols (→ SYMBOL) or labels that are useful for referring to objects or concepts. Given that the lexicon is not organized in a taxonomic way, prototype theory, whose postulates are based on such an organization, cannot be readily applied to it. This was François Rastier's rationale for introducing the concept of *paragon* as a replacement for prototype. The paragon of a lexical category is its most "powerful" term, the most prized. It can be used to refer to other members of the category or even to the category itself as a whole. In Chinese, for example, the word for *jade* has been extended to all gems, and in Italian, the word for *pasta* has come to also mean meal.

The utility of categorization in language is that it alleviates the need for a speaker to enumerate the properties of an object of discussion by situating it in a class. All categorization operations have a purpose within a specific framework. The taxonomist categorizes to generalize; the terminology specialist categorizes to define with concision; the technician has some operation in mind. Categorization is also subject to individual variations and cross-cultural or community differences.

GABRIEL OTMAN

SELECTED BIBLIOGRAPHY

Benveniste, É. (1971). *Problems in general linguistics* (M. E.. Meek, Trans.). Coral Gables, FL: University of Miami Press. (Original work published 1966–1974.)

Bruner, J. S., Goodnow, J. J., & Austin, A. (1956). *A study of thinking.* New York: Wiley.

De Rijk, L. (2002). *Aristotle: Semantics and ontology. General introduction: The works on logic.* Leiden, The Netherlands; Boston: Brill Academic Publishers.

Forde, E., & Humphreys, G. (Eds.). (2002). *Category specificity in brain and mind.* New York: Taylor and Francis.

Gelman, S. (2003). *The essential child: Origins of essentialism in everyday thought.* Oxford, England; New York: Oxford University Press.

Houdé, O. (2000). Inhibition and cognitive development: Object, number, categorization, and reasoning. *Cognitive Development, 15,* 63–73.

Inhelder, B., & Piaget, J. (1964). *The early growth of logic in the child* (E. A. Lunzer & D. Papert, Trans.). New York: Harper & Row; London: Routledge. (Original work published 1959.)

Lamberts, K., & Shanks, D. (Eds.). (1997). *Knowledge, concepts, and categories.* Cambridge, MA: MIT Press; Hove, England: Psychology Press.

Rastier, F. (1991). *Sémantique et recherches cognitives* [Semantics and cognitive research]. Paris: Presses Universitaires de France.

Rosch, E. (1983). Prototype classification and logical classification: The two systems. In E. K. Scholnick (Ed.), *New trends in conceptual representations: Challenges to Piaget's theory?* Hillsdale, NJ: Erlbaum.

Rosch, E., & Lloyd, B. (Eds.). (1978). *Cognition and categorization.* Hillsdale, NJ: Erlbaum.

Taylor, R. (1995). *Linguistic categorization: Prototypes in linguistic theory* (2nd ed.). Oxford, England: Clarendon Press.

CAUSALITY AND MENTAL CAUSATION

Psychology. — *Causality* is a relationship between two elements, one of which, the cause, produces an effect on the other. In Jean Piaget's theory, understanding causal relations is a crucial point in the development of intelligence (→ COGNITIVE DEVELOPMENT). The relations that interest infants first are the ones in which they are the causal agent. At the age of five months, infants have a "magical," phenomenalistic understanding of causality. They grasp relations of succession between their own action (→ ACTION) and phenomena occurring around them, and ascribe the latter to the former. After a long decentering and objectivation process, the two-year-old child has a clear grasp of causal relations.

Albert Michotte stressed another form of causality: *perceptual causality* (→ PERCEPTION), where the subject, neither the actor nor the acted upon, is the spectator of an event. Perceptual causality is based on a spatiotemporal contiguity relation between two distinct elements. It is accompanied by an illusion: when we look at object A moving at a uniform speed toward object B, which starts to move in the same direction when A arrives near it, we see A "push" B. This perception also makes us believe that the speed of A increases in the vicinity of B. According to Michotte, perceived causality is a *gestalt*, in the sense of the term described in Gestalt theory, where a gestalt is a basic, innate organizing principle of perception. Although today's cognitivists (such as Elizabeth Spelke) have demonstrated an early understanding of the laws of physics in infants (→ INFANT COGNITION), and in doing so, have cast doubt on Piaget's theory, there are still no studies proving that causal relations are perceived right from birth. The *contiguity principle* (spatiotemporal adjacency of elements in a perceived causal chain) is not acquired until the age of about six months.

ARLETTE STRERI

Philosophy. — Interpreting the concept of causality is a controversial issue. According to the dominant, *nomological* theory, two individual events A and B are connected by a cause-effect relation if and only if they obey a law of nature that connects event type A to event type B. This is a key theory in the philosophy of mind. According to Donald Davidson's *anomalous monism* (→ DUALISM/MONISM), the intentional properties of the mind (→ INTENTIONALITY, MIND)—which are called upon in rational explanations of actions (→ ACTION, REASONING AND RATIONALITY)—are unfit for figuring in causal explanations, because causal explanations require strict laws, that is, laws that can be applied without exception, under all circumstances. But the laws that govern intentional states are not strict in this sense: to be valid, they must be covered by a *ceteris paribus* (other things being equal) clause. The main drawback of nomological theory is that it makes a single causal relation depend on a general condition. This is counterintuitive because intuitively, causality is a local phenomenon. *Singularist* theories of causality strive to do justice to the constraint of locality (→ *mental causation* below; PHYSICALISM, REALISM).

Both common sense and the human sciences assume that certain behaviors of individuals can be explained by the content of their beliefs and desires (→ BELIEF, DESIRE). Can the content of people's beliefs and desires contribute to causally explaining certain bodily movements they make? This is the problem of *mental causation*. If, as René Descartes claimed, an individual's mind is an immaterial entity, if his/her beliefs are not physical states of the brain, then mental causation is a mystery: How can nonphysical entities act upon physical entities? If, as the *physicalist* viewpoint holds, an individual's beliefs are the states of his/her brain, the problem raised by mental causation is the problem of explanatory exclusion: Isn't the content of a belief rendered causally ineffective by the physical properties underlying the state of the brain? Don't these properties suffice for producing the bodily movement? Isn't the content of a belief epiphenomenal in the movement production process (→ EPIPHENOMENALISM)? Two strategies are available to physicalists for handling this explanatory exclusion problem: *functionalism* (→ FUNCTIONALISM) and the *dual-explanandum strategy*.

The following example illustrates the functionalist approach. An aspirin tablet has a chemical property: it is composed of acetylsalicylic acid. It also has a functional property: it is a pain reliever. If an object is red (determined property), it has color (determinable property). An object exemplifies a determinable (or functional) property by virtue of the fact that it exemplifies a determined property. Suppose the content of my belief was to the physical properties of my brain what the exemplification of a determinable property is to the exemplification of a determined property. Under this hypothesis, a physicalist is not condemned to regarding the content of my belief as epiphenomenal in the movement production process. By swallowing an aspirin tablet, I relieve the pain of my migraine headache. The tablet relieved the pain by virtue of the fact that it contained acetylsalicylic acid; this fact is a causal explanation of why the pain disappeared. But it being so does not take the causal effectiveness away from the fact that the tablet was an analgesic; had I swallowed a pain-relieving tablet with some other chemical composition, I would also have rid myself of the pain.

The dual-explanandum strategy is based on the idea that unlike a physical property, the content of my belief is not an intrinsic property of my brain: it is an extrinsic property that depends on my historical relationship with the environment. Can an extrinsic property have a causal effect in a local process? Suppose there is a vending machine that dispenses a beverage every time it receives two quarters. A quarter has intrinsic physical properties and a monetary value. The monetary value is an extrinsic historical property of the coin. Can a physicalist say that the monetary value of an object has a causal effect? Let us make the distinction here between the dropping of the beverage and the behavior of the vending machine: the former is a constituent of the latter. If what has to be explained is the mechanism by which the beverage is dropped, then only the intrinsic properties of the coin have a causal effect. If what has to be explained is why the machine dispenses a drink every time it receives two quarters, then the monetary value of the coin plays a role in the explanation. The fact that there is a reliable correlation between the monetary value and the intrinsic properties of certain metallic objects explains why the machine dispenses a beverage every time it receives two such objects. A physical movement is not a behavior; it is a constituent of a behavior. Hence, an extrinsic property of my brain—the content of my belief—does not explain the occurrence of my movement, but the structure of my behavior, that is, the consistent correspondence between the states of my brain and a type of physical movement.

PIERRE JACOB

SELECTED BIBLIOGRAPHY

Bunge, M. (1979). *Causality and modern science* (3rd rev. ed.). New York: Dover.
Davidson, D. (1980). *Essays on actions and events* (2nd ed.). Oxford, England: Clarendon Press.
Dretske, F. (1988). *Explaining behavior: Reasons in a world of causes*. Cambridge, MA: MIT Press.

Dretske, F. (2000). *Perception, knowledge and belief: Selected essays*. Cambridge, England; New York: Cambridge University Press.

Heil, J., & Mele, A. (1992). *Mental causation*. Oxford, England; New York: Oxford University Press.

Jacob, P. (1997). *What minds can do: Intentionality in a non-intentional world*. New York: Cambridge University Press.

Kim, J. (1998). *Mind in a physical world: An essay on the mind-body problem and mental causation*. Cambridge, MA: MIT Press.

Michotte, A. (1946). *La perception de la causalité* [The perception of causality]. Louvain, Belgium: Éditions de l'Institut de philosophie.

Pearl, J. (2000). *Causality: Models, reasoning, and inference*. Cambridge, England; New York: Cambridge University Press.

Piaget, J. (1954). *The construction of reality in the child* (M. Cook, Trans.). New York: Basic Books. (Original work published 1937.)

Piaget, J. (1951). *The child's conception of physical causality* (M. Gabain, Trans.). New York: Humanities Press; London: Routledge & Kegan Paul. (Original work published 1927.)

Spelke, E., Vishaton, P., & von Hofsten, C. (1995). Object perception, object-directed action, and physical knowledge in infancy. In M. Gazzaniga (Ed.), *The cognitive neurosciences* (pp. 165–179). Cambridge, MA: MIT Press.

Thinès, G., Costall, A., & Butterworth, G. (Eds.). (1991). *Michotte's experimental phenomenology of perception*. Hillsdale, NJ: Erlbaum.

COGNITIVE DEVELOPMENT

Psychology. — A mandatory reference for studying cognitive development is Jean Piaget's *structuralist theory*. All psychologists who attack the problem of the genesis of cognition refer to this theory, in areas as diverse as object construction, number, categorization, and reasoning, either to emphasize its contributions or to question its validity (→ CATEGORIZATION, NUMBER, OBJECT, REASONING AND RATIONALITY). The originality of Piaget's theory lies in its triple roots in epistemological, biological, and logicomathematical foundations (→ EPISTEMOLOGY, LOGIC). Whether in the development of scientific knowledge (historical-critical perspective) or in ontogeny (the psychology of intelligence), mental models are devised to reconstruct reality based on increasingly powerful logicomathematical frameworks that constitute the optimal form of biological adaptation (→ CONSTRUCTIVISM, LOGICISM/PSYCHOLOGISM, REALISM). In this way, the child, like the logician or mathematician, "models" objects, their properties, and their relations through a succession of cognitive frameworks. From infancy to adolescence, the child progresses from early assimilation and accommodation processes and action schemes (→ ACTION) (sensorimotor stage from birth to eighteen months) to the coordination and internalization of concrete operations (eighteen months-two years to eleven-twelve years) and then formal operations (eleven-twelve to sixteen years).

Intelligence is defined in Piagetian terms as the most general form of coordination of actions and operations. The mechanisms of its development are *equilibration* (regulation in response to external disruptions) and *reflective abstraction* (abstraction of the properties of actions and their co-ordination). While consistently relating to the issues raised by the contemporary logicomathematical setting, Piaget described the organizations or structures underlying the development of intelligence in terms of grouping (*concrete operations stage* at about age seven to eight years), combinatorics and groups (*formal operations stage* at about age eleven to twelve years), and, in his later work where he revised some of his earlier formalizations, in terms of the "logic of meanings" (or *intensional logic;* → REL-EVANCE), morphisms, and categories.

Piaget's powerful theoretical framework was accompanied not only by ingenious experimental tasks, including conservation (conservation of number, substance, etc.), class inclusion, and seriation (used to study concrete operations), but also by an original method of clinical interrogation consisting of conversing freely with the child about targeted themes (for example, for conservation of number and substance, respectively: *Are there more tokens when we spread them apart? More clay when we flatten the ball?*), and then following up on the child's response by requests for justifications and countersuggestions.

Posterity has retained Piaget's structuralist and constructivist theoretical approach and also, perhaps especially, his experimental situations (the "Piagetian tasks"), now famous around the world. Although Piagetian theory rapidly established itself as a mandatory reference, it also triggered many criticisms, mostly concerning the excessive amount of power granted to action (and to operational development in general), its exclusive interest in the logicomathematical structures of the "epistemic" or "epistemological subject" rather than in the "psychological subject" (note that the meaning of the term *epistemic* is different here from the one defined in logic and in the philosophy of mind), and the inability of the theory to explain the large variations in performance observed across situations and individuals (intra- and interindividual variability; → DIFFERENTIATION). Criticisms have also been directed at Piaget's failure to take into consideration the social factors of cognitive development (→ INTERACTION, SOCIAL COGNITION).

Some of these objections were overcome by the Piagetian School itself. The most striking comeback was the approach proposed by Bärbel Inhelder and Guy Cellerier, where a shift was made from studying general structures in the epistemic subject to studying the processes of invention and discovery in the psychological subject. The emphasis was now on the procedures children use to fulfill the immediate adaptation function of behavior, thereby situating adaptation leading to local cognitive equilibrium at the level of *microgenesis* (problem solving) and adaptation leading to overall equilibrium at the level of *macrogenesis* (development). This marked the first step toward bridging the gap between Piagetian structuralism and *cognitivism* (the cognitive psychology of information processing; → COGNITIVISM). In Cellerier's analysis, Piagetian structuralism deals with the long-term epistemic transformation of action into knowledge, whereas cognitivism studies the short-term, pragmatic transformation of knowledge into action. These two approaches to psychology "work" in different time spans: the former perspective is diachronic (macrogenesis or development); the latter is synchronic (microgeneses at a given development stage). The challenge for neo-Piagetian psychology has been to interrelate these two perspectives.

The research trend that most clearly took up this challenge in the 1980s was *neostructuralism*, principally represented by Juan Pascual-Leone, Robbie Case, Graeme Halford, and Kurt Fischer. These authors retained Piaget's aim to devise a general theory of development that could account for the construction of cognitive structures in any domain. The innovative part of neostructuralism lies in its attempt to come up with a synthesis of structuralism and cognitivism. A wide range of models emerged describing the cognitive functioning of the child "problem solver" in terms of "silent operators" in a modular system of *mental attention* (Pascual-Leone) (→ ATTENTION), *executive control structures* and *central conceptual structures* (Case) (→ CONCEPT, CONTROL), levels of *structure mapping* (Halford) (→ SYMBOL), or *structures of skills* (Fischer). With these new concepts in hand, so radically different from Piaget's logicomathematical structures, the neostructuralists redefined the stages and substages of development from infancy to adolescence (following a breakdown in fact quite close to Piaget's) and the processes that ensure the transition from one stage to the next.

Pascual-Leone "quantifies" cognitive development in terms of a mental attention operator in charge of activating relevant schemes in working memory during problem solving (→ MEMORY), with the magnitude of the operator being an index of the stages and substages of development (→ ACTIVATION/INHIBITION). Case describes a hierarchical sequence made up of sensorimotor, interrelational, dimensional, and vectorial stages—each subdivided into unifocal, bifocal, and elaborated coordination—in the course of which executive control structures and central conceptual structures become increasingly complex. The transition between substages is linked to the increased capacity of working memory (itself a function of operational efficiency or scheme automatization) (→ AUTOMATISM), and the transition between stages is ensured by a hierarchical integration process. For Halford, development is a series of levels involving element mapping, relational mapping, system mapping, and multiple-system mapping, with the transition from one level to the next being defined by the processing capacity increase. Finally, Fischer's model describes development in terms of structures of skills in four tiers, reflex, sensorimotor, representational, and abstract, interconnected by a coordination process, with each tier being subdivided into four levels: single sets, mappings, systems, and systems of systems. In all of these neostructuralist models, psychological structures are no longer reduced to mere logicomathematical structures in an epistemic subject, and the focus is on information processing (and the constraints imposed by how these processes function in working memory) rather than solely on the subject's actions. It became clear that neostructuralism was better able—that is, better than Piagetian theory—to account for the substantial variability observed in performance, through its precise analysis of the task characteristics, the goals and strategies adopted by the child, and the cognitive load incurred in each strategy.

Neostructuralist models benefited from advances made in several areas during the 1990s, including a finer articulation with cognitive neuroscience (for example, the link demonstrated by Pascual-Leone between attentional operators and the prefrontal cortex) (→ LOCALIZATION OF FUNCTION), the contributions of nonlinear dynamic systems (Fischer and Case, based on Paul van Geert's work), which introduced less regular developmental curves containing perturbations, bursts, collapses, and so forth (→ DYNAMIC SYSTEM), and the implementation of connectionist models to analyze tasks and understand the levels of cognitive complexity needed to perform them (Halford) (→ CONNECTIONISM).

One of the criticisms currently directed at neostructuralist models is that, like Piagetian theory, they all describe the *coordination-activation* of structural units and not *selection-inhibition*. Many authors, including Adele Diamond, Frank Dempster, Katherine Harnishfeger, and Olivier Houdé, have shown in a variety of areas, including object construction, number, categorization, and reasoning, that cognitive development should not be regarded solely as the gradual acquisition of knowledge (or of increasingly complex structures), but also as resting on the capacity to inhibit reactions that hinder the expression of knowledge already present. In this approach, where the emphasis is on executive functions, the new neurocognitive models of development essentially revolve around the idea of inefficient/efficient inhibition (Diamond, Harnishfeger, Houdé) and resistance to interference (Dempster). This approach is in line with *neural Darwinism*, represented in particular by Gerard Edelman and Jean-Pierre Changeux; that approach explains the dynamics of neural and cognitive ontogeny in terms of a *variation-selection* mechanism (→ NEURAL DARWINISM).

Another criticism aimed at neostructuralism is that its models of development are always very general. Hence the need for a complementary approach that is more local and more functional. Precisely such an approach, *developmental cognitivism*, began to develop after Piaget at the same time as neostructuralism. Research in this trend has a local orientation, since specific domains are studied at specific age ranges (for example, early object permanence in four- to five-month-old infants, mental rotation in preschoolers, etc.; → MENTAL IMAGERY). It is also *functional* (as opposed to structural in the Piagetian sense), in that cognitive functioning is described without resorting to the concepts of structure and stage.

One of the most striking examples of research in developmental cognitivism, which led to a radical revision of Piaget's theory, is the study of early abilities in infants (this line of study was also developed by the neo-Piagetian School itself, under the impetus of Pierre Mounoud) (→ INFANT COGNITION). The most important advances here were associated with a change in methodology (made possible by the use of videotapes and computers). Instead of analyzing infant action schemes, as advocated by Piaget, the infant's gaze behavior was examined (→ PERCEPTION). Experiments using the visual habituation technique and recordings of visual fixation time were conducted to study infant reactions to novelty and the detection of unexpected (or "impossible") events. This led to the discovery of early abilities unknown to Piaget, such as object unity and object permanence by the age of four or five months (along with other physical principles; Elizabeth Spelke and Renée Baillargeon), the existence of numerical abilities by that same age (Karen Wynn), and categorization by the age of three months (Roger Lécuyer). Other studies have dealt with neonatal imitation during the first few days of life and crossmodal perception in the early months (Andrew Meltzoff and Arlette Streri). This body of data as a whole suggests that infant capacities are either innate (Spelke's theoretical stance) or constructed through physical reasoning mechanisms (Baillargeon) in conjunction with a very early faculty to learn through perception (especially visual perception), thought to be the only preprogrammed faculty (Lécuyer) (→ LEARNING). The first position goes against Piagetian constructivism; the second remains constructivist but sees intelligence as originating in perception (in connection with reasoning) rather than in action. Other authors, such as Annette Karmiloff-Smith (and recently, Spelke) have taken an interest in the relationships between early infant abilities, the modularity of the mind (Jerry Fodor; → MODULARITY), and development processes throughout childhood: representational changes, flexibility and creativity of the mind, domain-specific or domain-general processes, and so forth (→ CREATIVITY, DOMAIN SPECIFICITY, REPRESENTATION). To resolve these issues, attempts have been made by Karmiloff-Smith to integrate Fodor's nativism and Piaget's constructivism.

In addition to the study of infant cognition, developmental cognitivism has explored the many facets of psychological functioning at different ages (even into old age, through life-span developmental studies of the elderly; → AGING). Some examples are the study of mental images, number, categorization, and theories of mind (→ THEORY OF MIND) during the preschool and school years. A currently thriving topic of particular interest to philosophers of the mind (→ BELIEF) is the study of theories of mind in two- to six-year-old children, where the cognitive, emotional ($\rightarrow$ EMOTION), and social aspects of development are combined. These studies look at the construction of "naive" metarepresentations of psychological function, based on situations like visual perspective-taking and the appearance-reality distinction (John Flavell), or false-belief attribution (Josef Perner and Henri Wimmer). If Piaget's subject was the logicomathematician, the subject studied here is of another kind, the psychologist.

Among the important new approaches that should be interrelated with neostructuralism and developmental cognitivism in the years to come are *nonlinear dynamic systems, connectionism,* and *cognitive neuroscience* (see recent advances in neostructuralism). In nonlinear dynamic systems, mathematical equations are used to formalize the more turbulent and chaotic forms of development based on growth parameters. In connectionism, formal neural networks are implemented to model the relationships between maturation and learning: the features of the network's basic architecture correspond to maturation, and the changes that occur when a network with a given architecture interacts with its environment constitute learning. Connectionism thus leads us to rethink innateness. In cognitive neuroscience, new functional brain imaging techniques should make it possible to compile an image bank of developing brain functions, an indispensable tool to complement the behavioral study of cognitive functions ($\rightarrow$ FUNCTIONAL NEUROIMAGING).

Other new theoretical trends are now also taking shape, including the return to the study of action, or more exactly, *agency* (a broader concept than Piaget's action, in that it also includes selective-attention mechanisms), with authors such as James Russell in the areas of object construction and theories of mind.

Although not an exhaustive inventory, this overview of cognitive development examines the various models or approaches that attempt to capture the complexity of this dynamic process. Unlike the days when Piaget reigned, it is no longer possible today to give a single definition of cognitive development. The challenge for future research will be to determine the conditions for the structural and functional coexistence of these multiple ways of gaining insight into intelligence.

OLIVIER HOUDÉ

SELECTED BIBLIOGRAPHY

Astington, J., Harris, P., & Olson, D. (Eds.). (1988). *Developing theories of mind.* Cambridge, England; New York: Cambridge University Press.

Baillargeon, R. (1995). Physical reasoning in infancy. In M. Gazzaniga (Ed.), *The cognitive neurosciences* (pp.181–204). Cambridge, MA: MIT Press.

Casey, B., & de Haan, M. (2002). Brain imaging and developmental science [Special issue]. *Developmental Science.*

Demetriou, A. (Ed.). (1988). *The neo-Piagetian theories of cognitive development: Toward an integration*. Amsterdam; New York: North-Holland.

Dempster, F., & Brainerd, C. (Eds.). (1995). *Interference and inhibition in cognition*. San Diego, CA: Academic Press.

Diamond, A. (1991). Neuropsychological insights into the meaning of object concept development. In S. Carey & R. Gelman (Eds.), *The epigenesis of mind: Essays on biology and cognition* (pp. 67–110). Hillsdale, NJ: Erlbaum.

Elman, J., Bates, A., Johnson, M., Karmiloff-Smith, A., Parisi, D., & Plunkett, K. (1996). *Rethinking innateness: A connectionist perspective on development*. Cambridge, MA: MIT Press.

Fischer, K., & Kaplan, U. (2003). Piaget, Jean. In L. Nadel (Ed.), *The encyclopedia of cognitive science* (Vol. 1, pp. 679–682). London: Nature Publishing Group, Macmillan.

Houdé, O. (2000). Inhibition and cognitive development: Object, number, categorization, and reasoning. *Cognitive Development, 15*, 63–73.

Johnson, M. (2001). Functional brain development in humans. *Nature Reviews Neuroscience, 2*, 475–483.

Karmiloff-Smith, A. (1992). *Beyond modularity: A developmental perspective on cognitive science*. Cambridge, MA: MIT Press.

Meltzoff, A., & Prinz, W. (Eds.). (2002). *The imitative mind: Development, evolution, and brain bases*. Cambridge, England; New York: Cambridge University Press.

Nelson, C., & Luciana, M. (Eds.). (2001). *Developmental cognitive neuroscience*. Cambridge, MA: MIT Press.

Russell, J. (1997). *Agency: Its role in mental development*. Hove, England: Erlbaum.

Siegler, R. (1996). *Emerging minds: The process of change in children's thinking*. New York: Oxford University Press.

Spelke, E., Vishaton, P., & von Hofsten, C. (1995). Object perception, object-directed action, and physical knowledge in infancy. In M. Gazzaniga (Ed.), *The cognitive neurosciences* (pp. 165–179). Cambridge, MA: MIT Press.

Van Geert, P. (1994). *Dynamic systems of development: Change between complexity and chaos*. New York: Harvester.

Wynn, K. (1998). Psychological foundations of numbers: Numerical competence in human infants. *Trends in Cognitive Sciences, 2*, 296–303.

COGNITIVE PSYCHIATRY

Psychology. — Although *cognitive psychiatry* designates a set of theories and methods that has been expanding considerably since the 1970s, the term is still rarely employed. It refers to the branch of psychiatry where the study of the mechanisms of information processing and decision making is applied to the mental disorders observable in a psychiatric clinic (→ COMPUTATIONAL ANALYSIS, INFORMATION). It is based on the principle that alterations in these mechanisms can partially account for psychiatric disorders.

It is important to make the distinction between cognitive psychiatry and *cognitive therapy*. Cognitive therapy is a derivative of behavior therapies and shares their principles: treatment deliberately keyed on symptoms, the use of prescriptive methods, and reference to conditioning and social learning (→ LEARNING). It differs from cognitive psychiatry by how far away it is from the behaviorist doctrine and the importance it places on beliefs (and secondarily on desires) conveyed by cognitions (→ BELIEF, DESIRE). Cognitive therapy can be included in cognitive psychiatry, provided the theoretical assumptions and methods are clearly distinguished from the study of the elementary cognitive mechanisms likely to be altered in mental illness.

The use of the term *cognitive neuropsychiatry* (often taken to be a synonym of *cognitive psychiatry*) should also be clarified here. This term sounds like neuropsychology, and both fields use the same methods and attempt to localize the brain mechanisms responsible for altered functions (→ FUNCTIONAL NEUROIMAGING, LOCALIZATION OF FUNCTION, NEUROPSYCHOLOGY). However, the term *cognitive neuropsychiatry* is more suitably employed for attempts to localize the neural pathways and centers responsible for the observed alterations, whereas *cognitive psychiatry* (or *cognitive psychopathology*) applies solely to attempts to describe those alterations and to compare them with normal cognitive mechanisms.

There are two ways of defining what the word *cognitive* adds here to the terms *psychiatry* and *psychopathology*. The first is rooted in an intellectualistic leaning that places the cognitive approach to phenomena in opposition to the conative and affective approaches. The second is methodological, and represents a fundamental breakaway from the study of symptoms and the syndrome- and nosology-based perspectives.

The intellectualist trend has always been present in the study of insanity. An early example is Immanuel Kant's works. Kant's idea of *proton pseudos*, or initial error, taken up by a very active trend in the nineteenth century, was thought to explain the chain of reasoning disorders that ensued (→ REASONING AND RATIONALITY). Work by Philippe Pinel in France and by Johann Herbart in Germany are clear illustrations of this view of insanity (or "mental alienation"), that is, as a disease of reason. Current resistance to the cognitive approach often stems from this intellectualistic leaning.

In today's understanding of the field, cognitive psychiatry is in fact aimed primarily at defining a basic level for studying cognitive operations, one likely to be better at accounting for mental disorders than the study of the behaviors and judgments alleged to be their symptoms. Psychopathology thus had to break away not only from behaviorist assumptions, but also from the somewhat naive claim made in biological psychiatry—based on the discovery of psychotropic drugs—that symptoms could be directly explained in terms of altered neural mechanisms. But more than anything else, the cognitive approach to psychiatry has thrived because it applies the methods used in cognitive science (particularly cognitive psychology) to the field of mental pathology, with psychiatry (or psychopathology) following in the footsteps of neuropsychology.

The principles are the same: (1) Lower the level of observation to a finer grain (from the molar study of symptoms to the molecular study of elementary, nondirectly observable operations). (2) Use indirect methods of observation (experimental method, search for mediating variables). (3)

Make the distinction between explaining the mechanisms and looking for antecedent causes, while placing priority on psychological models rather than on physiological data.

The methods are diverse: (1) Critically reassess traditional phenomenology based on theoretical speculations inspired by the philosophy of mind (for example, new definition of delusional belief). (2) Simulate mental disorders by applying the methods used in artificial intelligence (paradigmatic model of Kenneth Colby's PARRY program for persecutory delirium). (3) Study special cases (often using the single-case method) to find functional dissociations and sometimes even double dissociations, as is done in contemporary neuropsychology research (for example, observing discrepancies between identical twins, or studying theory-of-mind disorders in autistic children; → AUTISM, THEORY OF MIND). (4) Administer standard tests designed to assess cognitive abilities (for example, analysis of so-called frontal performance alterations in schizophrenic subjects using test batteries developed in neuropsychology; → CONTROL, SCHIZOPHRENIA), but also (5) use experimental methods that take advantage of most of the paradigms of cognitive psychology (merits of the additive method, measuring the processing load in terms of response time, etc.), while taking the necessary additional precautions: comparisons must be made with control populations, the effects of medication must be taken into account, and motivational factors must be neutralized, often by using devices that enhance the performance of these populations (reduction of contextual interference, for example) and by following certain ethical procedures (informed consent). Studies using these techniques have focused on attention, memory, and language processes (→ ATTENTION, LANGUAGE, MEMORY), and are usually run individually. Finally, (6) observe certain advantageous natural situations (communication processes, text corpora, and so on; → COMMUNICATION, TEXT).

All of the above approaches have been applied in a variety of pathological domains. Although one of the privileged fields of study is psychotic states (especially schizophrenia), depressive states (in which interesting within-subject comparisons can be made owing to the effectiveness and delayed action of medication) and neurotic disorders (anxiety, psychogenic amnesia, etc.) are also important areas of investigation. Autistic disorders and hyperactivity in children have benefited considerably from studies of this type.

Cognitive research must not be conducted separately from biological research. Indeed, biological studies based on brain imaging and genetic research offer an invaluable aid for understanding how medication takes effect. Electroencephalography, or EEG (late evoked potentials), provides additional insight into the links between processing steps.

Reservations about this type of research are grounded mainly on arguments derived from traditional clinical psychology, neurobiology, and psychoanalysis. It would seem, though, that a reductionist approach that attempts to explain symptoms in terms of a series of elementary operations runs the risk of overlooking both the specificity of the mental disorder and etiological considerations (→ REDUCTIONISM). The fact that certain cognitive alterations are found in various different diseases (certain memory disorders and dysfunctional decision making) or are manifested by particular symptoms (hallucinations, speech impairment) may mask the mechanism that in fact explains the syndrome or even the disease as a whole. This claim is supported by the observation that many cognitive abnormalities are not found in all subjects with a similar symptomatology.

The functionalist doctrine is sometimes seen as a refusal of the biological nature of the observed disorders (→ FUNCTIONALISM). Wry disapprovals are directed at its alleged overreliance on cognitive models, deemed to be cut off from all anatomical and physiological bases and liable to reproduce the error committed earlier in the study of aphasia.

Finally, cognitive psychiatry all too often looks like a return to an approach thought to undermine the role of emotional life and motivations (→ EMOTION), especially as a reaction against psychoanalysis. Pulling out of the debate led by both the opponents and the proponents of psychoanalysis calls for a theoretical reflection and empirical studies with an integrative approach (role of procedural and motivational memory, cognition and affect, cognitive description of unconscious processes, etc.; → AUTOMATISM, CONSCIOUSNESS), remembering that Sigmund Freud's very first psychoanalytic studies were considered by many to have set an example for neurocognitive psychopathology.

DANIEL WIDLÖCHER

SELECTED BIBLIOGRAPHY

Baron-Cohen, S. (1995). *Mindblindness: An essay on autism and theory of mind.* Cambridge, MA: MIT Press.

Frith, C. (1992). *The cognitive neuropsychology of schizophrenia.* Hove, England; Hillsdale, NJ: Erlbaum.

Frith, U. (1992). *Autism: Explaining the enigma.* Oxford, England; Cambridge, MA: Blackwell.

Halligan, P., & David, A. (2001). Cognitive neuropsychiatry: Towards a scientific psychopathology. *Nature Reviews Neuroscience, 2,* 209–215.

Kitcher, P. (1992). *Freud's dream: A complete interdisciplinary science of mind.* Cambridge, MA: MIT Press.

Mitchell, P. (1996). *Introduction to theory of mind: Children, autism and apes.* New York; London: Arnold.

Nelson, C., & Luciana, M. (Eds.). (2001). *Developmental cognitive neuroscience* (Section VII, *Neurodevelopmental aspects of clinical disorders*). Cambridge, MA: MIT Press.

Plomin, R., et al. (Eds.). (2003). *Behavioral genetics in the postgenomic era.* Washington, DC: American Psychological Association.

Posner, M., & Raichle, M. (1994/1997). *Images of mind* (Section IX, *Mental Diseases*). New York: Freeman.

Sharma, T. (2003). *Brain imaging in schizophrenia: Insights and applications.* London: Remedica.

Sharma, T., & Harvey, P. (Eds.). (2000). *Cognition in schizophrenia: Impairments, importance, and treatment strategies.* New York: Oxford University Press.

COGNITIVISM

Philosophy. — *Cognitivism* is a classic paradigm in cognitive science and can be defined as a combination of the *functionalist* and *computational-representational* theses (→ COMPUTATIONAL ANALYSIS, FUNCTIONALISM, REPRESENTATION). It acknowledges the existence of mental states, each of which is identical to a physical state (→ PHYSICALISM). However, the type of a mental state is determined by its functional role, that is, by its causal relations with other mental states, stimuli, and behaviors (→ CAUSALITY AND MENTAL CAUSATION).

Cognitivism postulates the existence of symbolic mental representations (→ SYMBOL) or statements in a formal internal language (→ LANGUAGE OF THOUGHT). Cognitive processes are conceived of as computational processes that operate on those representations and are governed by a system of formal rules.

This paradigm draws extensively from research on computability and formal systems, which gave birth to the computer. It sees the relationships between physical and mental entities as being analogous to those between a computer's hardware and software. Accordingly, it is generally considered that the level of description suited to the representational and computational properties of mental states and processes is independent of the level of description suited to the physical properties of the underlying substrate.

ÉLISABETH PACHERIE

SELECTED BIBLIOGRAPHY

Crumley, J. (1999). *Problems in mind: Readings in contemporary philosophy of mind*. New York: McGraw-Hill.

Descombes, V. (2001). *The mind's provisions: A critique of cognitivism* (S. A. Schwartz, Trans.). Princeton, NJ: Princeton University Press. (Original work published 1995.)

Fodor, J. (1980). *Representations: Philosophical essays on the foundations of cognitive science*. Montgomery, VT: Bradford Books.

Fodor, J. (2000). *The mind doesn't work that way: The scope and limits of computational psychology*. Cambridge, MA: MIT Press.

Haugeland, J. (Ed.). (1997). *Mind design II: Philosophy, psychology, and artificial intelligence* (Rev. ed.). Cambridge, MA: MIT Press.

COMMUNICATION

Neuroscience. — The term *communication* refers to all processes by means of which information is transmitted from one entity to another (→ INFORMATION). In cognitive neuroscience, two levels of communication can be distinguished. The first pertains to mechanisms that transmit information between neurons. These mechanisms are either *excitatory* or *inhibitory* (→ ACTIVATION/INHIBITION). The second pertains to mechanisms that transmit information between the cognitive subsystems of the brain's functional architecture, each of which can be seen as a neural network ($\rightarrow$ COMPUTATIONAL ANALYSIS, NEURAL NETWORK).

In general, neurons do not communicate in an arbitrary way. Many are prewired, so their connections do not change over time except in cases of cell death (which happens massively during childhood). Communication among neurons is achieved by neurotransmitters, and depending on the brain region involved, the same neurotransmitter can have excitatory or inhibitory functions. This is in fact contingent upon the characteristics of the neural receptor. In an artificial neural network ($\rightarrow$ CONNECTIONISM), the same unit can usually trigger excitatory and inhibitory connections. In the brain, it remains uncertain whether all neurotransmitters can have both an excitatory and an inhibitory action within the same network.

OLIVIER KOENIG

Psychology. — Opinions vary as to how human communication should be defined. Some authors accept an extensive definition that likens communication to all forms of interaction between living organisms ($\rightarrow$ INTERACTION), irrespective of their level or form. In this case, the communicated message may be chemical, sensory, or coded (the term's meaning can even extend to encompass communication among neurons within a single organism; see *neuroscience* above). If used in this broad sense, the exact meaning of the term should be specified, as François Bresson stressed, so that the structures and functions of the communication systems involved can be differentiated. Other authors restrict the definition to cases where the exchange is based on an *intent* to communicate. This narrower meaning is used in communicative *pragmatics* ($\rightarrow$ PRAGMATICS), where a speech act is taken to be any action carried out by means of language ($\rightarrow$ ACTION, LANGUAGE) that produces an effect on an addressee, whether intentional or unintentional. Even stricter (but complementary) is the definition proposed by authors such as Dan Sperber and Deirdre Wilson ($\rightarrow$ RELEVANCE), who contend that the messages must be emitted in view of obtaining an effect that is anticipated by the emitter. Such acts are driven by metarepresentations and involve planning of how to change the other person's mental state ($\rightarrow$ METACOGNITION, THEORY OF MIND).

The advantage of a definition based on reciprocal intentionality is its clarity ($\rightarrow$ INTENTIONALITY); a disadvantage is difficulty finding a valid and unequivocal criterion for establishing intentionality in nonverbal exchanges, one that can handle exchanges between individuals in nonhuman species as well as exchanges between young infants and the persons around them ($\rightarrow$ ANIMAL COGNITION, INFANT COGNITION). The findings on this matter are perplexing: studies on the beginnings of intentional communication using paradigms that experimentally render dysfunctional the "adult/infant system" (for example, the infant is presented with an unresponsive adult face) have shown, quite to the contrary, that the productions of eight-week-old infants are already active, predictive, and planned.

These considerations suggest that communication should be defined at several levels. The first level could be the *expressive communication* level, where effects are expected but not mentally planned. The second could correspond to *instrumental communication*, where specific effects of emitting a message are sought following the planning of tangible events, as in pointing to an object to obtain it (*protoimperative*). The third level could be the *pragmatic communication* level, where the effects of the produced message are sought and organized following mental-event planning, as when a child points to an object, not to obtain it but to get another person's attention (*protodeclarative*) (→ ATTENTION) based on the inference that pointing to an object will generate an interest in it. It is currently agreed that the capacity to initiate joint attention in this way is the earliest indication in children of an intent to influence the mental state of a partner.

In connection with these definition problems, an entire series of models of communication have been devised, sometimes in succession, sometimes coexisting. The *emit model*, advocated by ethologists for studying nonverbal communication, describes the different types of emissions and their frequency, although surprisingly without taking the effects on the addressee into account. The *telegraphist model* proposed in information theory (→ IN-FORMATION) defines communication in terms of messages circulating between an emitter and a receiver. It focuses on message processing and the management of speaker turn-taking, and one of its advantages is that it introduces a criterion for semantic coherence in communication (→ SEMANTICS). This criterion is not met by children until near the end of the second year, in gestures like giving and offering. The more recent *orchestra model* has added another essential component of communication, simultaneity, to the criteria stated in the telegraphist model. Timing is crucial in this case, and communication is studied as a dialogue coconstruction system, whether or not the content of the dialogue is referential, coded, or inferential.

JACQUELINE NADEL

Linguistics. — In everyday usage, many idiomatic expressions are employed to refer to communication. They can all be grouped under the general heading of *channel metaphor*. Communication is defined therein as an event or activity that entails transporting information from an emitter (speaker) to a receiver (listener) via words, sentences, or texts, which are regarded as containers for ideas (→ INFORMATION, LANGUAGE, TEXT). This view is reminiscent of the most common definition of communication—found in philosophy in John Locke's work—where communication means the transmission of information. Claude Shannon and Warren Weaver took this approach in proposing the *code model* of communication, wherein a message coming from a source is encoded as a signal and then transmitted via a channel to a destination, where the received signal is decoded.

The coding idea has been widely used, and seems to be a good model of what we know about animal communication (→ ANIMAL COGNITION). Animal communication relies on a wide range of channels, including auditory signals (bird songs, vervet monkey vocalizations, etc.), visual signals (bee dances), and, in insect societies like ants, olfactory signals (pheromones). The various signals animals send each other can be analyzed in different ways, depending on whether or not they are considered intentional. But there is one thing common to all animal signals: they have one and only one interpretation (that is, they are unambiguous).

A specific feature of human communication is that its medium is language, which differs in several important ways from the systems animal use to communicate. First, language has a highly strict and very rich structure or syntax (→ SYNTAX), whereas most animal signals are standalone messages that cannot be combined. Second, human language is an extremely flexible instrument of communication, owing both to its structure, which allows the same words to express different messages (*The mouse ate the cat* and *The cat ate the mouse*), and to the fact that its words, expressions, and sentences are often polysemous, ambiguous, or vague, and therefore depend largely on context (→ CONTEXT AND SITUATION, INTERPRETATION).

In addition to exhibiting these specificities, language can be considered a distinctive characteristic of the human species for at least two reasons. First, we are the only ones to possess it, and all attempts to teach the basics of human language to other species (for example, great apes) have failed. Second, it seems that language is a faculty of human beings in the same way that visual perception is a faculty (→ PERCEPTION), in that the linguistic capacity can be impaired without damage to other mental capacities, or on the contrary, can be spared when the rest of a person's mental capacities are severely disabled.

This does not mean that communication and language amount to the same thing. There are communication systems that are not language, as in animals (and infants; see *psychology* above). However, much if not most of human communication relies on language, and because of this, it cannot be understood in terms of the code model. Paul Grice's distinction between *natural senses* and *nonnatural senses* is useful here (→ MEANING AND SIGNIFICATION). According to Grice, natural and nonnatural senses differ in the same way that *to signal* or *indicate* differs from *to mean*. A rash on a child's body indicates a childhood disease. But when Pierre says *I am sick*, his sentence does not signal his disease but the fact that he wants to indicate that he is ill. In other words, nonnatural senses—which are specific to language—

imply a reflexive intention: the intention to transmit information, and the intention to do so via the acknowledgment of that intention. On the basis of Grice's distinction, then, we can differentiate animal communication systems and human language by saying that the former is based on natural meaning, whereas the latter is based on nonnatural meaning.

Although the code model seems more or less adequate in accounting for animal communication, it fails to explain human communication, especially communication by means of language. This is because intentions and the acknowledgment of those intentions are at stake in human communication; it implies, in short, what has been called a *theory of mind* ($\rightarrow$ THEORY OF MIND) or the capacity to mentally represent the thoughts, feelings, and intentions of others. Taking this approach, Grice proposed a theory of communication that rests on a *principle of cooperation* between interlocutors ($\rightarrow$ PRAGMATICS). This essentially inferential theory has been frequently taken up and amended since its proposal. In the same vein, *relevance theory* ($\rightarrow$ RELEVANCE), which relies on a similar approach but with an original theoretical development, has the advantage of combining the code-based and inferential aspects of linguistic communication.

JACQUES MOESCHLER

Artificial intelligence. — Artificial intelligence (AI) addresses the question of communication in terms of man-machine communication in which a human user is interacting with an automated system. It strives to make this type of interaction as natural and efficient as possible.

The use of natural languages in AI has been an important topic since the 1960s. Human beings are endowed with a faculty for natural-language processing that far surpasses that of any machine ($\rightarrow$ LANGUAGE, TEXT). However, for many applications, systems with a limited processing capacity are sufficient, and in certain cases, they afford substantial improvement over traditional means (such as graphic interfaces).

In practice, man-machine communication occurs within a universe of applications known a priori. This somewhat simplifies the problem of language understanding because the task becomes searching for "deep representations" of statements that fit with the general knowledge the machine possesses about the universe in question ($\rightarrow$ DOMAIN SPECIFICITY, REPRESENTATION). A critical but delicate problem nevertheless remains: that of how to process ambiguities, both those inherent in natural language and those introduced by the indeterminacy of written and spoken speech recognition systems ($\rightarrow$ PATTERN RECOGNITION). Specialized multiagent computer architectures must be designed to manage the interactions among the different levels of knowledge involved in language processing: phonetic and phonological (description of the basic sounds and their deformations in context;

→ CONTEXT AND SITUATION), morphological and lexical, syntactic, semantic, and pragmatic (→ LEXICON, MORPHOLOGY, PRAGMATICS, SEMANTICS, SYNTAX).

Natural language is approached in AI from a number of angles, some of which overlap.

1. *Text processing* research treats language as a series of presumably errorless character strings. The areas of study here include sentence understanding and sentence generation, machine translation or machine-aided translation, and text generation. The products currently available have a limited capacity, but development of interfaces with data banks or information centers should be expanding rapidly in the near future.

2. *Speech processing* research (→ ORAL) deals with speech synthesis (making a machine talk), automatic speech recognition (talking to a machine) using pattern recognition methods, and speaker identification. Speech processing can be broken down into (a) isolated word recognition (words pronounced separately and thus in an artificial way) based on stochastic models (*hidden Markov models*) and neural networks (→ CONNECTIONISM), and (b) continuous speech recognition, which includes phonetic analysis to determine the basic constituents, and syntactic analysis based on a language model (an n-gram statistical model that gives the conditional probability of sequences of n words, or standard models of syntax). Various products of both types are on the market today, for applications like dictation machines (with vocabularies of several tens of thousands of words), vocal commands (especially as aids for the physically handicapped), and voice-based telematic services (e.g., interactive voice-response systems, or IVRs). Current research is looking into the development of speaker-independent systems and the enhancement of recognition robustness (detection of out-of-vocabulary words, spontaneous speech processing, recognition in background noise).

3. Another area under development is *optical character recognition*. This is also a pattern-recognition task that takes advantage of the major models in the field: statistical models (again, hidden Markov models), neural networks, and structural models where characters are treated as concatenations of elementary figures (e.g., lines, curves).

4. *Recognition of multifont printed texts* is relatively well under control, and several products are now available on the market. On the other hand, recognition of handwriting is an unsolved problem analogous in difficulty to continuous speech recognition.

Multimodal man-machine communication is becoming increasingly important within the broader field of multimedia interaction, now expanding with today's ongoing technological progress and the development of hypermedia documents and virtual reality systems. Multimedia interaction involves several media: keyboard, voice, and pointing devices (mouse, touch screen, data glove). These media complement each other in the framework of multimodal communication, assuming a common representation of the messages exchanged. An elaborate form of communication would be a natural-language dialogue between a human being and a machine, either in writing or in speech (→ WRITING). Current research in this line deals with the semantic and pragmatic analysis of dialogue, use of a dialogue's past, defining a model of the actor in a dialogue, and the ergonomic aspects of communication.

JEAN-PAUL HATON

SELECTED BIBLIOGRAPHY

Dennett, D. (1987). *The intentional stance*. Cambridge, MA: MIT Press.

Grice, H. P. (1989). *Studies in the way of words*. Cambridge, MA: Harvard University Press.

Hausser, R. (2001). *Foundations of computational linguistics: Human-computer communication in natural language* (2nd rev. ed.). Berlin, Germany; New York: Springer.

Knapp, M., & Daly, J. (Eds.). (2002). *Handbook of interpersonal communication* (3rd ed.). London; Thousand Oaks, CA: Sage.

Knapp, M., & Hall, J. (2001). *Nonverbal communication in human interaction* (5th ed.). Australia, US: Wadsworth/Thomson Learning.

Nadel, J., & Camaioni, L. (Eds.). (1993). *New perspectives in early communicative development*. London; New York: Routlege.

Pinker, S. (1994). *The language instinct: How the mind creates language*. New York: W. Morrow.

Shannon, C., & Weaver, W. (1949). *The mathematical theory of communication*. Urbana, IL: University of Illinois Press.

Shepherd, G. (1974). *The synaptic organization of the brain: An introduction*. New York: Oxford University Press.

Sperber, D., & Wilson, D. (1986). *Relevance: Communication and cognition*. Oxford, England: Blackwell; Cambridge, MA: Harvard University Press.

Yuen, P., Tang, Y., & Wang, P. (Eds.). (2002). *Multimodal interface for human-machine communication*. Singapore; River Edge, NJ: World Scientific.

Yule, G. (1996). *Pragmatics*. Oxford, England: Oxford University Press.

COMPETENCE/PERFORMANCE

Linguistics. — Humans acquire language and linguistic knowledge in a largely unconscious way (→ LANGUAGE). Ferdinand de Saussure made the distinction between *langue* (language, a system of linguistic signs considered in and of itself and shared by the members of a linguistic community) and *parole* (speech or word, the virtually infinite set of written or spoken utterances produced by the individuals of such a community; → ORAL, WRITING). Noam Chomsky took up this distinction in *generative grammar* (→ GRAMMAR), which he defined as a model of linguistic competence, or implicit knowledge, not of a community but of the ideal speaker-listener, independent of education, social class, or neurological state. *Competence* is what allows every native speaker of a language (that is, someone who has learned it "naturally" as his/her mother tongue, or at least very early in life) to have intuitions about the grammaticality of sentences, about whether or not they are ambiguous, about what sentences are paraphrases of each other, and so forth. For example, all native English speakers would agree that *The toves gimbled the holes* and *The holes were gimbled by the toves* are two ways of expressing the same thing, regardless of whether they know what *toves* are or what the verb *to gimble* means. Similarly, when given an unknown string of letters, a native speaker has a hunch about whether it could be a word in the language, and perhaps even what forms could be derived from it.

By contrast, *performance* depends on extralinguistic factors such as the speaker's personal history (the number of words to which he/she has been exposed) and his/her immediate state of mental attentiveness. The frequent speech errors, slips of the tongue, misunderstandings, and so forth, along with the many observed variations (in pronunciation, lexical knowledge, etc.; → LEXICON) are all related to performance, not competence, which is assumed to be identical for every native speaker of a given language.

Performance is what determines the fact that, in practice, the number of words employed in a language is limited, and that the average length of sentences actually produced is predictable for a given language. According to Chomsky, any model of language competence contains rules for generating an infinite number of possible words, and innumerable infinitely long sentences. Performance is also what prevents us from understanding sentences with more than one nested subordinate clause, such as *The thing (the mouse (the cat was chasing) was eating) was Swiss cheese*, even though such sentences should be considered grammatical.

The competence/performance difference has multiple implications. From a methodological standpoint, the study of competence does not make use of the corpus-based observations so dear to American structuralists. It relies on introspection if the language under study is one's own (→ INTROSPECTION) or, if not, on questioning native speakers. From a teaching standpoint, the rules that describe competence are not the ones that get taught; deliberate and conscious language learning necessarily deals with performance (→ CONSCIOUSNESS, LEARNING).

Chomsky reformulated this distinction in the 1980s using the terms *I-language* (internal language), which refers to the set of rules internalized by all speakers, and *E-language* (external language), the set of utterances generated by those rules. He dropped the idea of generative capacity, which only applies to the external aspect of language. He also extended the definition of competence to mean the faculty of language independent of any knowledge of a given language. It was his aim to define a universal grammar that was not an inventory of the invariants of all languages in the world, but a model of the types of parameterizable rules that allow any child to learn any language. Given the impoverished nature of the oral stimuli to which a child's perceptual system is exposed (limited number of sentences and vocabulary words, frequent mistakes, etc.) compared to the great complexity of the language system to be learned, the faculty of language is conceived of as an innate biological device specific to the human species.

This conception of language has been criticized on various grounds. For William Labov and most sociolinguists, variation is at the very heart of language competence, so the notion of *variable rule* needs to be defined. For many linguists, moreover, communication failures are an integral part of the faculty of language (→ COMMUNICATION).

ANNE ABEILLÉ

Psychology. — By extension, the competence/performance distinction is applicable to the analysis of any task in psychology where a discrepancy is noted between assessed competence (for example, a logicomathematical structure; → LOGIC) and observed performance, which is dependent upon context (→ CONTEXT AND SITUATION) and factors related to perception, memory, attention, and so forth (→ ACTIVATION/INHIBITION, ATTENTION, MEMORY, PERCEPTION). In psychology, competence is not necessarily innate but may be the result of cognitive (or social) skills constructed in the course of development (→ COGNITIVE DEVELOPMENT). These considerations have led to criticisms of Jean Piaget's structuralist and constructivist theory (→ CONSTRUCTIVISM), for it fails to consider the difference between the cognitive competence of the "epistemic subject" (Piagetian structures) and the actual problem-solving performance of the "psychological subject." In fact, some psychologists consider the competence/performance discrepancy to be the rule—and not the exception—in cognitive development.

OLIVIER HOUDÉ

SELECTED BIBLIOGRAPHY

Chandler, M., & Chapman, M. (Eds.). (1991). *Criteria for competence: Controversies in the conceptualization and assessment of children's abilities*. Hillsdale, NJ: Erlbaum.

Chomsky, N. (1969). *Aspects of the theory of syntax*. Cambridge, MA: Harvard University Press.

Chomsky, N. (1986). *Knowledge of language: Its nature, origin and use*. New York: Praeger.

Chomsky, N. (1995). *The minimalist program*. Cambridge, MA: MIT Press.

Demetriou, A. (Ed.). (1988). *The neo-Piagetian theories of cognitive development: Toward an integration*. Amsterdam; New York: North-Holland.

Fischer, K., & Kaplan, U. (2003). Piaget, Jean. In L. Nadel (Ed.), *The encyclopedia of cognitive science* (Vol. 1, pp. 679–682). London: Nature Publishing Group, Macmillan.

Hauser, M., Chomsky, N., & Fitch, W. (2002). The faculty of language: What is it, who has it, and how did it evolve? *Science, 298*, 1569–1579.

Labov, W. (1972). *Sociolinguistic patterns*. Philadelphia: University of Pennsylvania Press.

Piattelli-Palmarini, M. (Ed.). (1980). *Language and learning: The debate between Jean Piaget and Noam Chomsky*. Cambridge, MA: Harvard University Press.

Saussure, F. de (1965). *Course in general linguistics* (C. Bally, A. Sechehaye, & A. Reidlinger, Eds.; W. Baskin, Trans.). New York: McGraw-Hill. (Original work published 1916.)

COMPLEXITY

Artificial intelligence. — A clear line can be drawn—albeit not easily—between two major types of problem classes (→ PROBLEM SOLVING): *decidable problem classes* (there exists an algorithm that solves all problems in the class in a finite amount of time) and *undecidable problem classes*. However, from the standpoint of complexity, this opposition is not the most important one. The crucial distinction is the one that separates decidable problems into those that are "rapidly" solvable and those that are not. This may seem paradoxical, because it keys on a notion that is both contingent (sooner or later, won't technology find rapid solutions to all decidable problems?) and ill-defined (what is a meant by a "rapid" solution?). We shall see below that the situation is not really paradoxical after all.

Let A and B be two methods for solving the same problem, and let n be its magnitude (say, the amount of information needed to specify it among the members of its class; → INFORMATION). Let $fA(n)$ and $fB(n)$ be the number of instructions that have to be executed (on a real or idealized machine) to reach the solution using methods A and B, respectively. If $q(n) = fA(n)/fB(n)$ is a "moderately increasing" function of n (→ FUNCTION), then for all large values of n, the cost of solving the problem is in the same "neighborhood" whether we use A or B.

Now, two computation models can be distinguished: the *deterministic model* (computers) in which the execution of each instruction uniquely determines which instruction is to be executed next, and the *nondeterministic model*, where the execution of an instruction supplies a subset of instructions but no criterion for determining which one to choose. One can simulate a nondeterministic computation B on computer A by exploring the possible choices one by one, but $q(n)$ in this case is an exponential function of n.

Two types of problem classes are of interest here. (1) The first includes problem classes for which there exists a deterministic method A such that $fA(n)$ is bounded by a polynomial $p(n)$. If this property is true, it is true for all known deterministic models, and as such, it is an intrinsic property, denoted P, of the class. (2) The second includes problem classes for which this property is true for nondeterministic models; these classes are called *NP-problems*. The question of the equality of these two types of classes is still unanswered, but everything points to the conclusion that $P \neq NP$. If this were true, *NP*-problems would be intrinsically exponential.

This distinction is extremely important: a rough calculation (one human life $\cong 2^{31}$ instructions; 2^{50} instructions $\cong 350,000$ centuries) shows that no matter how much technical progress is made, an exponential problem of magnitude 50 (which is a "small" problem) will never be solved within a time period measurable on a human scale.

In 1971, Steven Cook showed that one of the simplest problems, the satisfiability of a formula in propositional logic (→ LOGIC), was *NP*. This result forces us either to find *P* subclasses of *NP* problems—and there are many—or to settle for approximations, say, by estimating the probability that the answer to a question is *yes*. These two lines of research are currently thriving.

DANIEL KAYSER

SELECTED BIBLIOGRAPHY

Ausiello, G., et al. (1999). *Complexity and approximation: Combinatorial optimization problems and their approximability properties*. Berlin, Germany; New York: Springer.

Barthélémy, J.-P., Cohen, G., & Lobstein, A. (1996). *Algorithmic complexity and communication problems* (C. Fritsch-Mignotte & M. Mignotte, Trans.). London: UCL Press. (Original work published 1992.)

Bossomaier, T., & Green, D. (Eds.). (2000). *Complex systems*. Cambridge, England; New York: Cambridge University Press.

Hochbaum, D. (Ed.). (1997). *Approximation algorithms for NP-hard problems*. Boston: PSW.

Jansen, K., Leonardi, S., & Vazirani, V. (Eds.). (2002). *Approximation algorithms for combinatorial optimization: 5th International Workshop, APPROX 2002, Rome, Italy, September 17–21, 2002: Proceedings*. New York: Springer.

Kárn[yacute], M., Warwick, K., & Kurková, V. (Eds.). (1998). *Dealing with complexity: A neural networks approach*. London; New York: Springer.

Papadimitriou, C. (1994). *Computational complexity*. Reading, MA: Addison-Wesley.

Vazirani, V. (2001). *Approximation algorithms*. Berlin, Germany; New York: Springer.

COMPUTATIONAL ANALYSIS

Neuroscience. — A *computational analysis* is a logical analysis (→ LOGIC) of the qualities required of any system, whether biological or artificial, to accomplish a given task. David Marr was among the first to stress the importance of this type of analysis. A computational analysis thus requires a clear, step-by-step description of the different information-processing operations involved in the task (→ INFORMATION). In vision, for example, figure-ground separation is one of the unavoidable steps that any visual recognition system must carry out to identify an object (→ PERCEPTION).

Computational analysis should not be confused with computer simulation. However, the processing-step descriptions drawn up in computational analyses are explicit enough to serve as a basis for building artificial models that simulate human behavior (→ MODEL).

The *computational approach* (which uses computational analysis) is a key element of cognitive neuroscience. A basic postulate is that each particular processing *subsystem* is dedicated to executing one of the steps specified in the computational analysis. The subsystems are organized into a coherent whole that forms what is called a *functional architecture*. In such an architecture, each subsystem represents a functional processing unit that receives information from another subsystem and sends information to still another. A subsystem can be seen as a group or *network* of neurons (→ NEURAL NETWORK) working together to transform a given input into a given output. The existence of the alleged subsystems has been validated by a large body of experimental data from a variety of disciplines including cognitive psychology, neurocognitive psychology, neurophysiology, and neuroimaging (→ FUNCTIONAL NEUROIMAGING, NEUROPSYCHOLOGY). The fact that the conclusions converge, despite their being grounded on different types of observations from a range of paradigms and disciplines, lends additional credibility to the underlying theoretical model.

The computational approach in cognitive science thus merges the contributions of neuroscience and psychology; it can also be articulated with computer simulation.

OLIVIER KOENIG

SELECTED BIBLIOGRAPHY

Abbott, L., & Sejnowski, T. (Eds.). (1999). *Neural codes and distributed representations: Foundations of neural computation.* Cambridge, MA: MIT Press.

Fodor, J. (2000). *The mind doesn't work that way: The scope and limits of computational psychology.* Cambridge, MA: MIT Press.

Kosslyn, S., & Koenig, O. (1992/1995). *Wet mind: The new cognitive neuroscience.* New York: Free Press.

Marr, D. (1982). *Vision: A computational investigation into the human representation and processing of visual information.* New York: Freeman.

Pylyshyn, Z. (1984). *Computation and cognition: Toward a foundation for cognitive science.* Cambridge, MA: MIT Press.

CONCEPT

Philosophy. — *Concepts* are the constituents of thoughts. For example, the concept [bald] is a constituent of the thought [Socrates is bald]. One important feature of concepts is that they are shareable, both by different people and by the same person at different times. Consequently, they need to be distinguished from the particular ideas that pass through the mind at a particular time (→ MIND). In much of the psychological literature, where the concern is often with an agent's system of internal representation (→ CATEGORIZATION, REPRESENTATION), concepts are regarded as internal representation *types* that are *tokened* on different occasions (in the way that the type word *cat* can have many different inscriptions as tokens; → TYPE/TOKEN). But many philosophers argue that these internal representation types are not concepts any more than are the type words in a natural language (→ LANGUAGE). One person might express the concept [city] by the word *city*, another by the word *ville*, and still another perhaps by a mental image of bustling boulevards (→ MENTAL IMAGERY); for all that, however, they might have the same concept [city]. Moreover, different people might employ the same representation to express different concepts (→ DIFFERENTIATION): one person might use an image of the Eiffel Tower to express [the Eiffel Tower], while another person might use that image to express [Paris], and still another to express [France].

Some philosophers think that the common objects of people's thoughts are simply the *referents* of their thoughts. However, at least in the case of general concepts, there are at least three different candidates for their referents: (1) the *extension*, or sets of actual objects that satisfy the predicate (for example, the particular cities New York, Paris, etc.); (2) the *intension*, or *function* from possible worlds to sets of possible objects that satisfy the predicate in a given world (thus, for example, [city] would be the function that takes us in the real world to the set containing New York, Paris, etc., and in another world to a set of possible cities, such as North Polis); and (3) the *causally efficacious property* (for example, cityhood) that all the (possible) objects have in common. Extensional logicians such as Willard Quine (→ LOGIC), eschewing all talk of properties and nonactual worlds, prefer the first option; modal logicians and formal semanticists such as Richard Montague, interested in accounting for the semantics of natural languages (→ SEMANTICS), tend to prefer the second; and many philosophers of mind such as Jerry Fodor, interested in causal interactions between representations and the world (→ CAUSALITY AND MENTAL CAUSATION), tend to prefer the third.

Moreover, in addition to the referent of a general term, many (for example, Gottlob Frege and Christopher Peacocke) have argued for the existence of the term's *sense* or *mode of presentation* (sometimes term *intension* is used here as well) (→ SENSE/REFERENCE). After all, *is an equiangular triangle* and *is an equilateral trilateral* refer to the same things not only in the actual world, but in all possible worlds. They seem to have the same actual and possible extensions, and are perhaps subsumed under the same causal laws, but they are arguably still different concepts (it seems informative to learn that all and only equilateral triangles are equiangular ones). Such senses or "concepts" are often regarded as internal rules that determine a concept's extension of any of the above sorts.

GEORGES REY

SELECTED BIBLIOGRAPHY

Fodor, J. (1990). *A theory of content*. Cambridge, MA: MIT Press.
Frege, G. (1997). *The Frege reader* (M. Beaney, Ed.). Oxford, England: Blackwell.
Lamberts, K., & Shanks, D. (Eds.). (1997). *Knowledge, concepts, and categories*. Cambridge, MA: MIT Press.

Montague, R. (1974). *Formal philosophy*. New Haven, CT: Yale University Press.
Peacocke, C. (1992). *A study of concepts*. Cambridge, MA: MIT Press.
Quine, W. (1960). *Word and object*. Cambridge, MA: MIT Press.

CONNECTIONISM

Artificial intelligence. — *Connectionism* originated in the field of cybernetics. Founders of cybernetics such as Warren McCulloch and Walter Pitts were the first to model artificial neurons. This line of research was interrupted in the late 1960s, however, when Marvin Minsky and Seymour Papert demonstrated that the "perceptron" (the first connectionist pattern-recognition system; → PATTERN RECOGNITION) could solve only a small class of simple problems. Connectionism regained its position in the cognitive sciences in the mid-1980s, as an alternative to the *symbolic paradigm* (→ COGNITIVISM, SYMBOL).

The connectionist paradigm retains the idea of representation (→ REPRESENTATION), but the states of the world are no longer represented by symbols, but instead by the states of a *connectionist network*, within which knowledge is distributed across the *connection weights*. Cognition is no longer seen as the manipulation of symbols but as parallel distributed processing over the whole network. Connectionism can be considered as the computational branch of cognitive neuroscience (→ COMPUTATIONAL ANALYSIS, MODEL, NEURAL NETWORK; see also *neuroscience* below), and as such, it participates in the general tendency of modern science to add a computational branch to disciplines that model and simulate complex dynamic systems (→ DYNAMIC SYSTEM). Because it abstracts the fundamental dynamics of natural neural networks, connectionism, a subdivision of the artificial sciences, can also be regarded as a broader discipline whose purpose is to study learning (→ LEARNING) in both artificial and natural systems. This feature is inherited from the cybernetic tradition, which attempts to study both natural and artificial systems using the same theoretical framework.

Connectionism is situated between the symbolic paradigm and the *constructivist paradigm* (→ CONSTRUCTIVISM). It contributes to the symbolic paradigm by supplying solutions to the problem of how symbols originate in perceptions (→ PERCEPTION). Although it attempts to model the fundamental dynamics of "pure mind," it paves the way for the constructivist paradigm, where the cognitive system is studied as a system incorporated in a sensorimotor apparatus having to satisfy viability constraints in complex environments (→ ARTIFICIAL LIFE, EMERGENCE).

A connectionist network has *dynamic* and *metadynamic* properties. In its most generally accepted usage, the term refers to a body of coupled *functions* (→ FUNCTION), where each *unit* or *node* in the network is assigned a function that computes its own *state* at any time from the states of neighboring units at the preceding point in time. The overall dynamics of the network are well defined: via its units working in parallel, the network's current state is a function of its former state. At this level of abstraction, a connectionist network can model some of the large interactive systems studied in the physical and social sciences. But it can also provide a variety of models of neural activity, depending on the specifications of the network structure and the type of function assigned to the units.

The structure of the connections can be described by *directed graphs*. In general, the units are *layered*. A signal is *input* into the first layer and the desired result is *output* by the last layer. However, connection graphs differ considerably across models. In multilayered networks, the connections go only from nodes of one layer to nodes of the next layer: input (a signal) can be clearly distinguished from output (the result), and the network performs only *bottom-up processing*, proceeding from the signal to its interpretation (→ INFORMATION, INTERPRETATION). In other types of networks (such as those designed to approach the cortical column structure of the brain), connections are also introduced between units of the same layer; these networks are still basically bottom-up. In *recurrent networks*, which are biologically more plausible, connections can also go from higher- to lower-level layers, so processing is both bottom-up and *top-down;* it is difficult to distinguish input from output, and dynamic phenomena are more complex. Recurrent networks provide a universal formalism for Bernoulli machines—that is, Turing machines (→ TURING MACHINE) equipped with Bernoulli's register (heads or tails).

For a given network, the choice of the type of function is uniform across the network: all units aggregate the output of neighboring upstream units and compute their own output in the same way. As a general rule, *linear aggregation* is chosen, with weighting that depends on the connection weight w_i^j of neighboring upstream unit connections, such that if Γ represents the connection structure, the neighboring upstream units of unit i belong to Γ_i. Each unit transforms the aggregated input using the sigmoid function σ:

$$x_i^t = \sigma(\sum_{j \in \Gamma_i} w_i^j x_j^{t-1}) \tag{1}$$

There are several sigmoids that need not be presented in detail. Only their generic property matters: a sigmoid function is a nonlinear, increasing, function of $R \to R$ with finite bounds, whose role is to limit the output value when the input value becomes too large in absolute value. More important is the issue of aggregation linearity: sigma links in the above expression can be generalized as sigma-pi links, which have biological plausibility. This amounts to adding $w_i^{jj'} x_j x_{j'}$ terms to the sum, making the effects of upstream units no longer independent but joint.

Equation (1) defines the system dynamics as a function of the network's structure and connection weights. At the same time, it helps us understand how a network can support learning: all it takes to change its weights or even its structure is to endow it with another set of dynamic properties. These new dynamic properties modify the network dynamics and therefore define the network's metadynamic properties. The metadynamics of learning are slow compared to the fast dynamics of the connectionist network. Three major metadynamic families have been studied, corresponding to the following three learning modes: *autonomous learning, supervised learning*, and *learning by reinforcement*.

Autonomous learning allows a cognitive system to *categorize* its perceptions by autonomously building prototypes of the different classes of objects in its environment (→ CATEGORIZATION). This categorization process is purely internal and self-driven: there is a signal on the network's input layer, but there is no output. Teuvo Kohonen's *topological maps* have played an instrumental role in the study of this learning mode. Even though they do not enter directly into the framework described above, the dynamics and metadynamics of topological maps are very simple: (a) for the dynamic level, choose the closest prototype to the object to be categorized; (b) for the metadynamic level, "pull" the chosen prototype slightly toward the object. The metadynamics tend to distribute the prototypes equally over the space of encountered instances, and this uniform distribution acts as an attractor, a *meta-attractor*. Such equidistributions are known to have good properties in the categorization process: having some categories that are very frequent and others that are very infrequent is not particularly useful, at least not at the basic categorization level defined by Eleanor Rosch.

Categorization is a fundamental process for cognitive systems existing in complex environments. Without it, a cognitive system would be flooded with an overly rich flow of sensory information. The system must make use of redundancies in the information flow to build prototypes from perceptions. Current research is being conducted to study the structure of networks likely to model the networks of the cortex, where the metadynamic level is in charge of extracting statistical regularities in order to construct perceptual invariants, which, in the case of computational vision, are geometric in nature.

In supervised learning, the network receives a signal on the input layer and a signal on the output layer. It learns the function that allows it to go from the input signal to the output signal by gradually correcting its errors. The process is called *supervised learning* because the output signal is given to the network. This learning paradigm has given rise to a large body of research and a vast field of applications, in tasks ranging from pattern classification, case-based learning, and concept acquisition (→ CONCEPT), to system identification and prediction. In classification tasks where the instances are produced independently, a solely bottom-up multilayer network is sufficient. This is no longer true for system-identification tasks, where the entire dynamics must be learned, that is, the next signal has to be predicted from the current one. This requires a recurrent network, the most powerful formalism for connectionist machines.

The learning method most often studied here is *error backpropagation*. It is suited to both multilayer networks and recurrent networks. Given that the principle is the same and that the method is more difficult to explain for recurrent networks, the following description applies to a strictly bottom-up, multilayer network. The output of the network is a function $Y_W(X_0)$ that depends on state X_0 of the network's input layer and its weight vector W; the same holds for the error $E_W(X_0) = |Y_W(X_0) - Y_0|^2$ relative to supervised output Y_0. To reduce the error, it suffices to shift the weights slightly (small values of α) in the opposite direction to the error gradient $\nabla_W E_W$ relative to those weights:

$$w_{t+1} = w_t - \alpha \nabla_w E_w(x_0^t) \tag{2}$$

The error gradient is computed top-down, that is, by moving downwards from the network's output layer to its input layer. The gradient backpropagation rule is applied and reiterates the rule for the derivative of a composite function $[f(u)' = f'(u)\, u']$. While Equation (1) describes the network dynamics, Equation (2) precisely describes the metadynamics. If the number of examples increases indefinitely while the law of distribution remains the same, it has been proven that the metadynamics make the multilayer network converge to the minimal error: this gives the best estimator of the output value given the input values, that is, the *Bayesian estimator*. This estimator thus acts as the meta-attractor for the learning metadynamics.

For multilayer networks, the method is local, temporal, and spatial. The weights are modified at each instant by proceeding from node to node in the network, as in the above equation of the metadynamics. The localness condition, generally considered to be a precondition of biologically plausible mechanisms, is nevertheless insufficient since error gradient backpropagation is still far from achieving this goal. In addition, the method loses its localness in recurrent networks.

Finally, reinforcement learning is aimed at learning the expectation of upcoming rewards in a given situation and the action to choose in a given situation in order to maximize that expectation ($\rightarrow$ ACTION). This is a difficult task, because the consequences of current choices may not show up until much later. Moreover, the task is even harder, unless we assume that there are a priori known models of state transitions and their attached rewards. The additional difficulty lies in finding a subtle tradeoff between the utilization of well-known strategies and the exploration of new, less-familiar strategies. When a model of the transitions and their attached rewards is available, the problem is a *dynamic-programming problem*. The optimal solutions are obtained using *Bellman's equations*, which are local equations that solve the global optimization problem: to be optimal along an entire path, a solution must be so on every part of that path, no matter how small.

The learning method studied the most in this case is *Q-Learning*, which entails estimating the quality Q of each action in each situation. Many heuristics have been tested to incorporate the utilization-exploration tradeoff into Q-Learning. The meta-attractor of this learning method is the optimal dynamic-programming solution. The error under consideration is not a prediction error, as it was in supervised learning, but the error relative to the Bellman equations. Note that the Q-Learning algorithm converges to the dynamic programming solution, even though the cognitive system was not taught the transitions-and-rewards model at any time.

PAUL BOURGINE

Neuroscience. — Connectionist simulations of cognitive processes via artificial neural networks are a critical tool in cognitive neuroscience. Simulation studies are conducted to test the computational or logical validity of the proposed processing models (→ COMPUTATIONAL ANALYSIS, LOGIC, MODEL, VALIDATION). Through the complex interplay of network connections implemented in such studies, they are able to bring out results that would be difficult to imagine with common sense alone. A case in point is when a "lesion" is made in a network (deletion of units or connections) for the purpose of simulating possible cognitive dysfunction following brain damage (→ NEUROPSYCHOLOGY).

However, networks of real brain neurons are far more complex than artificial neural networks (→ NEURAL NETWORK). No computer model has yet been devised that can simulate something as complex as the networks of the human brain. A single neuron can have several thousand connections, and it is not certain whether the learning processes demonstrated in artificial networks of ordinary size (see *artificial intelligence* above) are of the same kind as those that would be observed if the artificial networks were life-size (→ LEARNING). Moreover, one of the learning principles currently used in connectionist networks, error backpropagation, is probably not a plausible learning mechanism for the neural networks of the brain. Backpropagation does not directly correspond to any known biological process, and there are no data that allow us to contend that information is fed back into the nervous system in order to enhance upcoming performance (→ INFORMATION).

Although connectionist models are only gross approximations of brain networks, they have nevertheless proven to be very useful for modeling functional architectures in cognitive neuroscience.

OLIVIER KOENIG

SELECTED BIBLIOGRAPHY

Bechtel, W., & Abrahamsen, A. (2002). *Connectionism and the mind: Parallel processing dynamics and evolution* (2nd ed.). Oxford, England: Blackwell.

Christiansen, M., & Chater, N. (Eds.). (2001). *Connectionist psycholinguistics.* Westport, CT: Ablex.

Elman, J., Bates, A., Johnson, M., Karmiloff-Smith, A., Parisi, D., & Plunkett, K. (1996). *Rethinking innateness: A connectionist perspective on development.* Cambridge, MA: MIT Press.

Kohonen, T. (1984). *Self-organization and associative memory.* Berlin, Germany; New York: Springer-Verlag.

Krogh, A., Palmer, R., & Hertz, J. (1991). *Introduction to the theory of neural computation.* Redwood City, CA: Addison-Wesley.

Marcus, G. (2001). *The algebraic mind: Integrating connectionism and cognitive science.* Cambridge, MA: MIT Press.

McCulloch, W. S., & Pitts, W. (1943). A logical calculus of the ideas immanent in nervous activity. *Bulletin of Mathematical Biophysics, 5,* 115–143.

Mira, J., & Prieto, A. (Eds.). (2001). *Connectionist models of neurons, learning processes, and artificial intelligence: 6th International Work-Conference on Artificial and Natural Neural Networks, IWANN 2001, Granada, Spain, June 13–15, 2001: Proceedings.* Berlin, Germany; New York: Springer.

Pinker, S., & Mehler, J. (Eds.). (1988). *Connections and symbols.* Cambridge, MA: MIT Press.

Plaut, D., & Shallice, T. (1994). *Connectionist modelling in cognitive neuropsychology: A case study.* Hove, England; Hillsdale, NJ: Erlbaum.

Quinlan, P., & Giannitrapani, M. (2003). *Connectionist models of development: Developmental processes in real and artificial neural networks.* Hove, England: Psychology Press.

Rumelhart, D., & McClelland, J. (Eds.). (1986). *Parallel distributed processing: Explorations in the microstructure of cognition* (2 Vols.). Cambridge, MA: MIT Press.

Tienson, J., & Horgan, T. (Eds.). (1996). *Connectionism and the philosophy of psychology.* Cambridge, MA: MIT Press.

CONSCIOUSNESS

Psychology. — Consciousness regained its position in the center of contemporary cognitive science after having been, if not overshadowed, at least set aside under the influence of behaviorism. Behaviorism had rejected consciousness, both as a methodological tool, once the limitations of the introspective method had become apparent (→ INTROSPECTION), and as a key subject in psychology, owing to the difficulty of gaining access to it with the techniques available at the time.

The "return of consciousness," however, is not so much the recovery of a topic once prohibited by the ideology underlying the leading paradigm as it is the result of converging pathways in the various disciplines of cognitive science. In the empirical realm, research in cognitive psychology and neurobiology has offered some answers to issues like the emergence and functions of consciousness ($\rightarrow$ EMERGENCE, FUNCTION), its oneness, and the mandatory or optional role it might play in various psychological processes. In the theoretical realm, studies in artificial intelligence (AI) have raised the disturbing possibility of building a machine that, no longer being confined to calculating, conversing, and reasoning ($\rightarrow$ REASONING AND RATIONALITY), would be endowed with a form of consciousness. It is not surprising that the renewal of these issues sparked a new philosophical interest and led to the reformulation of long-standing questions such as the possibility of ultimately accounting for subjectivity and the relationship between the mind (soul/consciousness) and the body (brain) ($\rightarrow$ DUALISM/ MONISM, MIND). The topic of consciousness is now at the core of the philosophy of mind and neurophilosophy (see *philosophy* below).

Among the many contributions of cognitive psychology, some of the more important ones are (1) the demonstration, through research in areas such as memory ($\rightarrow$ MEMORY) and decision making, that consciousness is not required for highly complex information processing ($\rightarrow$ INFORMATION) during operations like semantic categorization ($\rightarrow$ CATEGORIZATION, SE- MANTICS) or risk assessment, and (2) the refinement of the distinction between conscious and unconscious activities, for example, implicit versus explicit memory and automatic versus controlled processes ($\rightarrow$ ATTENTION, AUTOMATISM, CONTROL). Some particularly enlightening studies in the second category look at the *metacognitive* processes through which subjects grasp, describe, and interpret their own cognitive activity (whether related to memory, language, reasoning, or attribution, etc.) ($\rightarrow$ LANGUAGE, METACOGNITION, THEORY OF MIND). This line of research proposes an original approach to the construction of subjectivity and the functions of consciousness, in areas ranging from self-monitoring and self-control of one's own activities to the building of coherent representations and justifications of those activities ($\rightarrow$ REPRESENTATION), which brings us back to some of the notions formerly proposed in psychoanalysis.

Once they had shed light on the organism's levels of arousal, the neurosciences began to offer some intriguing data showing what is happening in the brain when a person becomes conscious of something, or when conscious activities are being carried out (see *neuroscience* below). Some of the phenomena studied are the evocation of highly specific memories by stimulation of certain cortical zones; split brains and the issue of the oneness of consciousness in relation to brain hemisphere specialization; residual vision and hemineglect, a testimony to dissociations between objectified sensorimotor function and consciousness ($\rightarrow$ SPACE, PERCEPTION); and the paradoxical lag between initiation of a voluntary act and awareness of the intention to act, with the latter following the former ($\rightarrow$ ACTION, WILL).

In the enthusiasm generated by the spectacular progress made in the neurosciences and in AI, new theories made consciousness an *emergent* property of brain matter or the thinking machine, and unduly ignored the role in that emergence of the subject's interaction with the environment (→ INDIVIDUALISM, INTERACTION), particularly with the linguistic milieu. What is needed, then, is to relate and merge the cognitive science research that brought the problem of consciousness back into the foreground with the much earlier contributions of the *interactionist* view that deemed consciousness to be subordinate to language, and in doing so made it into a psychosocial product constructed through ontogeny (→ SOCIAL COGNITION).

While drawing from the scientific data mentioned above, the philosophy of mind has not really broken away from the various theoretical options that continue to lend themselves to philosophical reflection. In a variety of forms and with different nuances, we find the entire range of classical positions, from the most blatant spiritualistic dualism to the most reductive materialistic monism (→ REDUCTIONISM). The problem of consciousness, here, is as inevitably tied as ever to problems of intentionality (→ INTENTIONALITY), subjectivity, and freedom.

MARC RICHELLE

Neuroscience. — Consciousness is one of the most complex domains of cognitive neuroscience, with the difficulty starting right at the definitional level. We shall therefore not venture to propose a precise definition of consciousness here, for it would be nothing other than too reductive. We might simply say that unlike other mental activities, consciousness apparently cannot be described as a functional architecture composed of information-processing subsystems (→ COMPUTATIONAL ANALYSIS, FUNCTION, INFORMATION). It would seem instead to "emanate" from the coordinated functioning of many specialized subsystems.

Note first of all that only some mental processes are accompanied by conscious experience (→ EXPERIENCE, METACOGNITION, MIND). While it is possible by sheer introspection to be aware of or "conscious of" the fact that we are rotating images of objects during mental visual imaging, we are not conscious of the fact that we built those images piece by piece (→ INTROSPECTION, MENTAL IMAGERY). Another example is in the area of memory, where *explicit learning* clearly occurs under conscious control, whereas *implicit learning* is beyond our awareness (→ CONTROL, LEARNING, MEMORY).

In neuropsychology, consciousness has been approached from at least three angles (→ NEUROPSYCHOLOGY). In studies on visual perception (→ PERCEPTION), residual perceptual capacities have been shown to exist even in the absence of the primary visual cortex. This phenomenon, which is referred to as *blindsight*, can be observed only by forcing such "blind" patients to locate stimuli they are unaware of perceiving. The many studies on patients who have undergone *commissurotomy* (surgical disconnection of the left and right brain hemispheres, generally following recalcitrant epilepsy) have revealed that each hemisphere can function more or less independently and would seem to possess a sort of conscious system of its own. Finally, certain neuropsychological disorders such as *hemineglect* (difficulty processing information situated in the half of the visual field located contralateral to the lesioned brain hemisphere) and *anosognosia* (unawareness of one's own neurological disability) show that brain lesions can alter a person's awareness of part of space ($\rightarrow$ ATTENTION, SPACE) or of a behavioral disorder obvious to other people.

Clearly, then, consciousness is tied to brain activity. Recordings have shown specific electrical activity appearing in the brain right before something comes to awareness, and synchronous neuronal spikes have been noted in separate areas of the brain that are processing the same stimulus at a given instant. The neurons of these regions apparently oscillate in phase at a frequency of about 40 Hz. Some authors have concluded from this that the emergence of consciousness is rooted in the interaction of electromagnetic rhythms ($\rightarrow$ EMERGENCE).

OLIVIER KOENIG

Philosophy. — The term *consciousness* encompasses several phenomena of mental life whose nature and relationships remain controversial. Its very existence is even questioned by some.

In the most common sense of the term, persons and animals are said to be "conscious" if they are in a state of arousal in which they are mentally receptive to signals coming from the environment. The expression *phenomenal awareness* refers to the qualitative aspects of our mental life, the way things appear to us subjectively, "what it is like" (Thomas Nagel) to feel a pain or to experience the sensation of red. *Introspective* or *reflexive awareness* ($\rightarrow$ INTROSPECTION) refers to the capacity we have of deliberately inspecting the course of our thoughts, and in particular, of having higher-level thoughts about the fact that we are in a given mental state ($\rightarrow$ METACOGNITION). *Self-consciousness* is the subject's possession of a self-concept and the capacity to use that concept to grant some degree of unity to his/her mental life ($\rightarrow$ IDENTITY). Finally, in *access consciousness*, proposed by Ned Block, a state is conscious if, by virtue of the fact that a person is in that state, a representation of its content is immediately poised for use as a premise in reasoning and for the rational control of action and speech ($\rightarrow$ ACTION, CONTROL, ORAL, REASONING AND RATIONALITY, REPRESENTATION).

René Descartes and John Locke stressed that our entire mental functioning is conscious, a claim contested by many today. To assess the true scope of validity of their affirmations, two main categories of mental states must be distinguished: *intentional states* such as beliefs and desires, which have *content* (→ BELIEF, DESIRE, INTENTIONALITY), and *sensory states* or *qualia*, such as pain or sensations of red (→ QUALIA). Determining whether a mental state is conscious is based on different things, depending on the category to which it belongs (intentional or sensory). Many philosophers agree that all sensory states are conscious in the phenomenal sense. They deem incoherent the idea of an unconscious sensation, insofar as the very fact of having a certain subjective quality would seem to be constitutive of what a sensation is. In contrast, many now believe that intentional states are not always conscious. In this case, however, the kind of consciousness at stake is not phenomenal awareness but access consciousness. The fact of entertaining a thought, say, that *3 is the square root of 9*, does not seem to involve a subjective experience of a particular quality (→ EXPERIENCE). Rather, one can say that this thought is "conscious" or "unconscious" on the basis of whether its representational content is or is not accessible at a given moment by one's reasoning and speech systems.

The most problematic kind of consciousness for the cognitive sciences is phenomenal awareness. We seem to be faced here with an explanatory gulf: there is no available theory of our physical or functional nature to explain subjective experience. Essentially three types of attitudes toward the mysterious character of subjective experience can be found. At one extreme, *eliminativists* such as Daniel Dennett deny the coherence of the traditional view of phenomenal awareness; they deny that our experiences possess the special properties traditionally ascribed to them and that render them mysterious, namely, the properties of being ineffable, intrinsic, private, and immediately accessible to consciousness. At the other extreme, unbending advocates of phenomenal awareness claim that it is irreducible and consider irreducibility to be a manifestation of the fundamental incompleteness of the *physicalist* or *functionalist* conceptions of the mind (→ FUNCTIONALISM, MIND, PHYSICALISM). Arguments referred to as *absent qualia* and *inverted qualia* are used to show that functional identity does not guarantee the identity of qualitative experiences, and accordingly, that functionalism is incapable of accounting for phenomenal awareness. The arguments set forth by Nagel and Frank Jackson more specifically doubt the possibility of coming up with a physicalistic explanation of phenomenal awareness. They contend that consciousness involves a subjective perspective that no physicalistic description in the third person can explain.

Between these two extremes is an intermediate view that recognizes the existence of phenomenal awareness, but, in refusing to grant it an irreducible nature, tries to show that it can be explained in functional, physio-logical, or representational terms. A possible strategy consists in claiming that phenomenal awareness does not constitute a sui generis category but can be reduced to other types of consciousness. David Rosenthal contends, for example, that a conscious mental state is simply a mental state of which we are conscious, that is, one that is accompanied by the thought that we are in that state. This view thus allows phenomenal awareness to be reconstructed in terms of reflexive or higher-level consciousness.

ÉLISABETH PACHERIE

SELECTED BIBLIOGRAPHY

Baars, B. (1997). *In the theater of consciousness: The workspace of the mind.* New York: Oxford University Press.

Block, N. (1995). On a confusion about a function of consciousness. *Behavioral and Brain Sciences, 18,* 227–287.

Block, N., Flanagan, O., & Güzeldere, G. (Eds.). (1997). *The nature of consciousness: Philosophical debates.* Cambridge, MA: MIT Press.

Damasio, A. (1999). *The feeling of what happens: Body and emotion in the making of consciousness.* New York: Harcourt Brace.

Davies, M., & Humphreys, G. (Eds.). (1993). *Consciousness: Psychological and philosophical essays.* Oxford, England; Cambridge, MA: Blackwell.

Dehaene, S. (Ed.). (2001). *The cognitive neuroscience of consciousness.* Cambridge, MA: MIT Press.

Dennett, D. (1991). *Consciousness explained.* Boston: Little Brown.

Edelman, G. (1989). *Remembered present: A biological theory of consciousness.* New York: Basic Books.

Edelman, G., & Tonomi, G. (2000). *A universe of consciousness: How matter becomes imagination.* New York: Basic Books.

Flanagan, O. (1992). *Consciousness reconsidered.* Cambridge, MA: MIT Press.

Gazzaniga, M. (Ed.). (2000). *The new cognitive neurosciences* (Section XI, *Consciousness*) (2nd ed.). Cambridge, MA: MIT Press.

Nagel, T. (1979). *Mortal questions.* New York: Cambridge University Press.

Penrose, R. (1994). *Shadows of the mind: A search for the missing science of consciousness.* Oxford, England; New York: Oxford University Press.

Searle, J. (1997). *The mystery of consciousness.* New York Review of Books.

Weiskrantz, L. (1986). *Blindsight: A case study and implications.* Oxford, England: Clarendon Press; New York: Oxford University Press.

Weiskrantz, L. (1997). *Consciousness lost and found: A neuropsychological exploration.* Oxford, England; New York: Oxford University Press.

CONSTRAINT

Neuroscience. — Constraint is a critical concept in cognitive neuroscience, as in psychology, where it is found in the expression *constraint satisfaction*. Constraint satisfaction corresponds to a process of matching against representations stored in memory (→ MEMORY, REPRESENTATION). The *input* to a memory subsystem that stores such representations is a complex signal containing different kinds of information output by other subsystems that have already processed some aspects of the stimulus (for example, variations in texture, line intersections, and color, in the case of a visual stimulus) (→ INFORMATION, PERCEPTION). This information is compared with that stored in memory, and the representation that best satisfies the different input constraints will be activated the most (→ ACTIVATION/INHIBITION). The memory subsystem's *output* specifies that representation, and sends it on to another subsystem in the functional architecture (→ COMPUTATIONAL ANALYSIS).

OLIVIER KOENIG

Artificial intelligence. — *CSP* (constraint satisfaction problems) is a very general problem-solving paradigm (→ PROBLEM SOLVING) with many applications, including computer-assisted design and decision-making systems, production scheduling and management, pattern recognition (→ PATTERN RECOGNITION), and other applications at the crossroads between artificial intelligence and operations research.

In the CSP approach, a problem is described by (1) a finite number of *state variables*, (2) the *definition domains* of those variables, and (3) a set of constraints the variables must satisfy in every solution to the problem. For example, suppose an audiovisual system is made up of seven components that one can choose from catalogues (amplifiers, tuners, CD or cassette players, recorders, antennas, speakers, and TV screens). The constraints to be satisfied involve compatibility, quality, and cost. A CSP solution to the problem assigns a value to each variable in its definition domain while complying with all problem constraints.

There are a variety of approaches for solving CSPs, depending on the domain and the type of constraint (→ DOMAIN SPECIFICITY). *Finite domains* and domains made up of numerical intervals are studied the most. Finite-domain CSPs rely on enumerative analysis. *Binary constraints* implicate two variables (for example, the electrical compatibility of two components), but a larger number of variables may sometimes be involved (for example, the cost of the whole system). The constraints are either explicit (list of possible antenna-tuner pairs) or implicitly defined by a relationship (for example, the total cost must not exceed the available amount of money). A binary-constraint CSP is represented by a graph: the nodes are the variables and the edges are the constraints.

For a given CSP, one might want to do various things, such as prove that there is a solution (that is, that the constraints are coherent), find any solution, list all solutions, choose a solution that optimizes a given criterion (for example, the system's quality-price ratio), or reduce the variable domains to only those values that necessarily enter into a solution. A finite-domain CSP generally corresponds to an *NP-complete problem*

($\rightarrow$ COMPLEXITY), so one often has to settle for partial approaches. *Filtering algorithms* are a good example of a partial approach. One can go through all pairs of variables and reduce their respective domains in accordance with the constraint they have in common (*arc consistency*). The problem can be further reduced by applying binary constraint propagation using composition relationships (*path consistency*). Reduction to an empty domain proves the incoherence of the initial constraints; however, the absence of a such a reduction does not prove coherence but simply shows that the algorithms are incomplete.

MALIK GHALLAB

SELECTED BIBLIOGRAPHY

Creignou, N., Khanna, S., & Sudan, M. (2001). *Complexity classifications of Boolean constraint satisfaction problems*. Philadelphia: Society for Industrial and Applied Mathematics.
Kosslyn, S., & Koenig, O. (1992/1995). *Wet mind: The new cognitive neuroscience*. New York: Free Press.
Yokoo, M. (2000). *Distributed constraint satisfaction: Foundations of cooperation in multi-agent systems*. Berlin, Germany; New York: Springer.

CONSTRUCTIVISM

Psychology. — One of the greatest figures of *constructivism* in the twentieth century was the Genevan psychologist Jean Piaget. His theory, which refuses empiricism as well as nativism, describes the intelligence as the most general form of coordination of a subject's actions and operations, constructed through the subject's logical (re)construction and (re)structuring of the environment ($\rightarrow$ ACTION, COGNITIVE DEVELOPMENT, LOGIC). Piaget's theory is one of the basic sources of inspiration for today's interdisciplinary constructivist trend in cognitive science.

In constructivism, knowledge is not a mere reflection of the outside world, nor the projection onto reality of innate transcendental structures of the mind ($\rightarrow$ MIND). The physical world must be shaped—"(re)invented," as Paul Watzlawick stated, or "made to emerge," in Francisco Varela's terms ($\rightarrow$ EMERGENCE). In other words, the physical world is recognized and broken down into interrelated single objects only by means of the actions and operations the subject exerts upon it. In Piagetian theory, then, objectivity and subjectivity are constructed jointly and complementarily, through constant action upon the real world. From infancy to adulthood, experiential information is assimilated into the subject's logicomathematical structures. These structures in turn coordinate the action (or *operatory*) schemes that generate objective knowledge of the world.

The *enaction* approach, advocated by Varela following his work on models of cellular automata in the neurophysiology of perception (→ ARTI-FICIAL LIFE, CONNECTIONISM, PERCEPTION), criticizes classical cognitivism (→ COGNITIVISM) for the very criterion it uses to assess cognition, which is always the "adequate representation" of a predetermined external world. In doing so, Varela is in fact challenging the philosophy of representation, which goes far beyond the scope of psychology and neurophysiology (*see also* Michel Foucault, Martin Heidegger, Maurice Merleau-Ponty, Michel Serres, and other contemporary philosophers). According to Varela, whose criticism is not confined to cognitivism but holds for Piaget too, "the endogenous" and "the exogenous" are mutually defined in the course of a long history that seeks only a viable mapping, not any sort of optimal fit. There is indeed a constructivism here, as in Piaget, but it is one where logicomathematical normativity (→ NORMATIVITY) is replaced by the flow of contextual meanings: relevance criteria are dictated by common sense, in a consistently context-based fashion (→ CONTEXT AND SITUATION, MEANING AND SIGNIFICATION). Although Varela's radically pragmatic constructivism (with its simple criterion of contextual viability) is applicable to the neurophysiology of perception, one can nevertheless doubt its relevance to the psychology of intelligence, where it takes a perhaps excessively antagonistic stance against Piaget's "solipsist-transcendental" constructivism (→ EXTERNALISM/INTERNALISM).

Still another variant of constructivism is *neural Darwinism*, proposed by Jean-Pierre Changeux and Gerald Edelman, who explain neurocognitive development and consciousness in terms of a *variation-selection* mechanism (→ CONSCIOUSNESS, NEURAL DARWINISM).

OLIVIER HOUDÉ

SELECTED BIBLIOGRAPHY

Changeux, J.-P. (1994). *Raison et plaisir* [Reason and pleasure]. Paris: Odile Jacob.

Changeux, J.-P., & Connes, A. (1998). *Conversations on mind, matter, and mathematics* (M. B. DeBevoise, Ed. and Trans.). Princeton, NJ: Princeton University Press. (Original work published 1989.)

Changeux, J.-P., & Ricoeur, P. (2000). *What makes us think?: A neuroscientist and a philosopher argue about ethics, human nature, and the brain* (M. B. DeBevoise, Trans.). Princeton, NJ: Princeton University Press. (Original work published 1988.)

Fischer, K., & Kaplan, U. (2003). Piaget, Jean. In L. Nadel (Ed.), *The encyclopedia of cognitive science* (Vol. 1, pp. 679–682). London: Nature Publishing Group, Macmillan.

Piaget, J. (1954). *The construction of reality in the child* (M Cook, Trans.). New York: Basic Books. (Original work published 1937.)

Piaget, J. (1970). *Genetic epistemology* (E. Duckworth, Trans.). New York: W. W. Norton. (Original work published 1970.)

Varela, F., Thompson, E., & Rosch, E. (1991). *The embodied mind: Cognitive science and human experience*. Cambridge, MA: The MIT Press.

Watzlawick, P. (1984). *The invented reality: How do we know what we believe?* New York: Norton.

CONTEXT AND SITUATION

Linguistics. — There is no fixed or universal definition of context. For some, the terms *context* and *situation* overlap or are even confounded—Bronislav Malinowski and John Firth spoke of "situational context" and "context of situation." Other investigators have attempted to make a clear-cut distinction between the two terms, for example, by defining *context* as a limited set of dimensions relevant to the current activity, and *situation* as the set of dimensions potentially available at the time the activity is taking place (→ TIME AND TENSE).

In other approaches, *context* is taken to mean the discourse that surrounds the linguistic entity under study (→ DISCOURSE) (the term *environment* is used as well), by opposition to *situation*, deemed in this case to be the scene in which the discourse is uttered (the term *circumstances* is also used here). This opposition was restated in text linguistics (→ TEXT) in terms of a dichotomy between *co-text* (the linguistic environment of a given text fragment) and *context* (the extralinguistic factors of the act of communication; → COMMUNICATION). However, the opposition between the *external* and *internal context* of a discourse does not define two disjoint domains. Take the case of two doctors who are conversing: their status (the external context) labels them as doctors, at the same time as their use of medical terminology in their dialogue (the internal context) reveals that same identity.

The external context can be granted a central or a marginal role, depending on one's conception of language and linguistic activity (→ LANGUAGE). Approaches that conceive of language as a system tend to undermine or even deny the role of context, whereas approaches based on speech acts or linguistic practices recognize its fundamental and structuring role (→ ACTION, PRAGMATICS). The role of context is minimal, for instance, in the opposition between intra- and extralinguistic: language is regarded as an independent object that can be detached and isolated from the actual practices of its speakers, its units are given autonomous definitions and descriptions, and context is only sometimes recognized as an outside, secondary factor that modifies literal senses and virtual, preestablished entities (→ SENSE). Yet the importance of context cannot be disregarded when we consider that not only usage but also the definitions of linguistic resources are structured in an essentially context-related way. Approaches where context is a peripheral dimension can thus be distinguished from those where it is constitutive, in which case the objects to be analyzed and how they are grasped must be redefined.

Moreover, context is not conceptualized in the same way when it is seen as a predefined set of parameters likely to unilaterally influence language usage, as when it is understood to be a set of dimensions generated during linguistic exchange, established by the participants at the same time as it structures their behavior in return. The first conception is static; the second is dynamic, and context is not reduced to physical, perceptual dimensions or to cognitive entities (knowledge, beliefs, shared or unshared goals; → BELIEF). Rather, it is formed by the participants' activity and is updated as their actions and interactions develop (→ INTERACTION). In the first view, the question becomes finding out what is part of context, and what is not. In the second, the problem is to describe the processes by which speakers identify, select, and configure the relevant facets of the context. In the first case, the aim is to come up with a systematic description based on a finite number of parameters that will isolate comparative variables (such as time, place, categories of speakers, degree of formality, types of events, etc.). In the second, a phenomenological description is called for, one that takes the speakers' points of view into account along with their interpretational and conversational strategies (→ INTERPRETATION).

The traditional way of treating context—as a set of external causal factors delineated a priori by an abstract analysis—poses a problem brought out by ethnomethodologists: the context in which an interaction develops can be described in multiple, concurrent ways, but this does not tell us a priori which description is the relevant one. This point can be illustrated using a parameter often taken to be a contextual factor, the speakers' occupations: the fact that a conversation takes place in a hospital between persons categorized as a doctor and a patient does not mean that it can legitimately be interpreted as being about medical issues—other ways of describing those same speakers are equally possible, based on, say, their age, their gender, their religion, their ethnic group, or other even more contingent characteristics. There are always a potentially infinite number of external a priori descriptions of any context.

One solution is to conceive of context as being reciprocally established by the persons participating in the current interaction. This means that context is not a given, but is constructed by the interlocutors in their efforts to make it available to all parties; it is utilized by the actors as a resource for organizing the ongoing activity in a mutually understandable way. At the same time, it is shaped, produced, and reproduced by that same activity in a way that is intelligible and relevant to it. In Emmanuel Schegloff's view, the question of context lies in knowing how participants decide to retain a given aspect of the context as relevant (and thus useful for producing and interpreting the rest of the interaction) and what makes that aspect relevant to the sequential organization of the ongoing interaction (→ RELEVANCE). In order to understand, and to make themselves understood, participants engage in a *contextualization* process whereby they interrelate relevant elements of the context. To do so, they rely on a number of verbal and non-verbal markers that John Gumperz called *contextualization cues*, by means of which they point to, identify, render relevant, maintain, or transform some facet of the context. Contextualization strategies, which are part of the communicational competence of speakers, are what link available cues, such as the fact of using a person's first name rather than last name, language switching, prosodic modifications, or particular gestures to their corresponding interpretations, inferences, and underlying expectations, and these links are what make the discourse meaningful.

The term *situation*—which, again, often overlaps with the notion of context—is used to refer to the social and spatiotemporal setting in which an utterance, an interaction, and more generally, an activity takes place (→ SPACE). The link between utterance and situation has been acknowledged in linguistics (by Roman Jakobson, for example) and in logic (Yehoshua Bar-Hillel) with regard to *deictic* or *indexical units* (first- and second-person personal pronouns, verb morphemes, adverbs of time and place, etc.), which are characterized precisely by the fact that the interpretation of their meaning is necessarily tied to the situation of utterance (for example, to understand the referent of *here*, one obviously has to know where the speaker is). Although these units cannot be understood outside of the circumstances in which they are used, they have been analyzed in two ways. The first, a weak version of indexicality, distinguishes deictic or indexical units from other linguistic units, thereby reducing the number of linguistic domains in which recourse to the situation is necessary. This position treats indexicality as an imperfection of natural languages, by contrast to formal languages, which are autonomous systems whose meanings are self-contained. The second, a stronger and more general version of indexicality, extends the analysis of deictics to any use of language: the sense of an expression is always contingent upon the circumstances of its utterance. This position thus sees indexicality as the very condition for the functioning of language. In this view, the indeterminacy of language is not a "flaw" but, on the contrary, a fundamental resource that guarantees flexibility of usage in the wide variety of situations where language is used.

LORENZA MONDADA

Psychology. — In the linguistic sense of the term, *context* is defined as the part of a discourse or text that precedes the utterance being processed (→ DISCOURSE, TEXT). The need to distinguish between this purely verbal information and other elements taken into account during language comprehension (→ INFORMATION, LANGUAGE) has led most authors to employ the term *co-text* to refer to the linguistic context proper and *context* to designate—as in any other cognitive process—all elements of the situation surrounding the to-be-processed object (the stimulus) (see *linguistics* above). *Context effects* (with context defined as such) have been found in many areas, although their interpretation remains controversial.

In psycholinguistics, context effects called *priming effects* are often used to study lexical access (→ LEXICON). A briefly presented prime word has been shown to affect the time it takes to decide whether or not a target word displayed after the prime belongs to the lexicon. The prime thus acts as the context. In a broader way, in Dan Sperber and Deirdre Wilson's *relevance theory*, the cognitive context chosen by the speaker in an exchange plays an essential role in accounting for language comprehension (→ COMMUNICATION, RELEVANCE). Another important context effect has been clearly demonstrated by Endel Tulving, who showed how compatibility between the *encoding* and *retrieval contexts* has a substantial impact on the probability of retrieving knowledge stored in memory (→ MEMORY). The encoding context is also an essential component of connectionist models proposed to simulate the acquisition of face recognition (→ CONNECTIONISM). Other types of context effects are *contrast and assimilation effects* in perceptual judgments and even in social judgments (→ PERCEPTION, SOCIAL COGNITION). Moreover, the fact that object categorization tasks are particularly context-sensitive—as manifested by the task-dependent differences in the magnitude of between- and within-individual differences—is claimed by Laurence Barsalou to be an essential argument for questioning the universality and stability of "natural" semantic categories (→ CATEGORIZATION, DIFFERENTIATION, SEMANTICS). Finally, in problem solving, the role of the cognitive context generated by *point of view*, which determines how a subject represents the problem space, has been thoroughly analyzed and demonstrated for logical and arithmetic problem solving, and in the study of cognitive functioning in aircraft pilots, for example (→ LOGIC, NUMBER, REASONING AND RATIONALITY, REPRESENTATION).

Although a large body of experimental data has proven the existence of context effects in cognitive processing, their role and importance have been understood differently. Two major views can be schematically opposed. In the first, the context acts mainly as a modulator: knowledge and processes are general, but the way they are implemented is context-dependent. In this case, the context is necessarily an external, situational one. This same modulating function is also found in classical Piagetian theory, where the characteristics of the situation are said to either "facilitate" or "complicate" the implementation of general cognitive structures, and procedural schemes are thought to act as mediators between the current situation and the subject's cognitive structures (→ COGNITIVE DEVELOPMENT, COMPETENCE/PERFORMANCE). In the second view, context is regarded instead as a constituent of knowledge, in such a way that the context is what determines the activation and validity limits of knowledge (that is, knowledge is valid only in a given context). Hence, there exists an internal context too. This approach is conceptualized in the now-growing theories of *situated cognition*, and has given rise to both symbolic models (→ SYMBOL) as well as connectionist ones. In this view, contextualization—which dictates the organization of human knowledge—is far from constituting a limitation, but appears instead as a condition for its effective use.

Claude Bastien

SELECTED BIBLIOGRAPHY

Clancey, W. (1997). *Situated cognition: On human knowledge and computer representations.* Cambridge, England; New York: Cambridge University Press.

Duranti, A., & Goodwin, C. (Eds.). (1992). *Rethinking context: Language as an interactive phenomenon.* Cambridge, England; New York: Cambridge University Press.

Kirshner, D., & Whitson, J. (Eds.). (1997). *Situated cognition: Social, semiotic, and psychological perspectives.* Mahwah, NJ: Erlbaum.

Light, P., & Butterworth, G. (Eds.). (1992). *Context and cognition: Ways of learning and knowing.* New York: Harvester Wheatsheaf.

Sperber, D., & Wilson, D. (1986). *Relevance: Communication and cognition.* Oxford, England: Blackwell; Cambridge, MA: Harvard University Press.

Sternberg, R., & Wagner, R. (Eds.). (1994). *Mind in context: Interactionist perspectives on human intelligence.* Cambridge, England; New York: Cambridge University Press.

Suchman, L. (1987). *Plans and situated actions: The problem of human-machine communication.* Cambridge, England; New York: Cambridge University Press.

Tannen, D. (Ed.). (1988). *Linguistics in context.* Norwood, NJ: Ablex.

Tulving, E. (1983). *Elements of episodic memory.* Oxford, England: Clarendon Press; New York: Oxford University Press.

Yule, G. (1999). *Pragmatics.* Oxford, England: Oxford University Press.

CONTROL

Neuroscience. — To control behavior, the central nervous system has about 10^{12} neurons at its disposal, all connected to each other in networks (→ NEURAL NETWORK).

In cognitive neuroscience, there are three fundamental questions related to control. The first concerns how the brain controls our behavior. Ultimately, control is achieved via commands that dictate the motor acts performed by the organism (→ ACTION).

The second question concerns where and how this control actually takes place in the brain. The brain has functional priorities that determine which neural responses are preferentially triggered (→ ACTIVATION/INHIBITION, ATTENTION, FUNCTIONAL NEUROIMAGING). In humans, there appear to be two major cortical regions that control behavior. The posterior cortical regions seem to be in charge of controlling behavior in routine situations at least. In more complex situations, the final behavioral decision is thought to depend on prefrontal structures. These two regions are closely tied to the limbic system, which is involved in personal motivation (value system, emotions; → EMOTION). Control thus seems to be supported by neural structures that form a hierarchical system. When one control area is damaged (→ NEUROPSYCHOLOGY), attentional deficits may arise and cause the patient to partially lose control over some of his/her behavior. A substantial number of psychopathological disorders where the individual has poor control over the situation (→ COGNITIVE PSYCHIATRY) appear to be rooted in dysfunction of either or both of these neural circuits.

The third question is trickier: What are the intimate control mechanisms that take effect at the neural level? It all seems to boil down to the interplay between neural *excitation* and *inhibition* (→ COMMUNICATION), although establishing the respective parts played by these two mechanisms is a difficult task. What we do know, at least at the cortical level, is that many excitatory potentials must be summed before a neuron becomes activated. On the other hand, there are cases where a single cell inhibits the response of another neuron. Neural control is clearly asymmetrical. The way these different types of neurons are organized is yet to be determined.

ÉRIC SIÉROFF

Psychology. — In cognitive psychology, the question of control goes back to the distinction established experimentally by Richard Schiffrin and Walter Schneider between two basic information-processing modes: *automatic processes* characterized by no attentional load, no control, unawareness, parallel operations, and fast execution (→ ATTENTION, CONSCIOUSNESS), and *controlled processes*, which are slower, serial, strategically determined, and therefore incur an attentional load in working memory (→ MEMORY) (→ AUTOMATISM for a description of Schiffrin and Schneider's original paradigm, along with an analysis of the automatic/controlled distinction). Controlled processes, at least those involved in complex cognitive tasks, are often said to depend on a higher-level cognitive system, like Alan Baddeley's *central executive* in working memory or Don Norman and Tim Shallice's *supervisory attentional system*, thought to be altered when the prefrontal cortex is damaged (see *neuroscience* above). Other forms of control are probably more highly distributed, as shown, for example, by the physiologist Alain Berthoz in his studies on movement.

Following John Flavell, controlled processes have been studied for their metacognitive function (→ METACOGNITION) in various activities including memory processing (*metamemory*), language acquisition (*metalanguage*), communication (*metacommunication*), and in the construction of *theories of mind* (→ COMMUNICATION, LANGUAGE, THEORY OF MIND). Analyses conducted in this framework have dealt essentially with the *metaknowledge* (knowledge about cognitive functions) used by the control processes.

In child psychology, neo-Piagetian models specifically emphasize the role of *executive control processes*, or *executive functions*, in accounting for the stages and mechanisms of cognitive development (→ COGNITIVE DEVELOPMENT). Robbie Case describes a hierarchy of stages between infancy and adulthood (sensorimotor, interrelational, dimensional, and vectorial), each divided into substages (unifocal, bifocal, and elaborated) in the course of which executive control structures become more and more complex. The transition between substages is a function of the greater working memory capacity, itself a function of operatory efficiency (*scheme automatization*); the transition between stages is ensured by the hierarchical integration of increasingly powerful control structures, both cognitive and social (→ DIFFERENTIATION).

Whether the control pertains to actions (→ ACTION), perceptions (→ PERCEPTION), or representations in memory (→ REPRESENTATION), one of the key questions in today's research, both in cognitive psychology and in neuroscience, concerns the respective roles of activation and inhibition in our multilevel functional architecture (→ ACTIVATION/INHIBITION), where control is exerted at every level, from communication among neurons, to executive functions in the prefrontal cortex.

Some neurophysiologists reject the idea of a controlling central executive, arguing instead for a *temporal synchronization* process (Wolf Singer, Rodolfo Llinas). In this view, the groups of neurons or cognitive modules involved in a given task become temporarily linked via the synchronization of their electrical activity (oscillating at a frequency of about 40 Hz). The momentary network that emerges captures all of the subject's available attention, consciousness, and resources to carry out the task (→ NEURAL NETWORK). For each new task, a new network is built, and so on. Here, the unity of the mind is the result of the transient association of specialized modules (→ MODULARITY), not of a high-level supervisor. This view definitively rules out the idea of a "Cartesian theater" (to borrow the philosopher Daniel Dennett's expression) at the core of the cognitive system. This issue is far from being resolved.

These two processes (selection by a central supervisor, temporal synchronization) could be involved in related or unrelated ways, according to the structure of the material and the task requirements.

OLIVIER HOUDÉ

Artificial intelligence. — For the tasks of interest to artificial intelligence (AI), there are usually no available methods that can simply be applied step by step (→ PROBLEM SOLVING). AI systems, whose reasoning processes are based on declarative knowledge (→ REASONING AND RATIONALITY), require elaborate mechanisms for controlling (or driving) the problem-solving process. The term *control* is used here to refer to the mechanism that decides what actions to carry out at each step of the solving process (→ ACTION), that is, what knowledge to use, how to use it, and what aspect of the problem requires attention (→ ATTENTION). A simple example is a *rule-based system* (→ KNOWLEDGE BASE): when the inference engine has to choose among several candidates, a control mechanism resolves the conflict by selecting an applicable rule.

Problem solving usually involves exploring a very large number of hypotheses. The exploration process can be controlled "in breadth" or "in depth." It brings heuristic knowledge to bear to help find a solution, but since there is no guarantee of success, backtracking may be necessary. At a more general level, control processes make use of metaknowledge that conveys experience acquired in a given application domain (→ DOMAIN SPECIFICITY, METACOGNITION). Control can also be exerted via an *action-planning mechanism* that determines a dynamically revisable sequence of problem-solving stages.

In some cases, especially in multiagent systems, two levels of control are defined, a tactical level that takes local decisions into account, and a strategic level that institutes an overall solving policy.

The direction of information flow defines two ways of proceeding cognitively in the face of a problem to be solved: via *bottom-up control*, which entails utilizing the available data and facts to figure out the answer (an inference engine's *forward chaining* mechanism), or *top-down control*, which, inversely, starts from the goal to be attained and proceeds by gradual refinement (*backward chaining*). In complex problem solving, these two methods are usually employed in conjunction with each other but at different times, particularly in control strategies based on *confidence islands*, which work from sure anchor points. This kind of control is frequently used in pattern recognition systems (images, speech, or signals) (→ PATTERN RECOGNITION).

An AI system can be controlled centrally by a single module, or hierarchically at the tactical and strategic levels. Or it may even be totally *distributed* (→ DISTRIBUTED INTELLIGENCE). In the last case, overall control results from a series of decisions made locally by different modules.

JEAN-PAUL HATON

SELECTED BIBLIOGRAPHY

Baddeley, A. (1986). *Working memory*. Oxford, England; New York: Oxford University Press.

Baddeley, A., & Weiskrantz, L. (Eds.). (1993). *Attention: Selection, awareness and control*. Oxford, England; New York. Clarendon Press.

Berthoz, A. (2000). *The brain's sense of movement* (G. Weiss, Trans.). Cambridge, MA: Harvard University Press. (Original work published 1997.)

Case, R. (1985). *Intellectual development: Birth to adulthood*. Orlando, FL: Academic Press.

Dennett, D. (1991). *Consciousness explained*. Boston: Little Brown.

Ferber, J. (1999). *Multi-agent systems: An introduction to distributed artificial intelligence* (Trans.). Harlow, England; Reading, MA: Addison Wesley. (Original work published 1995.)

Flavell, J. (1979). Metacognition and cognitive monitoring: A new area of cognitive-developmental inquiry. *American Psychologist, 34*, 906–911.

Miller, E. (2000). The prefrontal cortex and cognitive control. *Nature Reviews Neuroscience, 1*, 59–65.

Monsell, S., & Driver, J. (Eds.). (2000). *Control of cognitive processes*. Cambridge, MA: MIT Press.

Omidvar, O., & Elliott, D. (Eds.). (1997). *Neural systems for control.* San Diego, CA: Academic Press.

Schiffrin, R. M., & Schneider, W. (1977). Controlled and automatic human processing: II. Perceptual learning, automatic attention and a general theory. *Psychological Review, 84,* 127–190.

Schneider, W., Owen, A., & Duncan, J. (Eds.). (2000). *Executive control and the frontal lobe.* Berlin, Germany; New York: Springer.

Shallice, T. (1988). *From neuropsychology to mental structure.* Cambridge, England; New York: Cambridge University Press.

Singer, W. (1990). Search for coherence: A basic principle of cortical self-organization. *Concepts in Neurosciences, 1,* 1–26.

COUNTERFACTUAL

Philosophy. — In a *counterfactual conditional* proposition, one considers a situation that does not come to be, in order to derive from it the consequences it would have had in a world where it did come to be (→ LOGIC, MODALITY). An example of a counterfactual conditional is *If you had studied, you would have passed your exam,* which we denote $p \,\square\!\rightarrow q$ (if p had happened, q would have happened), where p is the antecedent and q is the consequent. This type of conditional is different from the *material conditional*, p implies q, which is true if p is false or if q is true. In other words, material conditionals are true when the antecedent is false and the consequent is true, whereas counterfactual conditionals are not.

Counterfactuals are indispensable for defining the concepts of dispositional property, law, and causality (→ CAUSALITY AND MENTAL CAUSATION), to the extent that these concepts presuppose an interest in noninstantiated properties or effects: the solubility of sugar in water is a property that applies not only to sugar that happens to be in water, but also to sugar that does not. Similarly, saying that cause c is necessary to produce effect e amounts to saying that if c had not occurred, then e would not have been produced.

JOËLLE PROUST

SELECTED BIBLIOGRAPHY

Jackson, F. (Ed.). (1987). *Conditionals.* Oxford, England; New York: Blackwell.

Lewis, D. (1973). *Counterfactuals: The social psychology of counterfactual thinking.* Oxford, England: Blackwell; Cambridge, MA: Harvard University Press.

Roese, N., & Olson, J. (Eds.). (1995). *What might have been.* Mahwah, NJ: Erlbaum.

CREATIVITY

Psychology. — *Creativity* is the capacity to produce something that is both new and *adaptive*. It can be an idea, a musical composition, a story, an advertisement, or a creation in any other form.

By definition, a new product is original and unexpected. It stands out from what its creator or any other individual has already produced. Its newness can vary in degree, but no new response can be considered creative unless it is adaptive, that is, unless it satisfies the constraints of some problem (→ CONSTRAINT, PROBLEM SOLVING). In judgments of creativity, the weight granted to these two criteria, novelty and adaptiveness, varies across individuals and also across tasks (→ DIFFERENTIATION). For example, adaptiveness is more important in the creative productions of engineers than in those of artists.

There are no absolute standards for assessing the creativity of a product. Because of this, judgments of creativity are subject to a social consensus. Whether the judging is done by a single individual, a committee made up of several persons, or a society as a whole, a creative piece is evaluated—and its degree of creativity is determined—with respect to others of its kind. In the same way, the creativity of a person (or group) is assessed relative to that of other persons (or groups).

Creativity tests have been developed by psychologists. In the best-known tests, devised by Joy Guilford and E. Paul Torrance, the subject has to come up with as many different solutions to a problem as possible in an allotted amount of time. For instance, the subject is asked to state all possible uses of a cardboard box. In tests of this type, creativity is evaluated in terms of *fluidity* (the number of different answers given), *flexibility* (the number of different categories into which the answers can be classified), and *originality* (which is inversely proportional to the frequency of the response in the reference population). These tests in fact assess variety, the "divergence" of thought. The current trend is to consider creativity as a multidimensional capacity involving not only the cognitive facet, but also personality and emotion-related dimensions (→ EMOTION).

The nature of the production process can also be a criterion for deciding whether a product exemplifies creativity on the part of its author. A work produced by chance, or by applying rules specified by some other person, is often deemed less creative than a work that is the outcome of a difficult, deliberate endeavor involving obstacles to be overcome (→ WILL). The creativity of artificial information-processing systems has been debated on this account, because although their responses are sometimes new and satisfy the constraints of the problem at hand, the processes employed to produce them are not necessarily the ones that are assumed to underlie human creativity.

Finally, conceptions of creativity vary across cultures and times. In some societies, creativity revolves around the product and the extent to which it breaks away from tradition; in others, more value is placed on the creative process than on its result, and novel ways of using traditional objects are prized.

The study of creativity in psychology has sparked a new interest in the *creative cognition approach*, where the idea is to understand creative processes using the methods and concepts of the cognitive sciences.

JACQUES LAUTREY AND TODD LUBART

Linguistics. — In linguistics, creativity is related to *generativity*. How many English words are there? How long is the longest sentence? It is impossible to answer these questions because of our linguistic creativity, that is, our faculty to understand or produce an apparently unlimited number of new words and new sentences.

In *generative grammar*, proposed by Noam Chomsky in 1957, linguistic creativity is governed by formalizable rules (→ GRAMMAR). A *formal grammar* (formal in the mathematical sense) is defined as a finite set of rules which, when applied to an equally finite set of vocabulary words, can generate a potentially infinite set of well-formed sentences. *Recursion*—a linguistic universal, as testified by the fact that recurrent subordination and coordination devices are found in every language in the world—is the property that enables the same rule to be used an unlimited number of times to generate innumerable sentences of limitless length. The set of all sentences produced or recognized by such a grammar is a subset of all possible combinations using a given vocabulary; this is its *weak generative capacity*, or the *language* (→ LANGUAGE). The set of all combinations of rules used to produce or recognize the sentences of the language, that is, the analyses associated with those sentences (generally represented in the form of syntactic trees; → SYNTAX) is the grammar's *strong generative capacity*. Two grammars can have the same weak generative capacity, that is, describe the same set of grammatical sentences, but assign them different structures (for example, for the same three-word sentence, one grammar will assign a binary left-branching tree, while another will assign a right-branching tree).

The generative approach to language was criticized by Maurice Gross, who characterizes languages in terms of finite combinatorics, and also by Jaako Hintikka, who rejects the idea of recursion on the grounds that the use of identical symbols in the rules of this approach masks the distinction he finds essential between the main and subordinate clauses of sentences. More generally speaking, it is clear that linguistic creativity cannot be reduced to syntax.

ANNE ABEILLÉ

SELECTED BIBLIOGRAPHY

Amabile, T. (1996). *Creativity in context*. Boulder, CO: Westview Press.
Boden, M. (1990). *The creative mind: Myths and mechanisms*. London: Weidenfeld and Nicholson.

Chomsky, N. (1969). *Aspects of the theory of syntax*. Cambridge, MA: Harvard University Press.

Gardner, H. (1993). *Creating minds: An anatomy of creativity seen through the lives of Freud, Einstein, Picasso, Stravinsky, Eliot, Graham, and Gandhi*. New York: Basic Books.

Gross, M. (1975). *Méthodes en syntaxe: Régime des constructions complétives* [Methods in syntax: The regime of complementary constructions]. Paris: Hermann.

Hauser, M., Chomsky, N., & Fitch, W. (2002). The faculty of language: What is it, who has it, and how did it evolve? *Science, 298*, 1569–1579.

Hintikka, J., Moravcsik, J. M. E., & Suppes, P. (Eds.). (1973). *Approaches to natural language: Proceedings of the 1970 Stanford workshop on grammar and semantics*. Dordrecht, The Netherlands; Boston: Reidel.

Hintikka, J. (1998). *Paradigms for language theory and other essays*. Dordrecht, The Netherlands; Boston: Kluwer.

Smith, S., Ward, T., & Finke, R. (Eds.). (1995). *The creative cognition approach*. Cambridge, MA: MIT Press.

Sternberg, R. (Ed.). (1999). *Handbook of creativity*. Cambridge, England; New York: Cambridge University Press.

Sternberg, R., & Lubart, T. (1995). *Defying the crowd: Cultivating creativity in a culture of conformity*. New York: Free Press.

D

DESIRE

Philosophy. — Actions are explained by saying that the agent desired something and believed it could be obtained by accomplishing the action in question (→ ACTION, WILL). A belief (→ BELIEF) is true if it corresponds to a state of affairs (if the mind fits with the world), whereas a desire is satisfied if the world corresponds to it (if the world fits with the mind) (→ MIND). A *behaviorist* view likens the intentional content of a desire to the behavior the desiring agent is disposed to have (→ INTENTIONALITY). This disposition can be specified only if the agent also believes that the action will satisfy his or her desire. Thus, a *functionalist* view defines desires in terms of the causal roles they play with respect to beliefs (→ CAUSALITY AND MENTAL CAUSATION, FUNCTIONALISM). But a desire is not just a disposition to do certain things; it is also a reason for acting. This reason may be independent of the agent's beliefs in the case of unmotivated desires like hunger and thirst, but it depends on those beliefs when the desire is motivated and is likely to undergo rational evaluation (→ REASONING AND RATIONALITY). A causal theory of the intentional content of desires relating the representations they produce to different types of primitive actions (→ REPRESENTATION) is probably possible for unmotivated desires (Fred Dretske), but it is inadequate for motivated desires because rational agents have more than just desires; they have desires about their desires.

PASCAL ENGEL

SELECTED BIBLIOGRAPHY

Dretske, F. (1986). *Explaining behavior: Reasons in a world of causes*. Cambridge, MA: MIT Press.

DIFFERENTIATION

Psychology. — The term *differentiation* has several acceptations that are related to each other but must not be confounded. Here, let us make distinctions among *intraindividual differentiation, differentiation of the perceived world*, and *interindividual differentiation*.

We owe the first description of a systematic relationship between differentiation and development to the English philosopher Herbert Spencer in the second half of the nineteenth century. Spencer noticed that all forms of development involve a gradual transition from homogeneity to heterogeneity of structure. He believed that this law applied to the evolution of the universe, as well as to that of animal species, social structures, and language. Spencer's ideas influenced several trends in psychology. In the field of psychopathology, his line of inquiry was carried on by the neurologist Hughlings Jackson, who, drawing from Spencer's work, made the connection between the dissolution process he observed in pathology and the differentiation and hierarchical integration process that characterizes development (→ NEUROPSYCHOLOGY). According to Jackson, three levels of organization were differentiated in the course of neurological development: elementary reflexes, middle centers, and highest centers. The function of the highest centers was to gradually coordinate the lower centers, controlling them by means of inhibition mechanisms (→ ACTIVATION/INHIBITION, CONTROL). Alterations caused by disease would affect the highest centers first, thereby releasing the uncoordinated responses of the lower centers that had previously been inhibited. In effect, Jackson assumed that the dissolution process triggered by pathological alterations followed the reverse pathway to that of development.

The hypothesis that differentiation is followed by a return to indifferentiation is also found in studies on the *factorial structure of intelligence*. Among psychologists who use factor analyses to study human intelligence, there is a fairly general consensus that the best model is a *factor hierarchy*. In such a model, factors from different levels of integration are defined: first, a general factor that accounts for the shared variance in the battery of intelligence test scores input into the analysis, and second, group factors that account only for the variance shared by certain groups of tests and thus correspond to relatively differentiated aptitudes, such as verbal, numerical or spatial aptitude (→ LANGUAGE, NUMBER, SPACE). This hierarchical model of the structure of intelligence was first proposed by Cyril Burt, who referred explicitly to Spencer and Jackson. Through comparisons of the respective amounts of variance explained by the general factor and group factors at different ages, Burt also attempted to show that abilities become increasingly differentiated with development (in the hierarchical factor model, ability differentiation is reflected by a decrease in the proportion of variance explained by the general factor and a concomitant increase in the variance of group factors). Because of certain delicate technical problems that arose, it is difficult to draw any firm conclusions from the many studies conducted since then to verify this idea. This reservation being made, there nevertheless appears to be a general tendency in the research to support the hypothesized differentiation of the factorial structure of intelligence during childhood and adolescence, with *dedifferentiation* (a relative increase in the amount of variance explained by the general factor, to the detriment of group factors) occurring during aging ($\rightarrow$ AGING).

The concept of differentiation was also critical for psychologists influenced by Gestalt theory, but for whom representations of forms (cognitive structures) nevertheless have a genesis. The idea of a transition from a state of indifferentiation to a state of increasing differentiation is found, for example, in Heinz Werner's developmental theory. This idea was to become a central one for Herman Witkin, one of Werner's disciples. Witkin's first interest was in individual differences in the perception of the upright ($\rightarrow$ PERCEPTION), which he explained in terms of a variable amount of differentiation in perceptual information processing, that is, between internal information (proprioceptive and gravitational) and information arriving externally (peripheral vision) ($\rightarrow$ INFORMATION). Witkin later generalized this understanding of differentiation to the separation of the self from the nonself, and to the differentiation of the various neurophysiological functions and psychological functions (specialized forms of defense, articulation of the body concept, etc.). In this way, he made differentiation the key explanatory principle of a general cognitive style he called *field dependence/independence*.

Witkin's theory of differentiation has been discounted, however, due to its failure to include the process of integration that ensures the coordination of the differentiated structures. By contrast, differentiation and coordination are indissociable in Jean Piaget's structuralist theory of cognitive development ($\rightarrow$ COGNITIVE DEVELOPMENT). For Piaget, new cognitive structures are built by an assimilation-accommodation process in charge of both the differentiation of previously undifferentiated action schemes and their coordination into a superordinate, integrated structure ($\rightarrow$ ACTION, CONSTRUCTIVISM). Piaget also insisted on the fact that subjects can differentiate between two stimuli only if they have differentiated two schemes likely to assimilate them. His theory thus closely ties intraindividual differentiation of the cognitive structures, the topic under discussion thus far, to differentiation of the perceived world, which is a consequence of it.

Although linked to intraindividual differentiation, differentiation of the perceived world is based on a different acceptation of the term. This expression is employed to speak of the case where modifying the stimulus changes the subject's response. The emergence in young children of the ability to differentiate between the various proprieties of the perceived world was studied extensively in France by Éliane Vurpillot.

Finally, differentiation can pertain to the process through which individuals become distinct from each other. The study of individual differences—which is the subject of differential psychology—requires devising sufficiently standardized situations to permit comparisons across individuals, as in the well-known psychometric tests. It also requires developing methods capable of isolating dimensions that are useful for classifying or ranking individuals in a relatively stable way, and for analyzing the relationship between the subjects' relative positions along those dimensions and their behavior in other situations. The factor analyses discussed above are a good example of the methods used in differential psychology.

How is interindividual differentiation related to intraindividual differentiation? The answer to this question lies in finding out whether intraindividual differentiation, a general process, takes the same form in all individuals. If so, interindividual differences show up only in the pace of intraindividual differentiation and thus, in development. If, on the other hand, intraindividual differentiation of cognitive structures can take forms that vary across individuals, then differences are manifested in the form assumed by that process (which does not mean that there cannot also be differences in the pace of development). The former position implicitly underlies most theories of cognitive development, whereas the latter, which recognizes the possibility of different developmental pathways, is an original line of research.

Jacques Lautrey

SELECTED BIBLIOGRAPHY

Duncan, J. (2003). Intelligence tests predict brain response to demanding task events. *Nature Reviews Neuroscience, 6*, 207–208.

Duncan, J., et al. (2000). A neural basis for general intelligence. *Science, 289*, 457–460.

Sternberg, R. (Ed.). (1982/2000). *Handbook of intelligence*. New York: Cambridge University Press.

Sternberg, R. (1997). *Thinking styles*. New York: Cambridge University Press.

Sternberg, R. (2000). The Holy Grail of general intelligence. *Science, 289*, 399–401.

Sternberg, R., Lautrey, J., & Lubart, T. (2003). *Models of human intelligence: International perspectives*. Washington, DC: American Psychological Association.

Vurpillot, É. (1972). *Le monde visuel du jeune enfant* [The visual world of the young child]. Paris: Presses Universitaires de France.

DISCOURSE

Linguistics. — *Discourse* is generally understood to mean any verbal production, whether written or oral, related to the context in which it was produced (→ CONTEXT AND SITUATION, ORAL, WRITING). In linguistics, it was not until recently that discourse was deemed to be a relevant unit of analysis. Traditional grammars do not go beyond the sentence and leave the study of discourse to rhetoric or stylistics (→ GRAMMAR). This distinction is found again in structural linguistics. For Roman Jakobson and Émile Benveniste, for example, the sentence is the cutoff point at which one leaves the realm of strictly coded entities and enters the realm of *parole*, or language performance, where subjects have full freedom to make use of the resources offered by the language, defined as a system (→ LANGUAGE). Similarly, for generative grammarians, any phenomenon that is not dictated by rules about the location of morphemes in the syntactic structure pertains to discourse (→ SYNTAX). Based on Noam Chomsky's *government-binding theory*, for instance, one would say that interpreting the reference of the pronoun in *Paul hit his head* is a question of discourse, insofar as the pronoun could refer either to Paul or to another referent present in the situation or co-text (→ INTERPRETATION). By contrast, in *Paul hit his own head*, the pronoun is necessarily coreferential with Paul, and its antecedent is necessarily found right within the short sentence that expresses it; this strictly predictable interpretation does not depend on the subject's knowledge of the entities in the sentence, nor on psychological factors like antecedent recency. It can be explained solely in terms of the specific structural constraints of the language used; linguistic analysis stops there.

Linguists who adhere to North American structuralism (like Leonard Bloomfield) never developed a line of research on discourse (except for Zellig Harris), arguing that no linguistic rule can be found for anything beyond the sentence. For these structuralists, this is the province of anthropologists or ethnologists, and more recently, for the generativists, the province of psycholinguists, who are the only ones in a position to determine the interpretation strategies preferentially used by subjects during comprehension or production.

European structuralists, on the other hand, attempted very early to extend the field of linguistics to include discourse, while nonetheless acknowledging that the aims and methods of analysis could not be the same as those used in phonology, morphology (→ MORPHOLOGY), or syntax. This was particularly true of Benveniste, for whom, once outside the realm of semiotics, where the combinatorial possibilities are strictly coded (→ SEMIOTICS), the question that arises is how speaking subjects utilize the resources for expression provided by their language in a way that fits with their communicative goals (→ COMMUNICATION). *Discourse analysis*, which strives to answer this question, looks at attested corpora and attempts to find linguistic markers of speaker involvement, for example, markers of subjectivity (first- and second-person pronouns, deictics, modal operators, etc.; → MODALITY) that indicate the speaker's attitude toward his or her statement and addressees. An inventory of all such markers found in discourses collected in comparable situations can be used in contrastive analyses to differentiate between two types of text: narrative (stories), in which the speaker is hidden, and discourse, where, on the contrary, the speaker is held accountable for what he or she is saying (→ TEXT).

The theoretical context today is quite different from the environment during the reign of structuralism: discourse analysis has earned a position as one of the major subdivisions of linguistics and entertains a privileged relationship not only with semantics and pragmatics (→ PRAGMATICS, SEMANTICS) but also with psycholinguistics, sociolinguistics, and artificial intelligence. Publications are abundant, spurred in particular by Teun van Dijk, with a large North American contingent, and the research perspectives are highly diverse. Among the most representative, two main lines of study stand out: analyzing *discourse cohesion markers*, and determining the overall organizing principles of discourse. The two themes of European structuralism are found again here, except for the fact that today's studies are aimed essentially at showing that at the discourse level too, there are regular principles governing how sequences of sentences or utterances are constructed and interpreted. Short of proposing a genuine "beyond-the-sentence grammar," researchers are working on figuring out what it is that makes texts more than just disconnected sequences of units.

Indeed, a discourse always has some degree of coherence, and even when that coherence is not explicit, the person interpreting the discourse makes inferences that reconstruct the relationships between the utterances (→ REASONING AND RATIONALITY). This inference-making process is based on more or less conventional background knowledge (scenarios, stereotypes, etc.) and is dictated by a general principal of relevance (Paul Grice, Dan Sperber, and Deirdre Wilson; → RELEVANCE). Languages have an entire gamut of markers that help speakers relate statements to each other. These markers—which grammars refer to as conjunctions, adverbs, pronouns, prepositional phrases, etc., and which are analyzed therein according to their morphosyntactic behavior—play an essentially semantic and pragmatic role in discourse. Although such cohesion markers, as they are called, are widely varied, they can nevertheless be classified into several major families, the most important being *connectives*, which indicate relations like consecution, justification, and opposition between denoted facts and/or speech acts (Oswald Ducrot); *anaphors*, which indicate relations between referents (Georges Kleiber, Francis Corblin, etc.); *introductory expressions* announcing the discourse domain (Gilles Fauconnier's "mental spaces"; → DOMAIN SPECIFICITY); and *metadiscursive organizers* like indentation.

The study of cohesion markers has become a key constituent of spoken and written discourse analysis. The descriptions proposed attempt to account for the interpretational guidelines these markers encode grammatically. As such, they are functional descriptions of a semanticopragmatic but also cognitive nature (for example, in research on anaphors, we find recourse to concepts like salience, prominence, etc.), and they play an essential role in so-called cognitive grammars (Ronald Langacker).

There are many interconnections between the above lines of study and the experimental psycholinguistic research on how subjects process these expressions in real time ($\rightarrow$ LANGUAGE). The most advanced work in this area concerns anaphor interpretation (Ann Morton Gernsbacher, Allan Garrod, Allan Garnham, and others), but studies on connectives are also available. Research on cohesion markers in descriptive linguistics is also of interest to computer scientists who are working to develop automatic speech-processing systems. No system today is yet capable of correctly resolving anaphors or of adequately processing relations marked by connectives, but new efforts are being made in this direction. One of the crucial problems that arises in this area is devising representation systems capable of formalizing, for example, in a machine-understandable language, the time course of the events and entities evoked in a discourse ($\rightarrow$ TIME AND TENSE).

Although cohesion markers play an important role in the local structure of discourse, their global organization also merits attention. This is where the concept of *type of text*—the second major branch of discourse research—enters the scene. Discourse is organized according to dispositional criteria that depend on the speaker's intentions (intent to tell, describe, persuade, etc.). The problem at this level is being able to define prototypical organization schemas that are consistently associated with these major types of communicative intent. Such schemas are necessarily updated inductively, and their normative power, even if it imposes constraints on discourse forms, does not hinge on the language used but on sociocultural criteria, themselves dependent upon the degree of codification, at a given time, of certain forms of interaction ($\rightarrow$ INTERACTION).

In continuation of structuralist analyses of narratives, research on text types—for example, narratives, descriptions, and argumentative text—has attempted to detect distinctive *superstructures* for different kinds of text (Walter Kintsch and Van Dijk). Text superstructures are made up of units (sequences, episodes, etc.) that, based on semantic and functional criteria (thematic, dialectic, dialogical, and tactical, according to François Rastier), group together strings of statements that fill preestablished slots in a given text schema. This research trend has become the basis for psycholinguistic studies, and the development of computer systems for processing specialized text corpora has made it possible to specify well-defined, type-specific text schemas (e.g., accident reports).

Many studies have also been devoted to dialogue and conversations. The aim in this case is to determine the principles that govern turn-taking and utterance chaining within and across speaking turns and conversational exchanges (Eddy Roulet, Jacques Moeschler, and others). More generally, these studies focus on the factors likely to have a bearing on what discourse devices speakers use, for example, to preserve the "face" of others (Catherine Kerbrat-Orecchioni). This line of research maintains close ties with (micro-)psychosociology, and in particular, with the ethnomethodological research trend. In addition, it has given rise to computer science projects aimed at modeling human-machine dialogue.

MICHEL CHAROLLES

SELECTED BIBLIOGRAPHY

Edwards, D. (1997). *Discourse and cognition*. London: Sage.
Koenig, J.-P. (1998). *Discourse and cognition: Bridging the gap*. Stanford, CA: CSLI Publications.
Van Dijk, T. A.(Ed.). (1985). *Handbook of discourse analysis*. Orlando, FL: Academic Press.
Van Dijk, T. A. (Ed.). (1997). *Discourse as structure and process*. London: Sage.

DISTRIBUTED INTELLIGENCE

Artificial intelligence. — Although the vast majority of studies in artificial intelligence consider intelligence to be an individual ability, a school of thought dating back to the 1980s questions this assumption and attempts to take the interactive and social components into account in explaining the complexity of allegedly intelligence-based activities ($\rightarrow$ INTERACTION, SOCIAL COGNITION).

This view initiated a research trend called *distributed artificial intelligence* that deals with the study and development of *multiagent systems*, that is, systems in which a set of computer entities, or agents, interacts in complex ways involving both cooperation and conflict in order to satisfy their individual goals. This field of study is multidisciplinary in nature and draws on work done in a variety of areas, including knowledge representation ($\rightarrow$ REPRESENTATION) and robotics ($\rightarrow$ ROBOTICS), biology in general and ethology in particular ($\rightarrow$ ANIMAL COGNITION), sociology, the philosophy of action ($\rightarrow$ ACTION), and the philosophy of mind ($\rightarrow$ MIND).

Two trends stand out from the others: the first focuses on the collective intelligence that emerges from the interaction of agents considered to be devoid of intelligence ($\rightarrow$ EMERGENCE); the second focuses on the collective construction of knowledge and skills by several agents, each of which already possesses a cognitive capacity of its own.

In the first case, the systems studied are called *reactive systems*. The paradigmatic example is the anthill, whose members self-organize and coordinate their actions with only minimal cognitive capacities (Éric Bonabeau and Paul Bourgine). It has been shown that relatively complex tasks such as exploring a terrain or building a dwelling place can be accomplished using techniques that do not require intelligence on the part of the agents (Luc Steels). These unintelligent agents coordinate their activities without building mental representations of each other and without awareness of the fact that they are cooperating (→ CONSCIOUSNESS). They communicate by means of simple signals they broadcast into the environment (→ COMMUNICATION). This form of communication is found in particular in mobile collective robotics, in simulations of animal societies, and, although much less often, in computer networks.

In the second case, the systems under study are *cognitive systems*, that is, systems in which the agents are endowed with intentions, have mental representations of their environment and of other agents, and are capable of making relatively complex plans to reach their goals. The behavior of these agents can be formally described in terms of relationships between mental states (basically, their beliefs, goals, and intentions) (→ BELIEF, CAUSALITY AND MENTAL CAUSATION, FUNCTIONALISM). These agents usually communicate by sending messages, or via the migration of communication agents called *messengers*. Their forms of communication are based on *speech act theory* (→ PRAGMATICS). Initiated by John Austin and John Searle's work in the philosophy of language (→ LANGUAGE), speech act theory describes the pragmatic dimension of communication in terms of the mental states of the sender and receiver of each speech act. This theoretical framework was taken up and formalized by Phil Cohen and Hector Levesque, and it lays the groundwork for many types of interaction protocols between communicating agents.

Cooperation is the most widely studied of the general forms of interaction in such multiagent systems. Stated simply, the idea here is to determine who does what, when, where, how, using what means, and with whom, in view of accomplishing a collective task. This involves dividing up the labor, resolving conflicts that arise, and, more generally, coordinating the tasks performed by the different agents.

The techniques implemented thus depend on whether the agents are reactive or cognitive. If they are reactive, then physical concepts such as forces or potential fields are brought to bear (Jacques Ferber). If they are cognitive, communication protocols are defined to describe their norm-based exchange sequences. A typical example of such a protocol is a *contract net protocol*, which is based on the notion of the marketplace (Reid Smith).

JACQUES FERBER

SELECTED BIBLIOGRAPHY

Austin, J. L. (1962). *How to do things with words*. Cambridge, MA: Harvard University Press.

Bonabeau, É., & Bourgine, P. (Eds.). (1994). *Intelligence collective* [Collective Intelligence]. Paris: Hermès.

Bonabeau, É., Dorigo, M., & Theraulaz, G. (1999). *Swarm intelligence: From natural to artificial systems*. New York: Oxford University Press.

Cohen, P. R., & Levesque, H. J. (1990). Rational interaction as the basis for communication. In P. R. Cohen, J. Morgan, & M. E. Pollack (Eds.), *Intentions in communications*. Cambridge, MA: MIT Press.

Ferber, J. (1999). *Multi-agent systems: An introduction to distributed artificial intelligence* (Trans.). Harlow, England; Reading, MA: Addison-Wesley. (Original work published 1995.)

Kennedy, J., Eberhart, R., & Shi, Y. (2001). *Swarm intelligence*. San Diego, CA: Morgan Kaufmann.

Searle, J. R. (1969). *Speech acts: An essay in the philosophy of language*. London: Cambridge University Press.

Smith, R. G. (1980). The contract net protocol: High-level communication and control in a distributed problem solver. *IEEE Trans. Computers, 29*, 1104–1113.

Steels, L. (1989). Cooperation between distributed agents through self-organization. In Y. Demazeau & J.-P. Müller (Eds.), *Decentralized AI*. North-Holland, NY: Elsevier.

Weiss, G. (2000). *Multiagent systems: A modern approach to distributed artificial intelligence*. Cambridge, MA: MIT Press.

DOMAIN SPECIFICITY

Philosophy. — According to a long-standing and widespread conception of how the mind works (→ MIND), humans are endowed with a set of general reasoning abilities that are called upon in all cognitive tasks, irrespective of their content (→ COGNITIVE DEVELOPMENT, REASONING AND RATIONALITY). A competing view contends that on the contrary, there are many cognitive capacities, each specialized in the processing of certain types of information (→ INFORMATION), and that every domain of knowledge has its own specific principles that dictate its organization and structure. A *domain*, then, can be defined as a body of knowledge that enables one to identify and interpret a set of phenomena assumed to share certain properties and to form a general type (→ INTERPRETATION); this knowledge serves as a guide when tasks involving perception, encoding, memorization, or reasoning are being performed on that class of phenomena (→ MEMORY, PERCEPTION).

Work in several fields has contributed to the development of this approach. In linguistics, Noam Chomsky contended that natural language grammars have particular properties that can be accounted for only if we assume that cognitive abilities specializing in language processing do indeed exist (→ GRAMMAR, LANGUAGE). Modular theories of perception also suggest that different types of sensory information are processed by means of specialized operations (→ MODULARITY). Developmental psychologists who study concept formation, such as Susan Gelman, have postulated the existence of specific organizing structures in order to explain how children, who have only inadequate and pluripotent experience to draw upon, are nevertheless capable of inducing the concepts they will share with adults (→ CATEGORIZATION, CONCEPT). Other findings support the hypothesis that domains have specific structures. This is true in neuropsychology—where certain brain lesions have been shown to cause a specific deficit in a particular cognitive domain, while sparing others (→ NEUROPSYCHOLOGY)—as well as in cross-cultural studies on the organization of conceptual domains in different societies.

Nevertheless, even for the proponents of the domain-specific approach, many questions remain unanswered or controversial, such as what criteria define domains, how many domains there are, whether the organizing principles underlying the domains are necessarily innate, how domain-specific cognitive abilities are related to general cognitive abilities, how the domains are related to each other, and what the nature of conceptual change is.

ÉLISABETH PACHERIE

Linguistics. — The term *domain* is used in two branches of applied linguistics: lexicology and terminology (→ LEXICON). In lexicology, domains are materialized in dictionary entries by domain labels. The introductory pages of every dictionary list the names of the domains, which refer either to broad, encyclopedic-type fields (didactics, history, literature, etc.) or to technical, more or less specialized areas (agronomy, cybernetics, falconry, zootechny, etc.). The breakdown into domains is designed to provide two kinds of information to dictionary users: descriptions of words (lexical information) and descriptions of the things the words designate (encyclopedic information) (→ INFORMATION). The use of domain labels makes it possible to present the different areas in which a polysemous term is employed by separating them into several monosemous frames of reference. Domains provide a way of removing any polysemous ambiguity.

In cognitive semantics, the notion of domain is extended to all semanticoconceptual classes (→ SEMANTICS). Ronald Langacker states that a domain can be any kind of conceptualization: a perceptual experience, a concept, a conceptual composite, or an elaborate knowledge system (→ CATEGORIZATION, CONCEPT, EXPERIENCE, PERCEPTION).

In terminology, where the goal is to achieve monosemy within any given terminological system, a domain is seen as a system of notions linked to each other by semantic relations (→ SEMANTIC NETWORK). As such, a term exists only in reference to a specialized, structured, and delineated domain (for example, the domain of artificial intelligence), within which it is defined by its similarities to, and differences from, the terms that surround it. The result is that a given word in a language (generally a noun) corresponds to as many concepts as there are specialized domains in which it is employed, being defined differently in each one. For example, in chemistry, water is a body whose molecules are made up of two hydrogen atoms and one oxygen atom;

opposing concepts are carbon, nitrogen, potassium chloride, and so forth. In physics, water is a body that freezes at 0° C and boils at 100° C; it can be opposed to alcohol, which boils at 78° C and solidifies at –112° C. The concept of domain is closely tied to the concept of ontology, and one of the roles of work in terminology is precisely to formulate the ontology of domains.

GABRIEL OTMAN

SELECTED BIBLIOGRAPHY

Forde, E., & Humphreys, G. (Eds.). (2002). *Category specificity in brain and mind*. New York: Taylor and Francis.

Hirschfeld, L. A., & Gelman, S. A. (Eds.). (1994). *Mapping the mind: Domain specificity in cognition and culture*. Cambridge, MA: Cambridge University Press.

Keil, F. C. (1989). *Concepts, kinds, and cognitive development*. Cambridge, MA: MIT Press.

Martin, A., Ungerleider, L., & Haxby, J. (2000). Category specificity and the brain: The sensory/motor model of semantic representations of objects. In M. Gazzaniga (Ed.), *The new cognitive neurosciences* (pp. 1023–1046). Cambridge, MA: MIT Press.

DUALISM/MONISM

Philosophy. — In metaphysics, the *monist* view holds that everything that exists can be reduced, derived, or explained in terms of a single thing or a single kind of thing (→ REDUCTIONISM). The existence of the mind constitutes one of the major challenges to monism (→ MIND): it must be conceded that mental phenomena do not "look like" any known physical entities or properties, and what is more, they are difficult to reduce or even explain in physical terms. For *dualists*, this dilemma is resolved precisely by relying on appearances: body and mind are fundamentally different things and each is equally fundamental. The strongest form of dualism, as with René Descartes's substance dualism, states that mind and body have independent existences: there can be bodies without minds, but also minds without bodies.

Today, substance dualism is no longer considered viable, insofar as it is incapable of accounting for the interaction between the physical and the mental, in particular in perception and action (→ ACTION, MODEL, PERCEPTION). However, extreme forms of physicalistic monism, such as logical behaviorism and psychophysical identity theory, have also been rejected (→ IDENTITY, PHYSICALISM). Against logical behaviorism, it is argued that higher forms of behavior (for example, the use of language) cannot be explained without positing the existence of mental states irreducible to behaviors (→ LANGUAGE). Identity theory has been repudiated for its failure to explain the qualitative nature of experience and consciousness, and the fact that the content of certain mental states, that is, propositional attitudes, depends on the properties of what they are about (externalism) ($\rightarrow$ CONSIOUSNESS, EXPERIENCE, EXTERNALISM/INTERNALISM, PROPOSITIONAL ATTITUDE, QUALIA).

In contemporary settings, the debate between monism and dualism no longer deals with the existence of a "thinking substance" but with the existence of mental properties. *Eliminativism* is a radical monism that denies the existence of mental properties. *Anomalous monism* (Donald Davidson) states that every single mental event is identical to a physical event. *Epiphenomenalism* interprets mental properties in terms of their supervenience on their underlying physical properties ($\rightarrow$ EPIPHENOMENALISM, SUPERVENIENCE). The most widely adopted stance today is *functionalism*, usually interpreted as a mental/physical property dualism ($\rightarrow$ FUNCTIONALISM).

MAX KISTLER

SELECTED BIBLIOGRAPHY

Davidson, D. (1980). *Essays on actions and events*. Oxford, England: Clarendon Press.
Descartes, R. (1979). *Méditations métaphysiques* [Metaphysical meditations]. Paris: Flammarion. (Original work published 1667.)
Gaukroger, S. (2003). Descartes, René. In E. Nagel (Ed.), *The encyclopedia of cognitive science* (Vol. 1) (pp. 947–950). London: Nature Publishing Group, Macmillan.

DYNAMIC SYSTEM

Artificial intelligence. — The concept of *dynamic system* was introduced by Henri Poincaré. Long forgotten, it was brought back into the limelight by René Thom, Steven Smale, and Vladimir Arnold, and is now benefiting from today's growing interest in chaotic phenomena ($\rightarrow$ EMERGENCE). This concept is used to describe the geometry of the behavior of a system.

In some ways similar to the concept of differential equation, a dynamic system differs from a differential equation in that it considers not just a single trajectory coming from an initial point, but the set of all possible trajectories within a given dynamic. A dynamic system is *continuous* or *discrete*, depending on whether the dynamic is defined by a differential equation (perhaps stochastic) or by a difference equation (in discretized time). To study a dynamic system, one begins by looking at its *attractors* and their *basins of attraction*. A trajectory's attractor is the set of topologically and infinitely recurring points (any neighborhood of such a point is crossed an infinite number of times by the trajectory from that point). The dynamic system perspective is less interested in a particular trajectory than in sets of trajectories: each attractor is associated with its basin of attraction, that is, the set of all points for which it is the trajectory's attractor.

There are three types of attractors. The simplest is a *fixed point*. The next is a *periodic orbit:* the attractor need only possess at least one point that gets crossed twice to have a periodic orbit. Finally, attractors that are much more complex are called *strange* (or *chaotic*) *attractors*, in which none of the points is crossed twice. *Linear* dynamic systems have only the first two types of attractors. One of the advantages of *nonlinear* dynamic systems is precisely that they can have the third, more complex type of attractor. Each of these attractor types has a corresponding type of sensitivity to the initial conditions: in the case of a fixed point, any two points in the basin will asymptotically become infinitely close; in the case of a periodic orbit, two points in the basin will reach the orbit and the gap between them will thus remain bounded; finally, in the case of a strange attractor, two points, even initially infinitely close ones, will exhibit large deviations. This sensitivity is measured by *Lyapunov's exponent*, which is positive in the case of large deviations, negative in the case of a fixed point, and null for a periodic orbit.

Sensitivity to the initial conditions in the case of strange attractors was observed long ago by Poincaré in three-body gravitation problems. It was rediscovered by Edward Lorenz for meteorological phenomena, where it was dubbed the "butterfly effect" on the climate. Initial-condition sensitivity leads us to rethink the relationship between deterministic systems and predictable systems: if there is the slightest uncertainty about the initial state, a chaotic deterministic system becomes unpredictable after a certain amount of time (whose magnitude is the inverse of Lyapunov's exponent). However, although one can no longer exactly predict the future state of the system, it is still possible to give a probability estimate of what that state might be.

A very useful concept for studying how a dynamic system will evolve (in terms of probabilities) is the idea of a *symbolic dynamic*. One starts with a partitioning of the phase space and a set of symbols to assign to the partitioned elements. From there, a trajectory can be described as a sequence of symbols (→ SYMBOL). One then considers the probabilities of occurrence of the symbols, at a given instant, as a function of the past, and of the entropy associated with the symbol sequence. It is easy to see that the entropy is null in the case of fixed-point or periodic attractors: beyond the period, the sequence reproduces a duplicate of itself and produces nothing new. The same does not hold true for a strange attractor; although deterministic, the dynamic system continuously generates something new. The production of novelty is not relative to the roughness of the observation, measured by the diameter of the partition: the limit remains positive when the dimension of the partition becomes infinitely small, and is called the system's *Kolmogorov-Sinai entropy*. Kolmogorov-Sinai entropy, like Lyapunov's exponent, is an invariant of a dynamic system. These two values can be used to distinguish between different types of attractors.

First used in physics, the concept of dynamic system is also a good tool for studying cognitive systems. Connectionist systems are dynamic systems ($\rightarrow$ CONNECTIONISM), albeit complicated ones due to the number of interconnected elements. An essential function of connectionist systems is categorization based on complex perceptions ($\rightarrow$ CATEGORIZATION, PERCEPTION). Because the categorization process sorts cognitive states into categories (perhaps fuzzy ones; $\rightarrow$ FUZZY), it produces a symbolic dynamic canonically associated with the connectionist system's dynamic.

PAUL BOURGINE

SELECTED BIBLIOGRAPHY

Abraham, F., Abraham, R., & Shaw, C. (1990). *A visual introduction to dynamical systems.* Santa Cruz, CA: Aerial Press.

Abraham, R., & Shaw, C. (1992). *Dynamics: The geometry of behavior.* New York: Addison-Wesley.

Anosov, D. A., Arnold, V. I., & Sinai, Y. G. (1988–95). *Dynamical systems.* (Vols. 1–9). Berlin, Germany, and New York: Springer-Verlag.

Hirsch, M. W., & Smale, S. (1974). *Differential equations, dynamical systems, and linear algebra.* New York: Academic Press.

Poincare, H. (2001). *The value of science: Essential writings of Henri Poincaré* (S. J. Gould, Ed.). New York: Modern Library.

Thom, R. (1975). *Structural stability and morphogenesis: An outline of a general theory of models* (D. H. Fowler, Trans.). Reading, MA: W. A. Benjamin. (Original work published 1972.)

Thom, R. (1983). *Mathematical models of morphogenesis* (W. M. Brookes & D. Rand, Trans.). New York : Halsted Press. (Original work published 1974.)

Van Geert, P. (1994). *Dynamic systems of development: Change between complexity and chaos.* New York: Harvester.

Zeigler, B., Praehofer, H., & Kim, T. (2000). *Theory of modeling and simulation: Integrating discrete event and continuous complex dynamic systems.* 2nd. ed. London: Academic Press.

E

EMERGENCE

Artificial intelligence. — Self-organized dynamic systems, which are composed of a very large number of interacting entities, exhibit global properties that the basic entities in them do not possess. These properties are called *emergent properties* ($\rightarrow$ DYNAMIC SYSTEM, HOLISM). They are generally dependent upon the spatiotemporal patterns generated by interactions between the basic entities. Examples of such patterns are spin-glass phenomena in physics, neural synchrony assemblies responsible for categorization in cognitive neuroscience ($\rightarrow$ CATEGORIZATION, CONSCIOUSNESS, NEURAL NETWORK), and epidemiological representation phenomena in anthropology ($\rightarrow$ REPRESENTATION).

In light of theories of nonlinear dynamic systems, it is not possible to contend that these spatiotemporal patterns and their morphodynamics can be predetermined on the basis of interactions between entities: even if the behavior of the entities is fully deterministic, a minute uncertainty in one of them can lead to a high degree of uncertainty in the future, as Henri Poincaré noted for three-body interactions. The best we can do is make predictions about the system's evolution in probabilistic terms, according to Ilya Prigogine, or in an even more minimal way, about its qualitative evolution, according to René Thom. The lack of sure predictability is an ongoing source of novelty unexplained by the system's history: an evolving dynamic system indefinitely produces positive marginal entropy in its chaotic phase; this remains true at the brink of chaos, even though the marginal entropy and the creation of novelty tend to cancel each other in this case.

PAUL BOURGINE

Philosophy. — The term *emergence* was first employed by evolutionist metaphysicians like Conwy Morgan and Samuel Alexander. It allowed them to get around the reductionistic consequences seemingly implied by Charles Darwin's theory of natural selection, which assumes that no new organisms can be created and no sudden modifications in their structure can occur in natural history. The emergentists contend on the contrary that evolutionary processes are not incompatible with the appearance of new, more complex mental and organic forms that emerge in the course of evolution (in particular, consciousness; → CONSCIOUSNESS), with the idea that there are distinct levels of organization that cannot be reduced—be it in nature or in the forces that produce them—to the physical and chemical mechanisms of causality (→ REDUCTIONISM). More or less radical versions of this doctrine exist, the strongest one being that the properties of organic wholes cannot be predicted from either the properties of their parts or their history (the biological thesis has its counterpart in holism in the social sciences, which argues, against atomism, that a social whole is not reducible to the sum of its constituent entities → HOLISM). In this radical version, emergentism seems to be compatible with a form of *dualism* or *vitalism*, which separates so-called high-level structures of living beings from low-level material structures, by creating an irreducible new vital principle (Henri Bergson's *élan vital,* or life force, seems to be a version of this type, and Alexander draws support from it for his temporal version of the existence of a deity) (→ DUALISM/MONISM). But, apart from its air of mysticism, this version falters in the face of the fact that emergent forms seem to disobey the principles of mechanical causality governing living beings, and to lead to epiphenomenalism (→ CAUSALITY AND MENTAL CAUSATION, EPIPHENOMENALISM). A weaker version proposed by Charlie Broad retains the idea that the evolution of higher-level properties (psychological ones in particular) depends on the lower levels, which would be compatible with their irreducibility. In this sense, the notion of emergence is close to that of supervenience employed by today's philosophers of the mind (→ SUPERVENIENCE). But that notion, too, runs up against the difficulties of epiphenomenalism. Contemporary philosophers of evolution such as Eliott Sober still make use of supervenience in contending that the fitness of organisms is a supervenient property relative to evolution and to gene selection, and dynamic theories of the morphogenesis of living forms may be tempted to adopt a version of emergentism.

PASCAL ENGEL

SELECTED BIBLIOGRAPHY

Alexander, S. (1920). *Space, time and deity*. London: Macmillan.
Broad, C. D. (1925). *The mind and its place in nature*. London: Routledge.
Morgan, C. L. (1925). *Emergent evolution*. London: Williams and Norgate.

Orzack, S., & Sober, E. (Eds.). (2001). *Adaptationism and optimality*. New York: Cambridge University Press.

Nicolis, G., & Prigogine, I. (1989). *Exploring complexity: An introduction*. New York: W. H. Freeman.

Prigogine, I., & Nicolis, G. (1977). *Self-organization in non-equilibrium systems: From dissipative structures to order through fluctuations*. New York: Wiley.

Prigogine, I., & Stengers, I. (1997). *The end of certainty: Time, chaos and the new laws of nature*. New York: Free Press.

Sober, E. (1990). *The nature of evolution*. Cambridge, MA: MIT Press.

Thom, R. (1975). *Structural stability and morphogenesis: An outline of a general theory of models* (D. H. Fowler, Trans.). Reading, MA: W. A. Benjamin. (Original work published 1972.)

Thom, R. (1983). *Mathematical models of morphogenesis* (W. M. Brookes & D. Rand, Trans.). New York: Halsted Press. (Original work published 1974.)

EMOTION

Psychology. — The human face is an important source of information for communication (→ COMMUNICATION). It tells us about inner emotional states such as happiness, fear, sadness, anger, or surprise, to mention only some of the so-called primary emotions. Expressing and understanding inner states of emotion is considered today to provide an early system of exchange between infants and adults (→ INFANT COGNITION, SOCIAL COGNITION).

The modern study of facial expressions has been made possible by the joint contribution of filming techniques and expression coding systems. Paul Ekman and Wallace Friesen's FACS (Facial Action Coding System) has the advantageous capability of differentiating the morphological features of facial expressions on the basis of their underlying muscle movements (→ ACTION). Studies using this system or Carol Izard's MAX system have shown that as early as the first few weeks of life, human infants possess a broad emotional repertory that is morphologically close to that of adults.

Habituation studies on infants' ability to discriminate emotions have shown that two and three month olds are already capable of distinguishing between expressions of happiness, sadness, and fear. The amount of visual attention infants pay to a slide showing a happy face decreases with repeated presentation (habituation), whereas visual fixation time increases when the same face is presented with a different expression. This does not mean that infants understand the semantics of these expressions (→ SEMANTICS); their discrimination scores do not decline, for example, when the faces are shown upside down (which is no longer true three months later). One can only conclude from the findings that infants are capable of discriminating between two facial patterns that vary along one dimension. At seven months, they appear to be able to categorize expressions, since they explore a new expression on a new face more than they do an old expression on the same new face (→ CATEGORIZATION). Other findings obtained using the habituation technique or the *pair-comparison* technique (comparison of two contrasting stimuli) have provided insight into the question of how the discrimination of morphological changes is related to the discrimination of meaningful emotional patterns.

This issue has been addressed directly in studies on *social referencing*, where subjects in ambiguous situations must process emotion information semantically in order to adapt their behavior accordingly (→ INFORMATION). For example, when separated from their mother by a false visual cliff, infants will cross it if the mother displays a happy expression but not if she expresses fear. Unfortunately, given that the criterion for semantic understanding in this situation is being able to walk unassisted, the emergence of this capacity cannot be located in time.

Colwyn Trevarthen, whose views are close to those of Henri Wallon and the Palo Alto group on this point, argues that the ability to grasp the meaning of emotions is innate and not inferential. Peter Hobson uses this theoretical framework to explain the development of autism as based on a primary disorder affecting the expression and decoding of emotions (→ AUTISM). A number of studies point in this direction and seem to indicate poor expressiveness in autistic subjects, accompanied by trouble distinguishing between facial movements that convey meaning and ones that do not. Yet, to the extent that emotions are observable mental states that can be shared directly, emotion understanding is considered by some authors to be a prerequisite to building a theory of mind (→ THEORY OF MIND). In addition, as Henry Wellman showed, these mental states are understood rapidly (at about eighteen months), and by the age of two years, are grasped and processed as being the result of an event-based causality (for example: she is sad because it was her birthday and no one gave her a present) (→ CAUSALITY AND MENTAL CAUSATION). Granted, it is not until children understand that beliefs are a necessary complement to information about desires that they can successfully predict or explain the actions of another agent (→ BELIEF, DESIRE): this is no doubt why surprise, which presupposes a failure of some knowledge or epistemic prediction (→ EPISTEMIC), cannot be verbalized by children until they are five.

JACQUELINE NADEL

In adults, as in children, the expression and discrimination of emotions are essential to information processing. The neuropsychologist Antonio Damasio published a noteworthy book entitled *Descartes' error: Emotion, reason, and the human brain*. For Damasio, pure reason does not exist: we think with both our bodies and our emotions. Denouncing not only Cartesian dualism (→ DUALISM/MONISM), but also the contemporary idea of a "computer brain," Damasio argues that the Cartesian view of the mind as "apart from" the body lies at the origin of the erroneous metaphor of the mind as a computer program proposed in the mid-twentieth century (→ COGNITIVISM, MIND). Going against this metaphor and referring to a coherent body of neuropsychological data, he defends a *somatic marker theory*. Based on the results of laboratory experiments on patients with lesions of the ventromedial prefrontal cortex (→ NEUROPSYCHOLOGY), Damasio noted that (1) these patients seem to no longer feel emotions and are incapable of detecting them in others (one of the measures used was the skin conductance response), and (2) their cold-blooded way of reasoning apparently prevents them from weighing the various possible solutions available to them, in such a way that the "landscape" upon which their decisions are made "is hopelessly flat" (→ REASONING AND RATIONALITY). According to the somatic marker theory, the ability to express and feel emotions is indispensable to the manifestation of rational behavior. The role of this faculty is to get subjects on the right track, to put them in the right place in the decision-making space, in a place where they can correctly apply the principles of logical reasoning (→ LOGIC).

From the neurobiological standpoint, the neural pathways thought to be responsible for emotional functions do not seem to be solely localized in the limbic system (the so-called emotional brain), as traditionally assumed, but also appear to reside in other parts of the prefrontal cortex and in brain regions where body signals are processed. The prefrontal cortex plays a critical anatomofunctional role in this respect, since it receives signals from all sensory areas where the images that underlie our reasoning processes are formed (→ MENTAL IMAGERY), including the somatosensory areas where representations of past and present bodily states are constantly being updated. This is the level where Damasio's hypothesized somatic markers enter into the picture.

Somatic markers are defined as connections between categories of objects or events, and pleasing or displeasing somatic states (→ CATEGORIZATION). They come from multiple individual experiences regulated by the homeostatic system. In the course of child development (→ COGNITIVE DEVELOPMENT), these connections, which become finer and finer over time, are thought to be stored in the brain in the form of simulation loops, which alleviate the need for direct references to real somatic states. According to Damasio, somatic markers bear emotional value and are integrated in the convergence zones of the prefrontal cortex, where they serve as a sort of automatic guide that orients the subject's decision making and reasoning. They are thought to act in a hidden way, that is, without necessarily being sensed by the subject, so that, by way of attentional mechanisms, some elements take precedence over others, and decision-making signals (on, off, and change-of-direction) are controlled (→ ACTIVATION/INHIBITION, ATTENTION, CONTROL). This is the level of cognitive integration where Tim Shallice's "supervisory attentional system" and Alan Baddeley's "central executive" come into play. Thus, the mind and its most complex operations would be rooted in the flesh, with the lack of body emotions preventing "true rationality." This is just one theory among others, but one that clearly illustrates a current desire in cognitive neuroscience (see *neuroscience* below) and psychology to break down the classic image of a "cold mind." A testimony to this is the proliferation of studies dealing with the so-called conative component of cognitive information processing (emotions, motivations, feelings, values, and so forth).

OLIVIER HOUDÉ

Neuroscience. — Cognitive neuroscience research into emotion is relatively recent compared to studies on the perceptual and motor mechanisms of cognition. Addressing the issue of emotion from a computational standpoint may sound surprising today ($\rightarrow$ COMPUTATIONAL ANALYSIS), but then, weren't some people surprised about twenty-five years ago when the study of visual mental imagery was approached from this same angle ($\rightarrow$ MENTAL IMAGERY)?

The study of the brain mechanisms involved in emotion is experiencing an upsurge, and it now seems that emotions can be approached in terms of a cognitive system made up of subsystems, just like vision, action, or language ($\rightarrow$ ACTION, LANGUAGE, PERCEPTION). Stephen Kosslyn and Olivier Koenig proposed a functional architecture of emotion composed of a *ventral system* and a *dorsal system*, after the fashion of the visual processing of form and location ($\rightarrow$ SPACE). The ventral emotion system, implicating the anterior part of the insula, is thought to enable recognition of bodily states, whereas the dorsal emotion system, situated in the posterior parietal lobe, would be specialized in locating the source of bodily sensations. Information processed by these two systems would be sent on to associative memory, thought to receive information from all perceptual modalities ($\rightarrow$ INFORMATION, MEMORY) and enable the subject to interpret the situation and select the most appropriate response.

But other subsystems, corresponding to subcortical structures or groups of structures, are also involved in emotional mechanisms. For example, there seems to be a subsystem responsible for making the connection between a perceptual stimulus and an emotional response. The striatum may be involved in this mechanism, and the amygdala as well. It has been amply demonstrated that the amygdala plays a critical role in the virtually automatic production of responses to potentially frightening or dangerous stimuli. The hypothalamus, activated by the amygdala, triggers the production of many neuromodulators, which facilitate certain kinds of cognitive processing while inhibiting others ($\rightarrow$ ACTIVATION/INHIBITION, CONTROL). Memory and attention mechanisms ($\rightarrow$ ATTENTION) appear to be particularly sensitive to these factors. Clearly, then, emotions are tightly intertwined with other cognitive functions.

OLIVIER KOENIG

Philosophy. — Emotions are mental changes correlated with physiological and hormonal changes. Beliefs can be regarded as causes or interpretations of emotions (→ BELIEF, CAUSALITY AND MENTAL CAUSATION, INTERPRETATION).

In the writings of William James, an emotion is essentially the perception of an involuntary physiological change (→ PERCEPTION). We do not cry because we are sad; we are sad because we cry: the interpretation is a secondary event with respect to the physiological reaction. The expression of emotion occurs within this feedback loop: at least in certain cases, one can deliberately trigger emotional reactions by manipulating the manifestations of the emotion: fleeing increases panic and sobbing increases pain. As James put it, "Refuse to express a passion, and it dies."

According to William Lyons, *appraisals* are what cause emotions. An emotion requires associating a feeling with a perceptual appraisal or even a conceptual judgment about the current situation (→ CONCEPT). The appraisal may be perceptual and nonconceptual (Kevin Mulligan, Christine Tappolet), which does not imply that access to values (which are different from appraised situations) is perceptual in nature. Perceptual procedures are fixed by evolution and are nonrevisable, whereas the stability of values lies in the fact that they are claimed to guide future *revisions* (to revise is to decide what must be changed in our representations in order to make them consistent with new information → INFORMATION, REPRESENTATION). Emotions can thus be seen as linked to situations in which we are led to reassess our beliefs, expectations, and even our preferences. Completing a revision process takes time, and the emotion remains activated until the revision is completed.

But this causes a perverse effect: the emotional state may attract and keep the subject's attention, to the detriment of the belief-revision process. Franz Brentano put this effect at the core of his theory of emotion in speaking of redundancy of feeling: when one likes wisdom, for example, one not only likes an object; one also has the immediate obvious experience of having the "right" emotion (→ EXPERIENCE). Similarly, in artistic emotion, we do not simply like the sensory quality of the appreciated object, we experience nonsensory pleasure in the fact of feeling pleasure, although this time, the pleasure is self-presenting (it is not referred to any content other than itself).

Emotions are not mere projections of subjective states about situations. They are at least partly objective. Regarded as dispositions, emotions refer to the tendency of individuals to respond to certain types of circumstances by exhibiting certain types of behavior. It is the properties of a given situation, when it occurs, that trigger the emotion that, among "normal" individuals, accompanies a given type of revision. These dispositions may be activated when a resemblance is perceived between the current situation and one or more prototypical scenarios acquired during development (see *psychology* above).

This raises the question of the relationship between emotions and beliefs. According to Ronald de Sousa, each emotion has a specific formal type that is irreducible to a combination of desires and beliefs (→ DESIRE). For Anna Wierzbicka, emotions are founded on beliefs: in an emotion, one feels something similar to what one normally feels when one has such beliefs. In the revision-based analysis of emotions, beliefs correspond to the information that survives the revision process. Our desires guide our expectations and our actions, in accordance with our preferences about changes induced by the world or by our actions (→ ACTION). Yet actions presuppose that we force all revisions to have goal attainment as one of their mandatory features. As such, emotions are affective resonances that fit with the various revision situations. *Cognitive emotions* are engendered by a revision of cognitive expectations (surprise, discovery, doubt, etc.); *affective emotions* are linked to cognitive revisions that do or do not fit with our preferences about the situation (happiness, sadness, etc.); *appreciative emotions* accompany revisions that are brought about by world-related or action-related change and that do or do not conform to our preferences about change (disappointment, relief, etc.); finally, *conative emotions* are linked to revisions involving actions (anger, fear, hope, etc.). Accordingly, anger comes along with situations where I am committed to carrying out an action but a change due to the world or to others' actions impinges upon or prevents that action and thereby forces me to execute other actions that go against my preferences: communicating what I feel in this case can promote the pursuit of the action (at least by maintaining my propensity to act).

The function of emotions may be more than just to focus our attention on important information (De Sousa); emotions may also serve to keep the revision process going until it is completed. They thus prepare us for an action when possible, and via the expressions that signal different types of revisions, they ensure coordination among individuals (Charles Darwin): the motor schema of my expressions helps me decode the expressions I perceive, by way of its permanent association with certain physiological changes. Emotions are essential to the attainment of unity in a personality, achieved through the revisions imposed upon us by our actions, those of others, and changes in the world (→ IDENTITY).

PIERRE LIVET

SELECTED BIBLIOGRAPHY

Damasio, A. (1994). *Descartes' error: Emotion, reason, and the human brain*. New York: Putnam.
Damasio, A. (1999). *The feeling of what happens: Body and emotion in the making of consciousness*. New York: Harcourt Brace.
De Sousa, R. (1987). *The rationality of emotions*. Cambridge, MA: MIT Press.
Gazzaniga, M. (Ed.) (2000). *The new cognitive neurosciences* (Section IX, *Emotion*) (2nd ed.). Cambridge, MA: MIT Press.

Houdé, O., et al. Access to deductive logic depends on a right ventromedial prefrontal area devoted to emotion and feeling. *NeuroImage, 14*, 1486–1492.

Izard, C. E. (Ed.). (1989). *Development of emotion-cognition relations*. Hove, Sussex, and London: Erlbaum.

Kosslyn, S. M., & Koenig, O. (1992/1995). *Wet mind: The new cognitive neuroscience*. New York: Free Press.

LeDoux, J. (1996). *The emotional brain: The mysterious underpinnings of emotional life*. New York: Simon and Schuster.

Luan Phan, K., Wager, T., Taylor, S. & Liberzon, I. (2002). Functional neuroanatomy of emotion: A meta-analysis of emotion activation studies in PET and fMRI. *NeuroImage, 16*, 331–348.

Lyons, W. (1980). *Emotion*. New York: Cambridge University Press.

Nelson, C., & Luciana, M. (2001). *Developmental cognitive neuroscience* (Section VIII, *Emotion and cognition interactions*). Cambridge, MA: MIT Press.

Panskeep, J. (1998). *Affective neuroscience: The foundations of human and animal emotions*. New York: Oxford University Press.

Rolls, E. (1999). *The brain and emotion*. Oxford, England; New York: Oxford University Press.

Trevarthen, C. The function of emotions in early infant communication development. In J. Nadel & L. Camaioni (Eds.), *New perspectives in early communicative development*. London, Routledge.

Wellman, H. (1990). *The child's theory of mind*. Cambridge, MA: MIT Press.

EPIPHENOMENALISM

Philosophy. — Traditional *epiphenomenalism* states that mental events have no causal efficacy and are mere epiphenomena relative to the physical events that cause them (→ CAUSALITY AND MENTAL CAUSATION). Another, now highly debated version gives mental events causal power, but only to the extent that they are identical to or exemplify physical properties (→ IDENTITY, PHYSICALISM), not on the basis of the fact that they exemplify mental properties. (For example: If my pain makes me scream, it is not by virtue of the fact that it is my pain, but because it is a certain neural state. Compare: If Castafiore's voice breaks the windowpanes in the living room, it is not by virtue of the fact that she is singing The Jewel Song, but by virtue of the high pitch of the sound she is emitting.) The objection to the effect that the doctrine is just epiphenomenalism in this second sense could be directed at any "occasional identity" theory of mental and physical events (as tokens, and not as types or properties), such as Donald Davidson's *anomalous monism* or some versions of functionalism (→ DUALISM/MONISM, FUNCTIONALISM, TYPE/TOKEN).

If only physical or neurophysiological properties of mental events have causal efficacy while the intentional or functional properties of those events do not (→ INTENTIONALITY), the latter are excluded from any causal explanations or at best appear redundant. This seems to be particularly true of so-called broad intentional properties that refer to distal or faraway traits in the outside environment, as opposed to the narrow, inner psychological properties of organisms (insofar as causality only seems to operate at a local level) (→ EXTERNALISM/INTERNALISM). But epiphenomenalism goes against folk psychology, which sees mental events as causing actions and physical events by sheer virtue of their intentional content (→ ACTION). Theorists who, like Jerry Fodor and Fred Dretske, want to retain the intuition that mental causality exists by acknowledging the reality and efficacy of intentional content, attempt to account for the causal efficacy of intentional properties on the basis of the physical or functional characteristics assigned to those properties; theorists for whom mental properties have causal relevance without being directly causally effective must specify the nature of the causal effect by showing how levels of intentional causality can supervene on levels of physical causality (→ EMERGENCE, SUPERVENIENCE) without competing with them or being redundant or epiphenomenal.

PASCAL ENGEL

SELECTED BIBLIOGRAPHY

Davidson, D. (1980). *Essays on actions and events*. Oxford, England: Clarendon Press.
Dretske, F. (1986). *Explaining behavior: Reasons in a world of causes*. Cambridge, MA: MIT Press.
Heil, J., & Mele, A. (1992). *Mental causation*. Oxford: Oxford University Press.

EPISTEMIC

Philosophy. — *Epistemic* concepts are such that their definition necessarily contains a reference to beliefs or knowledge (→ BELIEF, CONCEPT). For example, the concept a priori belongs to this category of concepts. The truth of a judgment can be known a priori if no experience is required to do so (→ EXPERIENCE, TRUTH). In the realist view, it is argued that definitions of ordinary concepts do not imply references to the subject of knowledge (→ REALISM). As such, they are not epistemic.

Moreover, there are concepts whose epistemic character is controversial. This is true of chance. For some, chance is a property possessed by some events independently of the presence or even existence of subjects who might know of those events. Chance is therefore considered nonepistemic. For others, this concept has no sense outside of its relationship to knowledge, in that the attribution of an event to chance merely means that the person lacks the necessary (and, in principle, available) information that would make the event appear determined.

An analogous controversy exists about information (→ INFORMATION). For some, an event has informative value only to subjects for whom it has a sense or is meaningful (→ SENSE). For others, information is a given entity that exists regardless of whether it is known to the subjects (Fred Dretske).

MAX KISTLER

SELECTED BIBLIOGRAPHY

Dretske, F. (1981). *Knowledge and the flow of information.* Cambridge, MA: MIT Press.

EPISTEMOLOGY

Philosophy. — The term *epistemology* has two different acceptations, one corresponding to the conventional French usage and the other to the English usage. In the French acceptation, the term is synonymous with the philosophy of science. Epistemology in this sense looks at the logical structure of scientific theories and at the methods used to assess them (→ LOGIC, VALIDATION).

In the English acceptation, the term is employed to refer to the theory of knowledge. Two questions are raised in this kind of epistemology: What is knowledge? And how does one acquire it (→ COGNITIVE DEVELOPMENT)? Traditionally, the answer to the first question is of the form "*S* knows *P* if and only if *S* has the true and justified belief that *P*" (→ BELIEF, TRUTH). All we need now is an appropriate definition of *justification*. In internalistic theories, the justification of a belief depends solely on its relationships to the subject's other epistemic states (→ EPISTEMIC), whereas in *reliabilism*, an externalistic theory, justification is grounded in the reliability of the belief-formation process (→ EXTERNALISM/INTERNALISM).

MAX KISTLER

EXPERIENCE

Philosophy. — The term *experience* is used to refer to the locus of an encounter between the mind and reality (→ MIND). It enables cognitive subjects to extract information from the signals that reach their sensory receptors (→ INFORMATION). It seems inevitable that we characterize our experiences in terms of what they are experiences "of." But one of the tasks of philosophers of perception is to construct a concept of perceptual experience that is compatible with nonveridical experiences (→ PERCEPTION): in an illusion, experience makes an object appear real, but it does not present that object with its real properties; in a hallucination, no real object corresponds to the experience. Accordingly, the distinction is made between the intentional or representational content of experience and its subjective or qualitative content (→ INTENTIONALITY, QUALIA, REPRESENTATION).

MAX KISTLER

EXPLANATION

Artificial intelligence. — One of the main reasons behind the success of the first *knowledge-based systems* (KBS), called *expert systems* at the time (→ KNOWLEDGE BASE), was their ability to furnish *explanations* to justify their results. Explanations are usually supplied to KBS users in text format, by means of a question-answer type of communication mode: the system produces sentences in response to a question asked by the user (→ COMMUNICATION).

An important feature of knowledge-based systems is their use of a non-computer formalism to represent expertise and store it in what is called a *knowledge base* (→ REPRESENTATION). The explicit representation of knowledge specific to a given application domain is an important tool for generating explanations (→ DOMAIN SPECIFICITY). The next step is easy: specifying the sequence of rules used by the expert system to produce a result. These *production rules* constitute a simple and uniform formalism thought to be powerful enough to translate expertise in a given domain, while still remaining understandable and readable by users. A trace of the reasoning path followed by the expert system and supplied to the user in the form of a sequence of rules was considered at first to be a satisfactory explanation (→ REASONING AND RATIONALITY).

Very quickly, however, it became clear that explanations limited to such traces were insufficient, due precisely to the uniformity of expert-system formalisms: the production rules could produce the very same code for pieces of knowledge of different natures and roles, making it impossible to distinguish between them. As a remedy, the uniformity of the knowledge and representations used by the initial expert systems to solve problems (→ PROBLEM SOLVING) was replaced by heterogeneity, both in the knowledge itself and in the formalisms employed to represent it. The new, enhanced knowledge-based systems included explicit representations of strategy and control knowledge (→ CONTROL) and now had the capability of displaying the goals pursued and the solving methods implemented to reach those goals. The enhanced systems could also display the domain knowledge used and state the role it played in solving the problem. More generally, the detailed specification of different models of a domain and the solving methods that utilize those models can point out various possible lines of reasoning whose explanatory power can be compared.

But specifying and distinguishing between the different types of knowledge used in reasoning do not suffice to produce adequate explanations. Additional knowledge proved necessary, namely, knowledge about the user, or *metaknowledge* (→ METACOGNITION). Metaknowledge is useful for understanding the importance of the domain concepts, situating the user's knowledge with respect to that contained in the KBS, and so on.

As the models of expertise represented in KBSs evolved, the explanation-generating process became increasingly elaborate and was finally seen as a problem-solving task in its own right, founded on its own knowledge and requiring its own models ($\rightarrow$ MODEL). Different explanation methods were then identified, such as explanation by summarizing a line of reasoning, negative explanation, explanation by analogy, and explanation by examples. A recent tendency is to no longer consider the user as a simple recipient of explanations, but as someone who plays an active role in explanation generation. In this view, the explanation-generation process is framed by real human-machine dialogue.

To perform the explanation-generation task, natural language must be formatted, and this requires text-generating techniques ($\rightarrow$ LANGUAGE, TEXT). Furthermore, explanation forms are likely to evolve further and will thus necessitate new modes for communicating with KBS users.

MARIE-CHRISTINE ROUSSET

SELECTED BIBLIOGRAPHY

Keil, F., & Wilson, R. (Eds.). (2000). *Explanation and cognition.* Cambridge, MA: MIT Press.

EXPRESSIVENESS

Artificial intelligence. — Some theoretical results have indicated that it is impossible to reason by means of an *expressive* language if one wants to be both valid and efficient ($\rightarrow$ COMPLEXITY, LANGUAGE, REASONING AND RATIONALITY). The expressiveness of a given language L is not measurable; attempting to assess it in terms of how many things are expressible by a formula in L is unsatisfactory. Indeed, propositional logic supports a countable but infinite number of proposition symbols, and one is free to interpret each symbol by whatever statement one wants. But it cannot account for ordinary syllogisms ($\rightarrow$ LOGIC, SYMBOL).

It is thus preferable to see the expressiveness of L as being related to the fit between what is legal in a deductive system operating on L, and the "natural" inferences drawn from the statements that the sentences written in L are supposed to express. For example, in propositional language L_0, the statements *All As are Bs* and *C is an A* translate into two atomic symbols, say p and q, and hence, no meaningful inferences can be drawn. On the other hand, translated into first-order language L_1 as

$$(\forall x)\ (A(x) \supset B(x))\ \text{and}\ A(C),$$

an ordinary deductive system infers $B(C)$, which is interpreted as *C is a B*. This is what authorizes one to regard L_1 as more expressive than L_0.

How much can we increase the expressiveness of a language while still staying inside a class of languages that exhibits "good" properties in terms of inferential efficiency? We know that a language has to be at least a second-order language (L_2) to express the properties of relations. For example, the symmetry of a relation R is expressed in L_2 as f_2:

$$(\forall R) \ (\text{symmetrical} \ (R) \equiv (\forall \ x, y) \ (R \ (x, y) \equiv R(y, x))).$$

But sentence f_1, which belongs to a first-order language L_1, tries to express the same thing:

$$(\forall R, x, y) \ (\text{symmetrical} \ (R) \equiv (t(R, x, y) \equiv t(R, y, x))).$$

In f_2, the variable R covers the set of all relations on objects, whereas in f_1, it encompasses only one universe of objects. Is this important? Yes, if one wants to express properties of all relations between objects, which, after all, is what symmetry is supposed to express. No, if one can settle for stating that certain properties, say, the ones found on a given list, are symmetrical.

How far can one go with this sort of reduction? Curiously, the results of probability calculations offer some partial answers to this question. For instance, it has been proven that any sentence in L_1 abides by a *0–1 law*, that is, the probability that it will be satisfied, when interpreted over universe U whose size approaches infinity, either tends toward 0 or tends toward 1. This suffices to prove that no sentence in L_1 can express the parity of U, since, when the size of U increases, its parity is alternately true or false but does not approach a limit.

DANIEL KAYSER

EXTERNALISM/INTERNALISM

Philosophy. — In what is commonly called *Cartesian internalism*, thoughts are understood to be subjective and internal, that is, independent of the world (→ INDIVIDUALISM). According to René Descartes, we could have the very same thoughts as we do now if the objective world were entirely different from what it is (or what we think it is), or even if the outside world did not exist.

The fundamental intuition behind internalism is that different causes can produce the same effects on our sense organs, and, by virtue of those effects, we can have the same subjective, inner experiences (→ CAUSALITY AND MENTAL CAUSATION, EXPERIENCE). From the subject's point of view, the experience of the world is the same, whether he or she is seeing a real apple, or hallucinating and "seeing" a qualitatively identical apple (thinking in both cases that it is green): either way, the subject has the impression of perceiving a certain green apple (→ PERCEPTION).

One of the reasons for rejecting Cartesian internalism lies in the discovery that there exist *indexical thoughts*, in the sense that there exist *indexical sentences*. The truth conditions for the utterance of an indexical sentence depend not only on the intrinsic meaning of the sentence, but also on the objective properties of the utterance context (→ CONTEXT AND SITUATION, MEANING AND SIGNIFICATION, TRUTH). Similarly, as shown for example by Hilary Putnam and John Perry, the truth condition of the thought *It's cold here* depends not only on the intrinsic content of the thought, but also on the context of the thinking episode. In our use of the same word *here,* my twin and I may be thinking of different places, while thinking about those places in exactly the same way (that is, we may have the same representations of the places in question: what happens in our heads when we think *It's cold here* may be strictly identical; → REPRESENTATION). Yet there is a difference between our thoughts as far as the referent and the truth conditions are concerned: my thought is about the place where I am, whereas my twin's is about the place where he is (→ SPACE). Thus, there is at least one aspect of the content of these thoughts, the *referential* aspect, that is not internal to the individual but depends on the external environment. As Putnam showed, the same holds true for thoughts about natural kinds of things (e.g., water). A thought whose referential content (truth conditions) depends on the context is sometimes called a *de re* thought.

Philosophers like Putnam, who showed that there are thoughts whose referential content depends on the outside environment, are only moderate externalists, however. They do not contend that all thoughts are *de re* thoughts, and they readily acknowledge the existence of another class of thoughts, made up of purely descriptive thoughts, that are Cartesian, that is, entirely internal and independent of the world. They seem to accept the Cartesian approach to one aspect of the content of *de re* thoughts: the fact that they have an internal, subjective ingredient that is unaffected by changes in the outside environment (for example, external changes that do not induce a corresponding change in the neurophysiological states of the thinking subject). According to these philosophers, a *de re* thought can be broken down into a subjective, inner constituent, and an objective constituent that determines the thought's truth conditions.

Examples of the following type lend intuitive plausibility to this two-constituent analysis. If I perceive a certain apple and think it is green, while my twin perceives an apple that is qualitatively indistinguishable from the one I am perceiving and thinks it is green, then our thoughts differ in their truth conditions (one thought is true if and only if apple A is green, and the other, if and only if apple B is green). But in one sense, they constitute "the same thought," as shown by the fact that they are brought about by the same sensory stimulations and trigger the same cognitive or behavioral reactions. What our thoughts have in common is called their *narrow content*, the subjective, internal aspect of the thought. Combined with the context, the narrow content determines a complete thought, a *broad content* that possesses both a subjective constituent and an objective constituent (the truth conditions, determined jointly by the narrow content and the context). In certain cases, like the one where my hallucinating twin "sees" an apple that is qualitatively indistinguishable from the one I see, the narrow content does not determine the truth conditions. In this particular case, the subject has not formed a complete thought; it has only a narrow content.

Radical externalism was initially proposed in response to the conception just presented. This conception is externalistic only with respect to broad content, but remains Cartesian as far as narrow content is concerned. Radical externalists like Tyler Burge, Gareth Evans, John McDowell, and, in his most recent studies, Putnam himself, go so far as to reject even this limited form of internalism. They think that the outside world fashions our thoughts in such a way that it is impossible to isolate any constituents of thoughts that might be internal and independent of the world. They present the following argument in support of their position: the alleged narrow content is, by definition, independent of the outside environment; a subject who perceives an apple and his twin who perceives (or hallucinates) a qualitatively indistinguishable apple are said to have thoughts with the same narrow content. However, the thing that makes a subject's internal state a content (or the thing that gives that state a content) is nothing other than the relationship between the state and something in the world. If this relationship is eliminated or disregarded, what remains no longer deserves to be called *content*: at best, it is a possible vehicle for carrying content, that is, a syntactic object (→ SYNTAX). Seen from this angle, narrow contents are not contents at all. At the very best, they are mental or neuronal "sentences." These sentences are interpreted (acquire content) solely through their relationships with objects and states of affairs in the outside world. The relationships in question constitute the content of thoughts, and there is no content, even narrow, that is not constituted by such relationships.

FRANÇOIS RECANATI

SELECTED BIBLIOGRAPHY

Evans, G. (1982). *The varieties of reference*. Oxford, England: Clarendon Press.

Kornblith, H. (Ed.). (2001). *Epistemology: Internalism and externalism*. Malden, MA: Blackwell.

Putnam, H. (1975). The meaning of meaning. *Philosophical papers: Vol. 2. Mind, language and reality*. New York: Cambridge University Press.

Putnam, H. (1988). *Representation and reality*. Cambridge, MA: MIT Press.

Sosa, E., & Bonjour, L. (2003) *Epistemic justification: Internalism vs. externalism, foundations vs. virtues*. Oxford, England: Blackwell.

F

FETAL COGNITION

Psychology. — Through the use of new ultrasound techniques for exploring the human fetus (echography, cardiotocography), along with studies on placental mammals and observations of premature infants, it has now become a well-accepted idea that abundant sensory input is available to the child even during the fetal period. Research on the learning capabilities of the human fetus (→ LEARNING) suggests that prenatal stimulation contributes to the development of the sensory system, and that sensory experiences during the fetal stage affect how postnatal behavioral responses will evolve (→ INFANT COGNITION).

The sensory systems begin maturing in the following predetermined order: the somesthetic system, the chemical senses (taste, smell), the vestibular system, the auditory system, and finally, the visual system (→ PERCEPTION). Behavioral data (such as changes in heart rate and motor reactions) obtained in response to appropriate stimulation are a testimony to the reactive capacity of each of these systems. All sensory systems exhibit reactive capacities in utero, well before they have reached structural and functional maturity. The fetus is capable of storing certain properties of its environment, especially auditory and chemical-sensory ones (→ MEMORY). Through its responses, it demonstrates its ability to detect incidental stimuli (loud noises); discriminate complex noises or spoken utterances on the basis of their pitch, loudness, or prosodic features; and recognize a complex utterance when subjected to daily exposure. While harmful stimulation is stressful, prenatal activation promotes the development of the peripheral systems and brainstem relays and keeps them anatomically and functionally intact during the maturation period.

Animal and human research has shown that through learning, fetal sensory experiences can modify postnatal behavioral responses to auditory or chemical-sensory stimulation. The newborn rat exhibits olfactory aversions or preferences that are based on prenatal acquisitions. Human newborns tend to prefer voices that exhibit features detected before birth. Because the mother's voice is neither attenuated nor masked by intrauterine background noise, infants manifest a preferential sensitivity to her voice and to the language she speaks (→ LANGUAGE). They have also been shown to prefer musical sequences or utterances sung or read daily by the mother or another speaker for several weeks before birth. In this way, the organism prepares itself in utero for detecting the sensory cues that will be relevant during postnatal life. If we assume that the fetus's immature brain is incapable of integrating the information it encounters, then we must acknowledge that fetal acquisitions are not the result of the conscious processing of sensory messages (→ CONSCIOUSNESS) and thus, that these "memories" cannot be retrieved later.

ARLETTE STRETI

SELECTED BIBLIOGRAPHY

Gazzaniga, M. (Ed.). (2000). *The new cognitive neurosciences: Vol. I. Development*. Cambridge, MA: MIT Press.

Jirásek, J. (2001). *An atlas of the human embryo and fetus: A photographic review of human prenatal development*. New York: Parthenon.

Lecanuet, J.-P., Fifer, N. Krasnegor, N., & Smotherman, W. (1995). *Fetal development: A psychobiological perspective*. Hillsdale, NJ: Erlbaum.

Schaal, B., Lecanuet, J.-P., & Granier-Deferre, C. (1999). Sensory and integrative development in the human fetus and perinates. In M. Haug & R. Whalen (Eds.), *Brain, behavior and cognition: Animal models and human studies* (pp. 119–142). Washington, DC: American Psychological Association.

FRAME PROBLEM

Artificial intelligence. — In 1969, while working on a logical formalism (→ LOGIC) called *situation calculus* for reasoning about the actions of a robot R (→ ACTION, ROBOTICS), John McCarthy and Patrick Hayes came up against the following difficulty, which they named the *frame problem*. Action a, say R *moves from A to B*, has preconditions (R *is in A*) and effects (R *is in B*). If a is performed in situation s, the result is situation $s' = exec$ (s, a), and if $t(p, s)$ means that proposition p is true in situation s, we have

(1) $(\forall s, s')\, (s' = exec\,(s, a) \supset (t(= (location\,(R), A), s))$
$\wedge\, (t(= (location\,(R), B, s'))).$

Suppose R is red in situation s, that is,

$$(2) \qquad\qquad t(= (color(R), red), s),$$

and one asks what color it is in situation s'. The frame problem lies in the fact that (1) and (2) do not allow us to answer this question. The list of a's effects would have to state that the color of R remains unchanged. Imagine the number of similar facts that would have to be included in the description of every action! One idea for avoiding such an enumeration would be to store in s' the truth value of propositions not listed among the effects of a. But this would not be suitable since one would conclude that in s', = $(location (R), A)$ was still true.

Several solutions based on nonmonotonic logic have been proposed in an attempt to maximize the inertia of propositions, that is, make it so their truth value persists unless proven otherwise. There are other problems of this type similar to the frame problem. The *qualification problem* (or, respectively, the *ramification problem*) is the problem of listing the preconditions (or, respectively, the effects) of an action. In the case of action a, for example, one would have to include among the preconditions that R is in working order and that it has enough energy to go to B, and among the effects, that its organs will be more worn out, that its movement will have generated vibrations, and so on.

DANIEL KAYSER

SELECTED BIBLIOGRAPHY

Ford, K., & Pylyshyn, Z. (1996). *The robot's dilemma revisited: The frame problem in artificial intelligence*. Norwood, NJ: Ablex.

McCarthy, J., & Hayes, P. (1969). Some philosophical problems from the standpoint of artificial intelligence. In B. Meltzer & D. Michie (Eds.), *Machine Intelligence 4*. Edinburgh, Scotland: Edinburgh University Press.

Shanahan, M. (1997). *Solving the frame problem: A mathematical investigation of the common sense law of inertia*. Cambridge, MA: MIT Press.

FUNCTION

Neuroscience. — The term *function* in neuroscience refers to a set of active, dynamic properties that competes to achieve the same goal in a living being. Since its beginnings, cognitive neuroscience has been attempting to establish a more or less direct correspondence between functions and brain structures ($\rightarrow$ LOCALIZATION OF FUNCTION, NEUROPSYCHOLOGY). The views on this issue have oscillated between a localizationist tendency and an antilocalizationist tendency. At the present time, studies using functional neuroimaging techniques ($\rightarrow$ FUNCTIONAL NEUROIMAGING) are often regarded as neophrenological (in reference to *phrenology*, the study of the "bumps of the skull" conducted around 1800 by Franz Gall), insofar as they relate brain activation patterns to a sensory, motor, or cognitive function. However, neuroimaging research sheds a new light on structure-function relationships. The *subtractive approach* (subtraction of images corresponding to different experimental conditions) has shown that elementary operations are localized in discrete brain regions. As a corollary, cognitive tasks are performed by broadly distributed neuron networks (→ NEURAL NETWORK). Rather than a simple serial model, some kind of nonlinear organization must be postulated, one where the activity of a brain region is a function of its own activity as well as that of other areas (→ ACTIVATION/INHIBITION). Indeed, a given region has many inputs, some of which originate in lower regions. And input regions also project into output regions.

In fact, a problem that arises, although it is rarely stated, concerns the breakdown into functions. Theoretical choices must be made, based on whatever paradigm is popular in the state of the art at the time. This is particularly true for cognitive functions, whose breakdown into attention, memory, and so on (→ ATTENTION, MEMORY) remains hypothetical.

JEAN DECÉTY

Psychology. — The functions of today's cognitive psychology are the functions studied in neuroscience research on structure-function relations (see *neuroscience* above). The new paradigm introduced by functional brain imaging (→ FUNCTIONAL NEUROIMAGING) is indicative of the close tie between the study of major psychological functions such as perception, attention, memory, mental imagery, executive functions, and so forth (→ ATTENTION, CONTROL, MEMORY, MENTAL IMAGERY, PERCEPTION) and the systematic analysis of the brain structures or networks they involve (→ LOCALIZATION OF FUNCTION, NEURAL NETWORK). This new interdisciplinary paradigm, which differs from the functionalist cognitivism initially proposed by Hilary Putnam and Jerry Fodor (→ FUNCTIONAL-ISM), should lead to a revision of the classical—and above all, theoretical—breakdown of psychological functions and thereby give rise to a new form of *neurofunctional modeling* (→ MODEL). In psychology as in other areas, a model is defined by a *syntax* and a *semantics*. Derived from computer systems during the 1980s (under the impetus of artificial intelligence), the model's syntax is now defined in cerebral terms: the physicochemical and neuroanatomical properties of the brain. Its semantics correspond to the spatial and temporal projection of that syntax onto a "psychologically meaningful" reality: the cognitive functions. New theoretical and methodological debates are already dealing with the various possible ways of achieving this projection and their validity.

OLIVIER HOUDÉ

Artificial intelligence. — In mathematics, when the value of a magnitude y is determined by the value of other magnitudes $x_1, \ldots, x_n$, y is said to vary as a *function* of the x_is. Formally, given n sets of values called *domains*, $X_1, \ldots, X_n$, and a set of values Y called a *codomain*, function f assigns, to all n-tuples $<x_1, \ldots, x_n>$ where each x_i belongs to set X_i, a unique value from set Y, denoted $f(x_1, \ldots, x_n)$. The x_is are the arguments of f. If the value of the function is defined over only part of the domain, the function is said to be *partial*. A function is not necessarily calculable: $f(x_1, \ldots, x_n)$ can be uniquely defined even if there is no known procedure for systematically computing its value.

In computer science, most programming languages have provisions for defining functions (in this case, of course, computable ones) ($\rightarrow$ LANGUAGE). The function *header* indicates the domains and the codomain, and its *body* gives the procedure for calculating its value. Some programming languages are called *functional,* that is, the body of the function is itself composed solely of function calls. LISP, a programing language created by John McCarthy in about 1960, is a functional language still widely used in artificial intelligence.

Function f is called *recursive* if it calls itself. For example, let function *anc* be a function that, when given the names of two persons x and y, calculates a truth value; it is true if and only if x is an ancestor of y. Now suppose we have functions *father* and *mother* (not stated here) and that after a certain number of generations, they output a value noted as "undefined," which is different from any real person. *Father* is called, with y as its argument. If the result is equal to x, then function *anc* is done and the final output value is *true;* the same occurs with *mother*(y) (x is thus an ancestor of y because x is one of y's parents). If not, and if *father*(y) is not undefined, function *anc* calls itself with the names x and *father*(y) as its input values. If the output of this function call is the value *true*, the function ends on that value (x is an ancestor of y's father and is therefore an ancestor of y). Otherwise, if *mother*(y) is not undefined, the desired result will be the output of a new call of *anc* with the names x and *mother*(y) as its arguments (clearly, x can then only be y's ancestor if x is an ancestor of y's mother). Finally, if *mother*(y) is undefined, the function *anc* outputs the value *false*.

As it is described above, the function *anc* is recursive since its execution may require calls to itself. For this description to be a genuine definition, the argument series used in the function calls must be finite. For example, the statement *A whole number greater than or equal to 0 is even if it is equal to 0 or if, when we subtract 2 from it, we get an even whole number* is part of a recursive definition; but if *add to* is substituted for *subtract from*, we obtain a mathematical truth that is unusable in a definition (in the first case, the arguments form a finite series, whereas in the second, the series is infinite).

In formal logic, languages use *function symbols*. Each function symbol is assigned a whole number, its *arity*, which is equal to the number of arguments in the mathematical function the symbol stands for ($\rightarrow$ LOGIC, SYMBOL). Except in the case of sorted logic, the same set acts simultaneously as the function's domains and codomain. Symbols of arity 0 are constants (the result of the function does not depend on an argument). While mathematics and computer science strive to define and calculate particular functions, logic is more interested in statements that are true for all interpretations of its function symbols ($\rightarrow$ INTERPRETATION, TRUTH). For example, let f and g be function symbols of arity 0 and 1, respectively, and let x be the symbol of a variable, then the formula $g(f) \supset (\exists x)\, (g(x))$ is true in every interpretation.

DANIEL KAYSER

Linguistics. — In linguistics, *functionalism* (not to be confused with cognitive functionalism; $\rightarrow$ FUNCTIONALISM) is a school of thought whereby the function of the elements of a system overrides their categorization and system modifications ($\rightarrow$ CATEGORIZATION). It argues that human culture, in all of its forms, is not a mere assembly of heterogeneous features but a set of complex elements linked into interdependent mechanisms. Syntactic functions are a good illustration of this ($\rightarrow$ SYNTAX). In syntax, the function of an element is defined by the role it plays in an utterance (examples of functions are subject, predicate, complement, etc.). The function of a word differs from its "nature" (its morphological category: noun, verb, adjective, etc. $\rightarrow$ MORPHOLOGY); that is, a word's role is not the same as its category. Some elements have function-specific forms (for example, *I* as a subject and *me* as a complement).

Ferdinand de Saussure stressed the role of language as a communication tool ($\rightarrow$ COMMUNICATION), based on the principle that communication is the primary function of language ($\rightarrow$ LANGUAGE). The Prague Linguistics Circle attempted to break down this function into components. Roman Jakobson established a typology of the six functions of language, related to the six factors inherent in any act of communication. He distinguished the *referential, expressive, poetic, conative, phatic*, and *metalinguistic* functions, which pertain respectively to the context, sender, message, receiver, contact, and code ($\rightarrow$ CONTEXT AND SITUATION, EMOTION, METACOGNITION).

The first functionalist research in linguistics was conducted in phonology. In this branch of linguistics, the function of the sounds of a language is to permit the distinction between units endowed with different meanings (for example, the phoneme /m/ in *mink* allows one to distinguish it from *think, rink, link, pink*, etc.) ($\rightarrow$ MEANING AND SIGNIFICATION). Relevant sounds (*phonemes*) are thus ones that change the meaning of the message. The device used to determine whether a given sound is a phoneme is *commutation*. The French linguist André Martinet, who studied functional syntax, considered every utterance to be composed of a subject or predicate (what one is talking about, asserting, or refuting) and possibly some complements aimed at supplying information about the predicate (place, time, etc.; → SPACE, TIME AND TENSE). With this information-based definition, the communicative function of language shifted to one of transmitting new information (the Prague Linguistics Circle spoke of the "functional perspective of the sentence") as determined by what information is old or given (theme/rheme or topic/comment opposition) (→ INFORMATION). Luis Prieto attempted to apply the principle of commutation to the semantic function of utterances and proposed the notion of relevant semantic features (→ SEMANTICS). When this concept did not suffice to specify the semantic function of utterances, he added the idea of contrastive features, which serve to express the viewpoint from which the feature is considered. This method remains only partially successful.

Another kind of function is defined in text analysis (→ TEXT). In this framework, a function is a typical interaction between actors. Vladimir Propp listed thirty-one functions for the folktale genre, including reconnaissance, rescue, solution, punishment, trickery, victory, and so forth. Following Propp, Roland Barthes distinguished three levels of narrative: functions, actions, and narration (→ ACTION).

It must be conceded that on the whole, functionalism is not very useful for studying language, because of the wide range of functions language has. We can agree with Oswald Ducrot in saying that it makes sense to study language "in its own right," as Saussure prescribed, but searching for its functions is not the right pathway.

GABRIEL OTMAN

Philosophy. — In philosophy, two ways of understanding the concept of function in the teleological sense (or *teleofunction*) have been clashing for two decades. The *etiological theory* argues that a structure possesses a function if, in the past, the structure in question had effects in analogous systems that causally explain its selection-reproduction (→ CAUSALITY AND MENTAL CAUSATION). *Propensity theory* contends that a structure possesses a function if it currently has the disposition to produce an effect that favors its capacity to be selected-reproduced.

The etiological theory of function, which is the most widely accepted since 1976 and Larry Wright's work, strives to explain causally the existence of the structure supporting a function. According to this theory, the function of an element (an object or a behavior) is always related to one of the effects brought about by elements of the same type, and it is this effect that explains why the element is "where it is." The theory thus makes having a function contingent upon two conditions, a *dispositional* condition and a *historical* condition. In the version proposed by Wright, the function of X is Z if and only if (1) X produces Z and (2) X exists because it accomplishes Z (has Z as its outcome). Condition 1 establishes the fact that Z figures among the consequences of the presence or form of X. However, the effect does not actually have to be produced for the disposition to exist; it suffices for X to be capable of producing Z. Condition 1 is a necessary but insufficient condition for X to have a function (it is the second step that permits identifying a relevant subset of consequences as constituting the function of a given structure). For an element to have a function, not only must elements of its type have the disposition to produce the functional effect (Condition 1), but the element must owe its existence to the capacity of past elements to produce that effect (Condition 2). Some present-day defenders of the etiological theory contest the importance of the dispositional condition (Condition 1) by insisting on the fact that having a function does not imply regular actualization of the disposition (Ruth Millikan).

The fundamental idea in the propensity theory of function is to make the selection of an element depend on existing dispositions, rather than making function depend on selection. In 1987 John Bigelow and Robert Pargetter contributed to popularizing the definition of a biological function as anything that confers a greater propensity to survive on an organism that possesses it. One can formulate the propensity-based definition of function in a somewhat more precise way in two steps analogous to those in the etiological theory: the function of X is Z if and only if (1) all other things being equal, X typically produces Z, and (2) Z confers a greater reproduction propensity on X. This definition can be extended to the ordinary usage of the term *function,* as it is applied to artifacts, via a minor modification to Condition 2 suggested by Bigelow and Pargetter: (2') a characteristic or structure has a certain function when it has a propensity to be selected by virtue of the relevant effects it produces.

One aspect generally said to distinguish this theory of function from the etiological theory is that it is forward looking rather than backward looking. Function does not have the same extension in the two theories. The etiological theory requires an effect to have been rewarded by natural selection for it to be deemed a function. Propensity theory requires only the present effect of a structure to contribute later to the reproduction of organisms that possess it—and to be selected accordingly. Thus, in the former theory, the appendix of the cecum still has a function (to decompose cellulose), whereas in the latter, it no longer has a function.

JOËLLE PROUST

SELECTED BIBLIOGRAPHY

Barthes, R. (1977). *Image, music, text* (S. Heath, Trans.). New York: Hill & Wang.

Bigelow, J., and R. Pargetter.(1987). Functions. *The Journal of Philosophy, 84*, 181–196.

Clarke, E., & Dewhurst, K. (1996). *An illustrated history of brain function: Imaging the brain from antiquity to the present* (2nd ed. rev.). San Francisco, CA: Norman.

Ducrot, O., & Schaeffer, J.-M. (1995). *Nouveau dictionnaire encyclopédique des sciences du langage* [New encyclopedic dictionary of language science]. Paris: Seuil.

Fox, B., Jurafsky, D., & Michaelis, L. (Eds.) (1999). *Cognition and function in language*. Stanford, CA: CSLI Publications.

Frackowiak, R., Friston, K., Dolan, R., Mazziotta, J., & Frith, C. (Eds.) (1997). *Human brain function*. San Diego, CA: Academic Press.

Frege, G. (1997). *The Frege reader* (M. Beaney, Ed.). Oxford: Blackwell.

Jakobson, R. (1995). *On Language* (L. R. Waugh & M. Monville-Burston, Eds.). Cambridge, MA: Belknap Press.

Martinet, A. (1964). *Elements of general linguistics* (E. Palmer, Trans.). London: Faber and Faber. (Original work published 1960.)

Millikan, R. (1984). *Language, thought and other biological categories: New foundations for realism*. Cambridge, MA: MIT Press.

Van Valin, R. D., & LaPolla, R. J. (1997). *Syntax: Structure, meaning, and function*. New York: Cambridge University Press.

Wright, L. (1976). *Teleological explanations: An etiological analysis of goals and functions*. Berkeley, CA: University of California Press.

FUNCTIONAL NEUROIMAGING

Neuroscience. — The term *functional neuroimaging* refers to a series of techniques used to draw up maps of the brain as it functions, and in this respect, it differs from methods aimed at supplying morphological information, that is, information about brain anatomy (MRI, X-ray scanner). The principal imaging techniques currently in use are *electroencephalography* (EEG), *positron emission tomography* (PET), *functional magnetic resonance imaging* (fMRI), and *magnetoencephalography* (MEG).

EEG (in the form of evoked potentials or EEG mapping) is a widespread technique in neurological research; it records brain-emitted electrical potentials using electrodes positioned on the scalp. This technique is frequently used in cognitive neuroscience because of its excellent temporal resolution (milliseconds) and its total noninvasiveness. However, it does not supply information about brain metabolism. In addition, the accuracy level for the spatial localization of electrical signals is still mediocre.

MEG is used to record magnetic fields generated by electric currents crossing cell membranes in the cerebral cortex. This technique is particularly useful when employed in conjunction with metabolic techniques (PET and fMRI) to follow the time course of brain activations.

PET is a method utilized in nuclear medicine to obtain images showing the distribution of radioactivity after injection or inhalation of a substance containing positron-emitting isotopes. The most common isotopes are oxygen-15, carbon-11, fluorine-18, and nitrogen-13, whose disintegration produces gamma rays that are detected and measured by sensors positioned outside the skull (*positron camera*). By nature, PET is a biochemical and physiological technique. Its powerfulness is rooted in the ingenuity of chemists who develop new molecules and the ability of physiologists to validate them. The parameters measured are brain metabolism, blood flow rate and volume, oxygen consumption, neurotransmitter synthesis, and receptor density. With today's positron cameras, one can obtain as many as sixty simultaneous cross sections with a spatial resolution of approximately 125 cubic millimeters. Brain activation studies use water marked with oxygen-15 to measure the blood flow in the brain. The very short half-life of this isotope (2 min) makes it possible to perform several tests on the same subject and then use the subtractive method to identify the neural bases of a given cognitive function ($\rightarrow$ ACTIVATION/INHIBITION, FUNCTION).

Conventional MRI gives high spatial-resolution images with contrast levels based essentially on differences between various tissue parameters, including water molecule density, transversal (T2) and longitudinal (T1) relaxation times of protons in water molecules, their diffusion properties, chemical shift between water protons and small lipid molecule protons, magnetic sensitivity of tissues, blood flow properties, and so forth. Only recently has it been possible with MRI to produce images of brain functioning during somatosensory or cognitive stimulation. In this case, MRI makes use of the hemodynamic properties of the brain, which are detected by observing the intravenous movement of the bolus of a paramagnetic contrast agent. This can be done only with extremely rapid MRI techniques (the first passage of the bolus lasts about ten seconds, and the required time resolution is a few hundred milliseconds) capable of discerning effects related to the presence or flow of the paramagnetic agent in the intravascular space. Fast acquisition is possible in instantaneous techniques (Echo Planar) or modified gradient-echo techniques (for example, Echo-Shifted Flash). The presence of the paramagnetic agent in the intravascular space can be detected using methods that rely on sensitivity to magnetic-field differences (T2 techniques): magnetic-field gradients are induced between the intravascular and extravascular spaces by differences between the magnetic sensitivities of these two spaces during the passage of the paramagnetic agent. The flow of the agent modifies the apparent relaxation time, T1, which can be measured using inflow-sensitivity techniques. One of the merits of measuring the passage of the paramagnetic bolus is that images representing the local cerebral blood volume can be deduced from calculations similar to those employed in nuclear medicine. An advantage of these MRI images is that their spatial resolution is far superior to that obtained using PET. This type of MRI is now being applied to functional brain imaging in cognitive neuroscience, where it is used to detect variations in the local cerebral blood volume during sensory stimulation.

Few centers are equipped with MRI techniques that meet the temporal resolution criterion for acquiring images of the cerebral blood volume (Echo Planar or Echo-Shifted Flash). Recently, a second functional brain imaging approach applicable to most clinical imagers was proposed. No contrast agent is injected, and modifications of MRI signals in cortical regions are recorded in real time. The modifications are induced by sensory stimulation (activation) and are linked to a local increase in blood flow. The MRI techniques used in this case (fast gradient-echo imaging sequences, with temporal resolution of a few seconds) make use of the local increase in the venous concentration of deoxyhemoglobin accompanying a local blood flow increase. Since deoxyhemoglobin is a paramagnetic molecule, the rise in the oxy- to deoxyhemoglobin ratio in the veins reduces the magnetic-sensitivity difference between the intravascular and extravascular spaces, hence the greater intensity of the nuclear signal in the implicated cortical regions. Inflow phenomena also seem to affect the functional images obtained using these techniques.

The merits of studying brain functioning using fMRI are obvious. This technique has the advantage of supplying images with spatial and temporal resolutions well above those obtained using PET. A second advantage is that fMRI is strictly noninvasive when contrastive products are not injected, and even when paramagnetic contrast agents are used, the procedures can hardly be considered invasive. The current approach in cognitive neuroscience is to combine a number of different functional brain imaging techniques, depending on the theoretical and experimental demands.

JEAN DECÉTY

Psychology. — Within the next few years, it will no longer be possible for any major laboratory to practice cognitive psychology or psychopathology (→ COGNITIVE PSYCHIATRY) without access to functional brain imaging techniques. To say that we are witnessing a technological revolution does not seem to be an exaggeration. In a 1993 issue of *Science*, Michael Posner, one of the pioneers of neuroimaging, wrote:

> The microscope and telescope opened vast domains of unexpected scientific discovery. Now that new imaging methods can visualize the brain systems used for normal and pathological thoughts, a similar opportunity may be available for human cognition.

Before the introduction of functional brain imaging, the two methods traditionally used in psychology and neuropsychology (→ NEUROPSYCHOL-OGY) to study cognitive functioning and its relationship to the brain were *mental chronometry* and the *lesion paradigm* (also, but less often, electroencephalography or EEG, the study of evoked potentials). Mental chronometry attempts to infer the "mental algorithms" of human beings by measuring their processing time and the errors they make. The lesion paradigm is used to investigate cognitive dysfunction among brain-damaged patients, in an attempt to determine what structures are involved in normal brain functions (→ LOCALIZATION OF FUNCTION). Considerable progress has been made with these methods and they are still being applied today. However, they suffer from a number of serious limitations, including difficulty interpreting the results due to their indirect nature.

Compared to these classical methods, functional brain imaging techniques offer a possibility never experienced in the history of psychology: the ability to directly visualize brain activity in normal human beings as they carry out cognitive tasks. The two main techniques used are functional magnetic resonance imaging (fMRI) and positron emission tomography (PET) (see *neuroscience* above). Today's psychologists must master the basic principles of these techniques in order to design suitable experimental protocols for interdisciplinary research programs (merging disciplines like cognitive neuroscience and psychology, for example, or even the philosophy of mind).

To visualize the brain in action, that is, the brain regions implicated when a subject executes a given function (whether the function in question is an elementary motor act or a more elaborate cognitive process), functional imaging techniques record the local effects of the neurons' electrical activity on blood circulation and energy consumption in the brain (→ ACTIVATION/INHIBITION, FUNCTION). When neuronal activation occurs, chemical and electrical signals are sent to the membrane of the brain capillaries that surround the synapses, and this modulates the regional cerebral blood flow (rCBF). This is how the brain rapidly and locally adjusts the supply of glucose to the needs expressed by the synapses. The resulting fluctuations in the cerebral blood flow are what neuroimaging techniques exploit. When a subject executes an experimental task (for example, preparing to move, reading a word, imagining a scene, or solving a problem; → ACTION, MENTAL IMAGERY, PROBLEM SOLVING, READING), neurons at rest are activated and the flow of blood to them increases. Given that activated neurons do not consume more oxygen than resting ones, it follows that the oxygen concentration in the blood vessels increases. The oxygen increase is detected by magnetic resonance imaging. In addition, when blood flow increases, the amount of water diffused outside the vessels to reach all brain regions also rises. In the case of positron emission tomography, the subject is first injected with radioactive water and the increase in the perfusion of marked water is detected by a positron camera.

In both of these techniques, the idea is to determine the locations in the brain where the blood flow changes in a statistically significant way during task execution. Special statistical techniques are applied (for example, Statistical Parametric Mapping [SPM] software), depending on the experimental design used by the psychologist: *subtraction maps* when two states are compared, *correlation maps* when a task is repeated while varying an experimental parameter, or *interaction maps* for protocols where several factors are varied in a systematic way. In this type of analysis, an area is considered activated when the value of a cluster of *voxels* (the units of three-dimensional images) goes above a certain threshold.

Thus, to study cognition today, that is, cognitive processes in operation, investigators have at their disposal genuine three-dimensional imaging methods that produce digital images containing the value—at every point in the brain—of a parameter correlated with synaptic activity (here, the regional cerebral blood flow). These images have a spatial resolution of about 5 mm for positron emission tomography and potentially less than 1 mm for functional magnetic resonance imaging. Their temporal resolution is less precise (at best a few seconds in MRI), but supplementary electro- and magnetoencephalography techniques (EEG and MEG) now being combined, despite their poorer spatial resolution, offer a temporal resolution on the order of a millisecond.

All of these technical feats are the fruits of knowledge and capabilities acquired in a number of disciplines ranging from medicine to computer science and including psychology and mathematics. If high-tech imaging now authorizes the in vivo observation of the structures and functions of the human brain, the production of the corresponding images has only become possible because of powerful computers capable of manipulating three-dimensional data files. Without knowing whether the history of science will dub functional brain imaging "the microscope of psychology," there is absolutely no doubt that, for this discipline, a real revolution is underway, not only technological but also paradigmatic (→ MODEL).

OLIVIER HOUDÉ

SELECTED BIBLIOGRAPHY

Cabeza, R., & Kingstone, A. (Eds.). (2001). *Handbook of functional neuroimaging of cognition.* Cambridge, MA: MIT Press.

Casey, B., & de Haan, M. (2002). Brain imaging and developmental science [Special issue]. *Developmental Science*.

Casey, B., Thomas, K., & McCandliss, B. (2001). Applications of magnetic resonance imaging to the study of development. In C. Nelson & M. Luciana (Eds.), *Developmental cognitive neuroscience* (pp. 137–147). Cambridge, MA: MIT Press.

Frackowiak, R., Friston, K., Dolan, R., Mazziotta, J., & Frith, C. (Eds.) (1997). *Human brain function*. San Diego, CA: Academic Press.

Kertesz, A. (Ed.) (1994). *Localization and neuroimaging in neuropsychology*. New York: Academic Press.

Posner, M. I. (1993). Seeing the mind. *Science, 262*, 673–674.

Posner, M., & Raichle, M. (1994/1997). *Images of mind*. New York: Freeman.

Roland, P. (1993). *Brain activation*. New York: Wiley-Liss.

FUNCTIONALISM

Philosophy. — *Functionalism* is the name of a popular philosophical strategy with regard to the proper analysis (or definition) of mental phenomena (mental terms, concepts, properties) (→ CAUSALITY AND MENTAL CAUSATION, CONCEPT, MIND). It is based upon a simple idea: many things in the world are what they are, not particularly by virtue of what they are made of, but by virtue of what function, or role, they serve in a system (→ FUNCTION). For example, something is money by virtue of its being the kind of thing that serves in a certain way to exchange commodities. Since Hilary Putnam's pioneering work, many philosophers of mind have argued that mental phenomena ought to be understood in this way. For example, a defining condition for something's being a belief might be that it issues in a certain way from perception and reasoning and, in combination with desires, forms the basis for decisions (→ BELIEF, DESIRE, PERCEPTION, REASONING AND RATIONALITY). A leading example of a functionalist theory, defended in particular by Jerry Fodor, is the *language of thought hypothesis*, according to which propositional attitudes are taken to consist of computational relations to representations encoded in the brain (→ COGNITIVISM, LANGUAGE OF THOUGHT, PROPOSITIONAL ATTITUDE, REPRESENTATION); however, many connectionist theories would count as well (→ CONNECTIONISM).

Functionalist proposals have a number of attractions. One technical attraction is that they permit many mental terms to be defined simultaneously by their roles with respect to one another. Thus, as in the previous suggestion, belief and desire might be defined together, in relation to each other and possibly still other mental states, as well as in their relation to stimuli and responses (this is done through the exploitation of "Ramsey sentences," as in the work of David Lewis). In this way, functionalism is an improvement on *behaviorism*, which tried to tie a mental state too closely to behavioral dispositions (for example, a belief as a disposition merely to utter something when stimulated in a certain way).

More important, functionalism allows us to capture the fact, ignored by behaviorism, that how behavior is produced is often as important as the behavior itself (one person's impassive expression might be indistinguishable from that of someone who feels nothing, but he or she might nonetheless be experiencing intense feelings). Different causal relations between internal states can distinguish different mental states that might be behaviorally indistinguishable.

Functionalism also captures what many regard as the important intuition of *multiple realizability:* just as the same functional process can be realized (actualized) in many different substances (money can be made of most anything), so too might a mind be composed of very different stuff than humans are (which allows for the possibility of computer and/or extraterrestrial intelligence). Functionalism in this way cuts across traditional philosophical discussions of the mind, materialism, and dualism, which focused on whether the mind involved a different substance than the body.

But perhaps the most important consequence of functionalism is a methodological one: it permits a level of psychological explanation that is relatively autonomous from the physiology that may realize it, but without denying the reality or underlying causal importance of that physiology. If functionalism is correct, then studying merely the physiology of mental states without an account of their organization would be as explanatorily blind as studying the chemistry of money to learn about business cycles; or, to take an analogy that has been tremendously influential in cognitive psychology, like studying the physics of transistors to learn how a word-processing program works. In this way, functionalism captures the widely felt intuition that psychology is not reducible to physiology, without needing to claim that it involves some special nonphysical substance (as Cartesian dualists urged) ($\rightarrow$ DUALISM/MONISM, REDUCTIONISM).

Such is the general strategy of functionalism. When we turn to supplying actual functional analyses, however, there is a surprising diversity of views, depending upon what relations one thinks are essential to our mental concepts. *Folk functionalists*, such as David Lewis or Frank Jackson, propose looking at the roles played by mental phenomena according to common platitudes about the mind. For example, pain might be a state that is caused by burns and blows that in turn cause people to avoid such stimulation. But many philosophers are worried that folk beliefs may turn out to be false (for example, there may be no immortal souls, and women might well be as smart as men). So *analytic functionalists* (such as Sydney Shoemaker) look instead at the relations specified by idea-reflective philosophical analysis. *Psychofunctionalists* (such as Georges Rey) look at the relations between states that might be postulated by an ideal empirical psychology, rather in the way that the proper functional definition of money might be provided by an empirical economics.

There is also disagreement about how many of the relations among mental states need to be included in the definition of any one of them.

Holistic functionalists (such as Lewis) would take the entire psychology of the organism (→ HOLISM); *molecular functionalists* (such as Rey) confine definitions to small groups of states involved in specific subsystems, such as perception, reasoning, decision making, and so forth (→ COMPUTATIONAL ANALYSIS).

Many philosophers have worried that a mere functional system of causally interrelated states in the brain would not suffice to capture how mental states can have meaning, or content (→ EXTERNALISM/ INTERNALISM). A famous example showing the difficulty is that of Putnam's "Twin Earth." Suppose there were a planet exactly like the earth except for having, wherever the earth has H_2O, a strange chemical XYZ, superficially indistinguishable from H_2O. Arguably, an earthling thinking about water would not be having thoughts with the same content as the thoughts that her Twin Earth twin would be thinking, even though she might be in exactly the same functional states. It would appear that a person's mind must somehow be properly "anchored" in the world for his or her states to possess specific contents. One way that many have claimed this latter anchoring could come about is by causal relations between an internal functional state and the phenomena in the external world that provide its meaning. Others have argued that this anchoring must come about by natural selection.

For many philosophers, however, only such external anchors to a mind do not seem to be enough. Many complain that functionalist definitions, even supplemented by external relations, are still so abstract as to include most anything as a mind. In his famous "Nation of China" argument, Ned Block points out that if the material in which a mental system is realized really is irrelevant, then a billion people might be organized to realize the mind of a conscious being—but, he claims, it seems wildly implausible that the resulting organization would actually *be* the mind of a conscious being. Block further argues that functionalism cannot rule out the possibility of functional isomorphisms: two states might involve all the same functional relations, and yet intuitively be different mental states. Take, for example, the traditional worry about spectral reversals: one person might see green, but have all the associations and other psychofunctional connections of someone else who sees red (→ QUALIA). One reaction to these worries is to claim that functional states need to be anchored not only in external phenomena, but in certain internal, physiological properties as well. Thus, for example, the actual experience of green, as opposed to red, may involve the specific physiological properties that are part of the realization of the functional state associated with it.

GEORGE REY

SELECTED BIBLIOGRAPHY

Bealer, G. (1985). Mind and anti-mind. *Midwest Studies in Philosophy, 9*, 283–328.

Block, N. (1980). Troubles with functionalism. In N. Block (Ed.), *Readings in the philosophy of psychology* (Vol. 1) (pp. 283–328). Cambridge, MA: Harvard University Press.

Block, N., & Fodor, J. A. (1980). What psychological states are not. In J. Fodor (Ed.), *Representations: Philosophical essays on the foundations of cognitive science*. Cambridge, MA: MIT Press.

Fodor, J. (1968). *Psychological explanation*. New York: Random House.

Fodor, J. (2000). *The mind doesn't work that way: The scope and limits of computational psychology*. Cambridge, MA: MIT Press.

Lewis, D. (1980). Psychophysical and theoretical identifications. In N. Block (Ed.), *Readings in the philosophy of psychology* (Vol. 1, pp. 207–215). Cambridge, MA: Harvard University Press.

Putnam, H. (1960/1975). Minds and machines. *Philosophical papers: Vol. 2. Mind, language, and reality* (pp. 362–385). Cambridge, England: Cambridge University Press.

Rey, G. (1996). *Contemporary philosophy of mind: A contentiously classical approach*. Oxford: Blackwell.

Shoemaker, S. (1984). *Identity, cause, and mind*. Cambridge, England: Cambridge University Press.

FUZZY

Artificial intelligence. — One of the difficulties ordinary logic has in representing knowledge comes from the fact that calculating a truth value necessarily ends with either a *true* or a *false,* even though many situations call for verdicts in shades of gray (→ LOGIC, REPRESENTATION, TRUTH). We know how to assign a gradual measure to propositions: their probability. However, while probability is considered suitable for representing uncertainty, other techniques are deemed necessary for imprecise knowledge, if for no other reason than because calculating probabilities is too complicated to be compatible with the cognitive processing of this kind of knowledge. Authors have been proposing other techniques for quite some time (for example, Jan Lukasiewicz in 1920). In 1965, Lotfi Zadeh introduced the term *fuzzy subset* to refer to the idea of a grade $\mu_E(e)$ of membership of element e in set E. Given that the interpretation of a unary relation is a subset, this idea can be extended by stating that the degree of truth of atomic proposition $P(A)$ is equal to $\mu_p(a)$, where a is the element that interprets constant A, and p is the subset that interprets relation P. A fuzzy logic is thereby generated.

The truth t of a formula is calculated as follows: for an atomic formula, it is the corresponding grade of membership; for a negation, it is $t(\neg f) = 1 - t(f)$; for a conjunction, it is $t(f \wedge g) = \min(t(f), t(g))$, from which we get $t(f \vee g) = \max(t(f), t(g))$. This implication poses a delicate problem: defining $f \supset g$ in the usual way as $\neg f \vee g$ strangely makes the truth of the tautology $f \supset f$ depend on the truth of f. There are several ways of avoiding this obstacle: Lukasiewicz's solution is to have $t(f \supset g) = \min(1, 1 - t(f) + t(g))$.

In view of drawing direct inferences from linguistic data (→ LANGUAGE), Zadeh took words in the language whose intuitive interpretation is gradual (*young*, *rich,* etc.) and assigned them functions of a base variable (*age*, *wealth*) in the interval [0, 1] representing the degrees of truth. To expressions that explicitly evoked graduality (e.g., *very*, *little*, *more or less*), he assigned values obtained by performing operations on those degrees (in particular, the square and the square root). Note that the fit between this one-dimensional representation and language is far from perfect.

A generalization of fuzzy logic, *possibility theory*, associates two values with each proposition: its degree of necessity and its degree of possibility. Fuzzy logic is mainly employed as a cognitive engineering technique. Expert systems make use of plausibility coefficients, which are sometimes considered to be part of fuzzy logic (→ KNOWLEDGE BASE). Fuzzy logic also supplies interesting tools for categorization, particularly for modeling the cognitive phenomenon of typicality (→ CATEGORIZATION). But these tools require determining degrees of truth, which poses both empirical and epistemological problems.

DANIEL KAYSER

SELECTED BIBLIOGRAPHY

Mukaidono, M. (2001). *Fuzzy logic for beginners*. River Edge, NJ: World Scientific.
Pedrycz, W., & Gomide, F. (1998). *An introduction to fuzzy sets: Analysis and design*. Cambridge, MA: MIT Press.
Zadeh, L. A. (1965). Fuzzy sets. *Information and Control, 8*, 338–353.
Zadeh, L. A. (1975). Fuzzy logic and approximate reasoning. *Synthèse, 30*, 406–425.

G

GOAL

Philosophy. — Intuitively, a *goal-directed behavior* is one that is executed in view of attaining a certain goal. The realm of living things exhibits innumerable examples of goal-directed behavior, such as web spinning by spiders, courtship rituals in birds, dam building by beavers, and so on (→ ANIMAL COGNITION). The difficulty inherent in this concept, however, is that it seems to imply a type of final causality in which the desired result is what orients and guides the action (→ ACTION, CAUSALITY AND MENTAL CAUSATION). Goal-directed behavior thus seems to necessarily involve the representation of a goal or purpose (→ REPRESENTATION). Yet a number of studies have shown that goal-directed behaviors can be manifested independently of any type of representation.

The first attempt to *naturalize* the idea of purpose dates back to the work of Arturo Rosenblueth, Norbert Wiener, and Julian Bigelow (→ NATURALIZATION). They showed that purpose can be understood without recourse to the idea of a final cause, and that it does not require considering the cause of a goal-oriented action to inhere in an event that comes after the action itself. They proposed seeing goal-directed behaviors as behaviors that require negative *feedback* coming from the goal. There is feedback when the system can use part of its output as input. It is positive when it has the same sign as the output, and negative if not. Negative feedback in goal-directed behavior consists of signals emitted by the goal that constrain the output in order to reduce the object's error margin as the goal is being pursued. Based on the analysis of Rosenblueth and his collaborators, the behavior of servomechanical devices (like the ones use to control torpedoes) can be defined as goal-directed (→ ROBOTICS).

However, this initial definition suffers from two shortcomings. First, one cannot distinguish a strictly physical system from a goal-oriented system; for example, a liquid in a vase that returns to a state of equilibrium seems to manifest a self-regulated behavior. Second, it seems to imply that a behavior cannot be goal-directed unless it makes use of information that enables the *target event* to be accomplished by means of adaptive corrections (the *target element* is the object upon which the action must be performed; the target event is the final phase of the behavioral process that must be reached for the action to be successful).

To remedy this state of affairs, one needs to bring to bear an additional set of conditions, which Gerd Sommerhoff analyzed as follows: (1) A goal-directed behavior continues to be executed until it reaches a certain state of completion. It is the attainment of this state, often called a *state of equilibrium*, that interrupts the behavior. (2) The agent must be in a certain physical nonnomological relationship with the target element at time *t* in the target event. In other words, physical system *A* (made up of the agent and its environment) is connected to physical system *B* (the target event and its possibility conditions) by a causality link, granted, but one that does not have force of law. (3) The agent must reach the target event at least in part by virtue of the way in which he, she, or it initiated and/or carried out the action. This condition guarantees that the action sequence is not the result of chance or of a physical causality that cannot help but produce the concerned effects. (4) If the properties that are causally relevant to the action exerted upon the target element had been different, the target event–directed action required by those properties would nevertheless have been accomplished. (5) Physical systems consisting respectively of the agent and the instrument of his, her, or its action, and the process that leads to the target event, share the causal determinants that affect the dynamic at certain crucial points in the unfolding of the goal-directed process (*correction devices*).

There are types of behavior that satisfy properties 1 to 5 only partially; they are referred to as *weakened* goal-directed behaviors. The most elementary class is the class of *goal-seeking behaviors* (David McFarland). The system engaged in this type of behavior does not achieve the target event by virtue of its own correction devices, nor can it determine whether the action succeeded or failed: it is designed to reach the goal without that goal being explicitly represented in the system. A second class, *goal-achieving behaviors* (McFarland), includes behaviors in which, like goal-directed behaviors, the system is capable of recognizing that the goal has been attained when it has, but is incapable of modifying the pathway of the action.

JOËLLE PROUST

SELECTED BIBLIOGRAPHY

McFarland, D. (1989). Goals, no-goals and own goals. In A.Montefiore & D. Noble (Eds.), *Goals, no-goals and own goals: A debate on goal-directed and intentional behaviour*. London: Unwin Hyman.

Rosenbleuth, A., Wiener, N., & Bigelow, J. (1943). Behavior, purpose and teleology. *Philosophy of Science, 10*, 18–24.

Sommerhoff, G. (1990). *Life, brain and consciousness: New perceptions through targeted systems analysis*. North Holland, NY: Elsevier.

GRAMMAR

Linguistics. — The term *grammar* refers to both a familiar object and an ancient activity (Panini's grammar of Sanskrit dates back to 500 B.C.E.). In its descriptive sense, the term refers to the set of all phonetic, morphological, and syntactic regularities observable in a given language, along with the representation of those regularities (→ MORPHOLOGY, REPRESENTATION, SYNTAX). When someone speaks of a language "with no grammar," the language in question can only be one whose rules have not (yet) been described. In its normative sense—generally criticized by linguists—grammar is the set of conventions defining a dialectal variant deemed by the society to be superior and chosen as the one to teach (don't say *with John and I,* say *with John and me,* or don't say *I just seen him,* say *I've just seen him*) (→ NORMATIVITY). In its linguistic senses, grammar is either the analysis of the observable regularities of a given language (e.g., the grammar of French anaphors), or the theoretical model used to conduct such an analysis (syntagmatic grammar, functional grammar, etc.; → FUNCTION). The advent of *generative grammar* added another meaning to the term: according to Noam Chomsky, a grammar is a model not of existing languages but of the faculty of language, that is, the ability of every child to learn and to speak any language (→ LANGUAGE). Although the term has been overextended (to refer to any system of regularities, as in the "grammar" of the cinema or the "grammar" of behavior), it should be reserved for linguistic entities.

Grammar is rooted in two traditions. On the one side, there is the tradition of Western philosophy, which makes the study of language into a privileged road for understanding things; on the other side, there are the traditions of rhetoric and religion, which conceive of grammar as a means of access to literary and sacred writings. The philosophical approach looks at the origin of languages, the reasons why words mean what they do (etymology), the fit between linguistic constructions and logical operations (→ LOGIC, MEANING AND SIGNIFICATION, SENSE): according to Aristotle, who proposed a binary breakdown of sentences into subject/predicate, the noun/verb opposition reflects the substance/accident opposition.

It was in the sixteenth century that grammar in the modern sense (as a means of access to new languages) came into being and that linguistic categories no longer had to be logical (→ CATEGORIZATION). Until the eighteenth century, when the literature began to proliferate, we find various trends coexisting, with writings in the descriptive, philosophical (including the plan to devise a universal grammar), and didactic or normative approaches. The nineteenth century brought the specialization of knowledge, and linguistics was recognized as a branch of knowledge that encompassed grammar. In comparative grammar, which was the prevailing focus at the time, the idea was to classify languages according to their lineage and to discover the laws that governed their evolution over time. In the twentieth century, along with the work on descriptive, historical, and comparative grammar, under the influence of Ferdinand de Saussure linguists began to direct their efforts toward studying a given state of a language, seen as a system in and of itself. Different levels of analysis were distinguished (phonetic, syntactic, semantic; → SEMANTICS). This led to the division of traditional grammar into several autonomous constituents, and, with progress in logic and computer science, to the development of formal logico-mathematical models of grammar.

Along with dictionaries, grammar books have always claimed to offer a natural means for learning to read and write (→ LEARNING, READING, WRITING). Schoolbook grammars generally mix descriptive and normative considerations, and they place more weight on the written language and literary style than on speech. The utility of teaching children the grammar of their native language has been contested, especially for English, where this type of knowledge does not appear to improve the writing skills of pupils. With French, however, the orthographic system cannot be mastered unless grammar is explicitly taught. As far as second-language learning is concerned, it is not clear whether grammar-based teaching yields better results than immersion methods.

Modern linguistics has attempted to distinguish itself from the traditional grammatical, philosophical, and pedagogical approaches by defining itself as the study of language for its own sake. The goal is not to attain a better understanding of thought processes, nor to achieve a better mastery of a particular language. As Jean-Claude Milner noted, linguists and grammarians agree that one can judge whether sentences are properly constructed (assess their grammaticality) without taking the context of utterance into account (→ CONTEXT AND SITUATION). A traditional grammar like Maurice Grevisse's for French, presented in *Le bon usage*, describes a single language without relating it to others and states its rules and their exceptions. This type of book usually includes as much morphology as syntax, and focuses on classification problems such as assigning words to parts of speech (→ DISCOURSE) and orthography (agreement). A linguist's grammar, which is based on a rational, hypotheticodeductive method, states the implicit, unconscious rules that govern the use of the language, and looks for rules common to all languages. It distinguishes between several levels of linguistic analysis and generally concentrates on syntactic problems, often using invented examples to demonstrate a given type of grammatical or agrammatical sentence.

Charles Morris distinguished three levels of linguistic analysis: syntax, semantics, and pragmatics (→ PRAGMATICS). When syntax is studied in a structuralist framework, questions of meaning are generally ignored, whereas the functionalist approach (Talmy Givòn, André Martinet) refuses to make the distinction between the syntactic and semantic levels. In Chomsky's generative grammar, the thesis of the *autonomy of syntax* is thoroughly developed, and grammar is viewed as a modular system with limited, one-directional interactions between modules (Jerry Fodor; → MODULARITY). The syntactic module is the core module; it is formally different from the others because it is the only one that is generative (→ CREATIVITY), the phonetic and semantic components being simply in charge of interpreting grammatical sentences (→ INTERPRETATION). As an alternative, Jerrold Katz and his collaborators defined a *generative semantics* in which the syntactic component does nothing but transform deep semantic structures into surface syntactic structures. *Unification grammars* usually follow the generative model, but in parallel, they generate phonetic, syntactic, and semantic representations within a single structure of features. Other theories, such as Maurice Gross's *lexicon-grammars* or certain unification grammars, conceive of syntax not as a set of generative rules, but as simply verifying the compatibility of the lexical properties of words when they are combined (→ LEXICON). The doctrine of the autonomy of syntax poses the problem of how syntax is learned: if very young children cannot guess the category or construction of words on the basis of their meaning, then there must be an innate formal system capable of detecting true syntactic regularities (Steven Pinker).

Chomsky and George Miller defined a formal grammar as an algorithm for deciding whether or not a particular combination of words belongs to the language: *a mean dog* is a phrase in the English language, but **dog a mean* is not. A grammar in the logicomathematical sense is a finite set of rewrite rules capable of starting from a set of vocabulary words that is also finite, and generating a potentially infinite set of well-formed sentences. Four types of grammar are distinguished, according to their generative capacity. The most restricted grammars, *Type 3 grammars* (also called *regular* grammars), can only describe a language where no two words occur the same number (n) of times ($a_n b_n$). *Type 2 grammars*, called *algebraic* or *context-free* grammars, are capable of characterizing such a language but solely by assigning it an embedded-dependency structure wherein the first a is connected to the last b, the second a to the next-to-last b, and so on. *Type 1 grammars*, or *context-sensitive* grammars, can assign cross-dependency structures to sentences in the same language and generate other languages (including, for example, copying phenomena). *Type 0 grammars*, or *unrestricted* grammars, can generate all recursively enumerable languages. This hierarchy is important not only in mathematical linguistics, which attempts to determine the correlations between the empirical properties of languages and the logico-mathematical properties of formal systems, but also in computer science for developing programming languages and compilers.

ANNE ABEILLÉ

SELECTED BIBLIOGRAPHY

Abeillé, A., & Rambow, O. (Eds.). (2001). *Tree adjoining grammars: Mathematical, computational and linguistic properties*. Chicago, IL: University of Chicago Press.

Chomsky, N. (1955/1975). *The logical structure of linguistic theory*. New York: Plenum.

Chomsky, N. (1995). *The minimalist program*. Cambridge, MA: MIT Press.

Damon, W. (1998). *Handbook of child psychology: Vol. 2. Cognition, perception, and language*. New York: Wiley.

Fodor J. (1983). *The modularity of mind*. Cambridge, MA: MIT Press.

Katz, J., & Postal, P. (1964). *An integrated theory of linguistic description*. Cambridge, MA: MIT Press.

Jackendoff, R. (2002). *Foundations of language: Brain, meaning, grammar, evolution*. Oxford, England; New York: Oxford University Press.

Milner, J.-C. (1989). *Introduction à une science du langage* [Introduction to a language science]. Paris: Seuil.

H

HOLISM

Philosophy. — *Holism* characterizes any theory whereby the properties of the whole cannot be predicted or explained from the properties of the parts. As such, holism is often associated with *emergentism*, in particular in biology and in the social sciences: the properties of the whole "emerge" in a manner that cannot be derived from the properties of the constituents (→ EMERGENCE).

Holism also applies to doctrines specific to a particular domain. Holism in theory confirmation is the doctrine, defended in particular by Willard Quine, according to which a statement is confirmed or refuted by the facts, not by virtue of its content alone but by virtue of the set of hypotheses and logical rules authorized by the theory (→ LOGIC, VALIDATION). *Meaning holism* is the thesis whereby the meaning of a sentence depends on how it is related to other sentences in the language (→ LANGUAGE, MEANING AND SIGNIFICATION, SENSE). *Belief holism* posits that the content of a given belief is determined by its relationships to the subject's other beliefs (→ BELIEF, FUNCTIONALISM, PROPOSITIONAL ATTITUDE). These diverse types of holism can be defended independently of each other.

JOËLLE PROUST

SELECTED BIBLIOGRAPHY

Fodor, J., & Le Pore, E. (1992). *Holism: A shopper's guide*. Oxford, England: Blackwell.
Peacocke, C. (1979). *Holistic explanations*. Oxford, England: Oxford University Press.
Quine, W. V. O. (1953). Two dogmas of empiricism. *From a logical point of view: Nine logico-philosophical essays*. Cambridge, MA: Harvard University Press.

I

IDENTITY

Philosophy. — *Identity* is generally understood to mean *numerical identity*: thing *a* is numerically identical to thing *b* if *a* and *b* are one and the same thing. Numerical identity must be distinguished from *qualitative identity*, which applies to two distinct things that share all of their characteristics except their spatiotemporal properties. This identity relation satisfies the *indiscernibility-of-identicals principle*, which stipulates that if *a* is identical to *b*, *a* and *b* have the same properties. Reciprocally, the identity-of-indiscernibles principle posits that if two things share the same properties, they are identical. Gottfried Leibniz's law states the equivalence of these two principles.

Leibniz's law has been challenged by saying that two identical things cannot be indiscernible from the standpoint of all possible qualities. This is particularly true of things that last and whose matter is altered over time, like the human body (→ TIME AND TENSE). Accordingly, Peter Geach contends that identity is always relative to the property that determines the class to which the concerned objects belong: *a* is the same *F* as *b*, but it can be a different *G* than *b*. David Wiggins proposed making this type of analysis compatible with Leibniz's law by saying that only *sortal* concepts can determine identity among a class of objects (*sortal dependency of identity* theory): *being a tree* is a sortal; *being brown* is not.

Ruth Barcan-Marcus demonstrated that the necessity of the identity relation between *a* and *b* follows from the indiscernibility of identicals. Clearly, one of the properties of *a* is being necessarily identical to *a*, which must therefore also be a property of *b*. This result became the grounds for Saul Kripke's theory of *rigid designators*, that is, proper nouns that designate the same individuals in all possible worlds where they exist. Kripke rejects the view that there is an identity relation between a mental state and the corresponding state of the brain, arguing that such an identity cannot be necessary. However, one can reply that our impression that such an identity is purely contingent is just as fallacious as the belief that the identity between heat and the kinetic energy of molecules is contingent.

The problem of personal identity raises some interesting issues since in essence, persons are constantly evolving and hence are not readily reducible to strictly spatiotemporal conditions. Three types of theories have been put forward. *Substantialism* views identity as founded on a substance, which can be either an individual soul (René Descartes) (→ DUALISM/MONISM) or a body that can be individuated spatiotemporally (Bernard Williams, David Wiggins). *Physicalism* differs from substantialism in that it makes personal identity supervene on each individual brain (→ PHYSICALISM). The third type of theory, initially proposed by John Locke, is founded on a criterion of *psychological continuity*. Continuity-based theories appear to many philosophers to be promising and better equipped to handle the counterexamples of brain transplantation, information transfer, and fission imagined by philosophers.

In one version of this last type of theory, being such and such a person means having certain partially overlapping memories about events observed or actions performed in the past (→ ACTION, MEMORY). In another version, continuity is built from intentions and plans for action. To avoid circularity in the criterion for psychological continuity, Sydney Shoemaker and Derek Parfit tempered the concept of psychological continuity by speaking of "quasi memory" or "quasi intention," acknowledging the possibility of psychological events experienced "from the inside" but not identifiable as "one's own." This approach is consistent with theories of cognitive psychopathology, which stress the importance of the sense of control over one's actions in representations of personal identity, particularly in autism or schizophrenia (→ AUTISM, COGNITIVE PSYCHIATRY, SCHIZOPHRENIA).

JOËLLE PROUST

SELECTED BIBLIOGRAPHY

Engel, P. (1991). *The norm of truth: An introduction to the philosophy of logic* (M. Kochan & P. Engel, Trans.). Toronto, Ontario; Buffalo, NY: University of Toronto Press. (Original work published 1989.)

Kripke, S. (1972). *Naming and necessity*. Oxford, England: Basil Blackwell.

Parfit, D. (1984/1987). *Reasons and persons*. Oxford, England: Clarendon Press.

INDIVIDUALISM

Philosophy. — *Individualism* is a doctrine that posits that the intentional mental states of individuals (→ INTENTIONALITY) can be characterized or defined without reference to their physical or sociolinguistic environment. Two forms of individualism must be distinguished: *ontological* and *methodological.*

Ontological individualism, also called *internalism*, is a doctrine about the nature of mental contents that sees those contents as being solely determined by facts pertaining to the subject, irrespective of his or her environment (→ EXTERNALISM/INTERNALISM). It is opposed to the *externalistic* theses of Hilary Putnam and Tyler Burge, according to which, even assuming that facts internal to a subject remain constant, modifications in the subject's relationships to the physical or social environment should cause changes in the content of his or her thoughts.

Methodological individualism, advocated by Jerry Fodor, acknowledges externalist arguments to the effect that people's mental states at least partly depend upon their relationships to their environment, but it also stipulates that scientific taxonomies must obey a principle of *causal relevance* (→ CAUSALITY AND MENTAL CAUSATION). According to this principle, the properties of a mental state, whether they are relational or nonrelational, need be taken into account in psychological taxonomies only if they are causally relevant. Methodological individualism thus argues that the (environmentally) relational properties of mental states, which define *broad content*, have no causal relevance, and that only nonrelational properties, which define *narrow content*, have to be included in psychology's scientific taxonomies. It is important to make the distinction between methodological individualism, which stresses that mental states are individuated relative to their causal power, from methodological *solipsism*, according to which their individuation is independent of their semantic evaluation (→ SEMANTICS).

One possible motivation for entertaining individualism in both of its forms is to preserve the intuition that each of us is a sort of firsthand authority about the contents of our own mental states: we know better than anyone else what our thoughts are. Another motivation is to guarantee the possibility of a scientific, intentional psychology. Insofar as mental states exercise causal power by way of the cerebral states that realize them, the attribution of causal efficacy to mental contents requires embracing the *supervenience* thesis, which posits that there can be no difference in mental content without a difference in the state of the brain (→ SUPERVENIENCE). No such supervenience would exist, however, if mental contents were characterized relationally.

ÉLISABETH PACHERIE

SELECTED BIBLIOGRAPHY

Burge, T. (1986). Individualism and psychology. *Philosophical Review, 95,* 3–45.

Fodor, J. (1987). *Psychosemantics: The problem of meaning in the philosophy of mind.* Cambridge, MA: MIT Press.

INFANT COGNITION

Psychology. — Capturing the mental states of infants and how they evolve and fluctuate, and knowing what part of adult conceptions infants share at a given time in development (→ COGNITIVE DEVELOPMENT)—these are some of the main driving forces of research on *infant cognition*. We owe the discovery of infant learning abilities (→ LEARNING) to a paradigm shift more than anything else. Contrary to Jean Piaget's theory, it seems that infants learn more through information about the outside world captured by their perceptual systems (→ PERCEPTION) than through motor skill development (→ ACTION). Infant cognition studies look at both the capacity to interpret sensory data and the faculty for understanding and reasoning about complex events (→ REASONING AND RATIONALITY). However, the extent of the knowledge infants can acquire is limited by their neural maturation speed and motor ineptitude.

Right from birth, infants notice regularities in the environment. Their ability to respond to objects rather than to their retinal projection already guarantees the newborn some degree of environmental stability (object-size and object-shape constancy). Although infants prefer looking at a real three-dimensional object than at a drawing of it, object recognition is not ensured until the age of four months, and only if the infant sees the object being rotated. Infants have trouble interpreting static spatial information, but they possess a perspective decoder that, even in monocular vision, enables them to detect objects on the basis of optical transformations governed by projective geometry rules.

Tactile-kinesthetic perception of objects reaches its full capacity within the first few months of life. Once vision-prehension coordination is well established, at about five or six months, the infant's hands become genuine tools in the service of vision, but their function is confined to holding and moving objects in space (→ SPACE). At this point, the capabilities of the two hands begin the differentiation process. The left hand is in charge of exploring and perceiving space and objects, whereas the right hand finds its true function in manual skills and fine motricity.

While auditory knowledge is already partially organized at birth by fetal imprinting (→ FETAL COGNITION), the change of medium in which sound events are transmitted is further complicated by difficulty detecting sound sources in what is now boundless space. Sound detection is contingent upon the infant's capacity to turn its head and body in the direction of the source. The analysis and processing of nonverbal auditory patterns depend largely on the infant's memory capacity for storing a flow of successive events (→ MEMORY). These abilities nevertheless emerge in infants well before they are capable of breaking down a sequence of verbal patterns into meaningful units.

All everyday activities rest on the simultaneous interaction and participation of the senses. Signals that are biologically important for responding appropriately to the problems posed by the environment are organized in an *intermodal* way and play a crucial role in the ontogeny of learning. The *perceptual* or *perceptuomotor integration process* shows up in infant behaviors as varied as intermodal transfer, visuoauditory matching, speech perception, early imitation, and reaching for and grasping objects. It is now well established that, right from birth, information processed by one sensory modality can be modified by another (→ INFORMATION). Research has shown that intermodal relationships cannot be understood as the sum of the abilities of each system, but as a function of their joint participation, at each stage of development, in producing a response that is adapted to the demands of the surroundings. Although the infant's integration processes are sometimes fragile and unstable, their existence invalidates the hypothesized early functional modularity of the perceptual and motor systems (→ MODULARITY).

These analytic processors, whose maturation is still incomplete at the end of the first year, are what enable infants to interpret sensory data. By the age of three months, babies are capable of detecting invariants in a series of different-shaped objects, and of classifying objects into genuine perceptual categories (→ CATEGORIZATION). But their intelligence goes beyond the mere analysis of unprocessed reality. Their ability to reason effectively about the environment also shows up very early. Reasoning is required whenever some important dimension for apprehending the world in a coherent way is missing or imperceptible and must be reconstructed by the infant based on immediately available data or information retrieved from memory. This capacity has mainly been assessed by studying the concept of object: its existence or permanence, the constraints that determine its motion in space and time, and its numerosity (→ NUMBER, OBJECT, TIME AND TENSE). Two experimental paradigms that differ in the learning phase have been used to test the reality of this reasoning ability in situations qualified as *possible/impossible*. The first, found in Elizabeth Spelke's research, is based on an invisible change in an object's location. This approach is used to figure out how infants reason with the representations they have of the world (→ REPRESENTATION). The second, found in Renée Baillargeon's studies, is used to assess the rapidity and accuracy with which infants learn a physical law by examining how they react when it is violated.

Research on *object permanence* has revealed that infants are capable of mentally evoking parts of the world they cannot or can no longer see. An object that is partly hidden by a screen preserves its oneness, its cohesiveness. While for Piaget, successful searching for a hidden object is the result of a slow and gradual, action-scheme-dependent acquisition, it has been shown that by the early age of three or four months, an infant's failure to search actively for an object does not imply that it no longer exists.

Three and four month olds are surprised to see a screen pass through a box located behind it, because they already know that objects are solid and that two objects cannot occupy the same space at the same time. Objects exist for the infant even when they are out of sight.

Because objects possess the properties of cohesiveness and solidity, their motion is constrained by the principle of *continuity* (all moving objects follow exactly one path in space and time), the principle of *gravitation* (all unsupported objects fall), and the principle of *inertia* (a moving object does not abruptly or spontaneously change direction). Physical laws also govern the relationships objects have with each other. The principle of *contact* implies that an object's motion is affected only if it is touched by a second object (→ CAUSALITY AND MENTAL CAUSATION). In situations where the movement of the object is not in sight, these laws become operational at different ages. The principle of continuity is applied by the age of two months, whereas inertia and gravity are not clearly understood until the infant is a year old. Reasoning in this case rests on an inference process, because only the object's initial and final states can be perceived, not its transformations. In conditions where infants are given the problem data and the chance to extract the rules from the materials, these three principles are applied at an earlier age, depending on whether deductive or predictive reasoning is at stake.

For example, the principle of gravitation becomes operational earlier in situations where the rule is presented during the learning phase. In these situations, infants who are three to five months old are shown a base on which an object is being pushed by the finger of someone's hand. The object is slid along the base and stops halfway. The entire situation is visible. Then on the test phase, two situations are presented, one possible and one impossible: (1) the object is pushed along the base until it just reaches the edge, and (2) the object goes past the edge but is still touching it. Young three-and-a-half month olds, who quickly understand the situation during the learning phase, are surprised and look longer at the suspended object in the impossible situation.

In research on number, newborns have proven capable of differentiating between sets of two or three elements (and even more in certain studies). Studies by Karen Wynn have shed new light on numerical abilities in young infants (addition and subtraction): using the possible/impossible event paradigm, she showed that four and five month olds are capable of adding and subtracting small numbers.

Baillargeon proposed a two-step model of the early development of physical reasoning, based on her infant cognition research. Infants are thought to be capable of qualitative, global reasoning at about three months, and then to evolve toward more precise, quantitative reasoning during the second half of the first year. This viewpoint goes against

Spelke's resolutely rationalist theory, which holds that a core of innate knowledge guides infant reasoning. If infants' responses are dependent upon the situation (or range of situations) they are viewing, then a precise analysis of the relationships between perception and reasoning should help articulate these two conceptions of development. What remains surprising about infant cognition is as much the findings obtained as the rapidity of learning during this brief period of life.

ARLETTE STRERI

SELECTED BIBLIOGRAPHY

Baillargeon, R. (1995). Physical reasoning in infancy. In M. S. Gazzaniga (Ed.), *The cognitive neurosciences*. Cambridge, MA: MIT Press.

Baillargeon, R., & Wang, S. (2002). Event categorization in infancy. *Trends in Cognitive Sciences, 6*, 85–92.

Bremner, G. & Fogel, A. (Eds.) (2001). *Blackwell handbook of infant development*. Oxford, England: Blackwell.

Damon, W. (Ed.). (1998). *Handbook of child psychology: Vol. 2. Cognition, perception, and language* (5th ed.). New York: Wiley.

Gopnik, A., Meltzoff, A., & Kuhl, P. (1999). *The scientist in the crib: Minds, brains, and how children learn*. New York: William Morrow.

Goswami, U. (1998). *Cognition in children*. East Sussex, England: Psychology Press.

Johnson, M. (2001). Functional brain development in humans. *Nature Reviews Neuroscience, 2*, 475–483.

Piaget, J. (1954). *The construction of reality in the child* (M. Cook, Trans.). New York: Basic Books. (Original work published 1937.)

Piaget, J. (1984). Piaget's theory. In P. Mussen (Ed.), *Handbook of child psychology* (pp. 103–128). New York: Wiley.

Spelke, E. S. (1994). Initial knowledge: Six suggestions. *Cognition, 50*, 431–445.

Spelke, E. (1995). Object perception, object-directed action, and physical knowledge in infancy. In M. S. Gazzaniga (Ed.), *The cognitive neurosciences*. Cambridge, MA: MIT Press.

Spelke, E. (2000). Core knowledge. *American Psychologist, 55*, 1233–1243.

INFORMATION

Neuroscience and psychology. — In cognitive neuroscience and psychology, all input or output to and from the subsystems of a functional architecture is *information* (→ COMPUTATIONAL ANALYSIS). The neuroscientist's task is to specify the nature of that information and the mechanisms that transform it within each subsystem. At the neural level, neurophysiologists have long assumed that the information content of a neuron is represented only by its *discharge frequency*, that is, the number of action potentials it sends to its axon within a given period of time. An alternative view today contends that it is the *temporal pattern of discharge* that contains the information. In other words, the different patterns generated by variations in the discharge frequency over time may themselves carry information.

Cognitive scientists often define concepts in terms of information processing. Their task is to study how information from the environment is encoded, selected, organized, stored, and retrieved by the sensory, perceptual, attentional, and memory systems (→ ACTIVATION/INHIBITION, ATTENTION, MEMORY, PERCEPTION, PSYCHOPHYSICS). Here, the term *information* has a broader meaning (in particular, it includes a semantic and a cognitive component → SEMANTICS) than in Claude Shannon's *information theory*, where it is employed in a strictly numerical, statistical sense (see *artificial intelligence* and *philosophy* below). Information theory has nevertheless provided psychology with a number of metaphors, including *communication or processing channel, limited capacity*, and the *noise* that interferes with information transmission.

An essential distinction for studying information processing in cognitive psychology opposes *bottom-up* and *top-down* processing. In bottom-up processing, assumed to be automatic (→ AUTOMATISM), the information processed comes directly from sensory stimulation: processing is stimulus-driven. In top-down processing, which is more controlled (→ CONTROL), information processing is concept-driven, that is, guided by cognitive representations in memory (→ CONCEPT, REPRESENTATION). Current research focuses on the complex interactions that take place between these two types of processing and how they are related to the task demands and the subject's individual characteristics. Some authors even stress the role of action (or representations of action) in information processing (→ ACTION). Accordingly, the physiologist Alain Berthoz argues that perception is a simulated action, in the sense that it is a judgment or a decision, a prediction about the action's consequences.

The notion of information is also related to the idea of the *modularity* of the mind: according to Jerry Fodor, the cognitive modules involved in perception and language are "encapsulated" in such a way that there is no information flow between them (→ LANGUAGE, MIND, MODULARITY).

JEAN DECÉTY AND OLIVIER HOUDÉ

Artificial intelligence.—The meaning of the term *information* in information technology is directly inherited from Shannon's information theory and does not have the same sense as it does in everyday language.

Suppose agents could communicate only by means of messages composed of symbols taken from a given alphabet A (→ COMMUNICATION, SYMBOL). The arrival of message M is likely to inform its addressee that one of N possible events has occurred. The amount of information, I, transmitted by M is considered to increase as N increases. It is customary to choose the base 2 logarithm of N as its increasing function, that is, $I = \log_2 N$. One can easily show that if A has n symbols and if the length of M is k, then N is at most equal to n^k, so $I \leq k \log_2 n$. If the alphabet has only two signs ($n = 2$, a common case in today's computer technology), we have $I \leq k$, that is, the amount of information contained in *M* expressed in a binary language is at most equal to its length (→ LANGUAGE). The unit for measuring information is the *bit* (abbreviation for *binary unit*).

This definition implies that any series of *k* symbols taken from the same alphabet carries the same amount of information; but this is counter-intuitive, for various reasons. First, agents will feel they have received more information if the answer announced in *M* was unexpected than if it was predictable. Shannon's theory offers a remedy to this drawback by authorizing messages of variable length, in such a way that the shortest ones denote the events that are the most probable. Second, a message formed by a million consecutive *a*'s is not as informative as a book of the same length. This difficulty can be overcome by considering, as Andrei Kolmogorov did, that the amount of information conveyed by *M* is dependent not upon the probability of what *M* announces, but upon the complexity of the simplest mechanism capable of generating *M*. Finally, and in particular, as far as the cognitive sciences are concerned, the definitions of information given by Shannon and Kolmogorov do not consider the effect produced on the receiver. Yet if *M* is written in Chinese, it will be judged less informative by an agent who does not understand that language than by one who does.

Defining the quantity of information, *I*, as the increase in knowledge brought about by interpreting *M* would be more consistent with intuition (→ INTERPRETATION). But this idea is impractical in information technology because it presupposes being able to quantify knowledge (such that *I* depends both on the message and its receiver). The quantity presented here is easy to measure and very useful for storage and transmission devices; the only unfortunate part is that it bears the name *information!*

DANIEL KAYSER

Philosophy. — One way of approaching intentionality in the philosophy of mind is to define the content of mental states (propositional attitudes) using the concept of information (→ INTENTIONALITY, PROPOSITIONAL ATTITUDE). Initially, this concept was approached from a probabilistic, quantitative standpoint in research on telecommunication systems (information theory; see *artificial intelligence* above). It was later adapted to the processing of individual messages.

According to information theory, all information reduces uncertainty. Three steps must be taken if one wishes to measure the amount of information contained in an event. How much information is there, for example, in a flipped coin that comes down *tails* (*T*)? First, one determines the set of possible events with respect to which *T* is considered. This set could be the set of all (nonrigged) coin tosses. Next one determines the set of all possible alternative types of events that could have occurred instead of event type *T*, along with the a priori probability of occurrence of each type. In our example, the only possible alternative event is *heads* (*H*), and its a priori probability is the same as the probability of *T*, namely 50 percent. Probability calculations supply the framework for information theory.

Information theory considers any event that reduces uncertainty to be a signal or message. This view of information has the following special properties. (1) It is insensitive to the content of the information whose quantity it measures. For a given receiver, the difference in content between two distinct messages may be crucial, but for information theory, the only interesting thing is the probability that a given sequence of signals will be produced. Equiprobable sequences coming from the same source convey the same amount of information. (2) One cannot apply it to the occurrence of an event independently of a series of events of the same type (→ TYPE/TOKEN). (3) The physical medium of the information-bearing events (taken to be the symbols that encode the message) plays no role, nor does the real context in which they are produced, or their causes and effects (→ CAUSALITY AND MENTAL CAUSATION, CONTEXT AND SITUATION, SYMBOL). (4) The informativeness of event *E*—that is, the amount of information it contains—is well determined only if the *reference class*, or the set of event types known a priori to be possible, and the set of events counted as equivalent to *E*, are well determined.

Information can be transmitted. For this to be possible, though, the source or sender must be connected to the receiver (that is, the input must be connected to the output) by an information channel. Information channel is a purely statistical concept: for such a channel to exist between two series of events *A* and *B* (in the sense defined in mathematical probability theory), it suffices that the probability that event A_i will occur, $p(A_i)$, be different from the conditional probability $p(A_i \mid B_j)$ that A_i will occur given that B_j occurred. The information channel does not have to be physically realized, for example, by a causal link. In this way, two series of events that are causally separate but triggered by one or more common causes may be statistically correlated. Hence, information flows between them.

The amount of information $T(x, y)$ transmitted from *x* to *y* is equal to the information contained in the input message minus the *ambiguity* generated by the transmission channel, or, equivalently, to the information contained in the output message minus the *equivocity* generated by the transmission channel. Equivocity and ambiguity are properties of the information channel. Together, they constitute the noise in the message. Equivocity measures the uncertainty that persists in the input message given a certain output message. Ambiguity measures the uncertainty that persists in the output message once the input message has been determined.

Fred Dretske adapted the concept of information to defining the content of mental states. Dretske's definition involves a relation between two individual events: the fact that r is G (G is, say, the state of an internal indicator) conveys the information that s is F (F is, say, a property of the environment) if and only if $P(F(s) \mid G(r)) = 1$. The requirement that the conditional probability be equal to 1 is equivalent to the requirement that the transmission channel be free of noise. This theory opposes the factive character of the information relation (which can be applied only if it is realized: in this view, there is no false information) to the normative character of the representation relation (which can be true or false) ($\rightarrow$ NORMATIVITY, REPRESENTATION, TRUTH). If $G(r)$ is an internal state of a cognitive system that carries information about fact $F(s)$, then it can be said to *indicate* it. For indicator $G(r)$ to be a representation of $F(s)$, it must also be true that its function is to indicate a certain type of event or property ($\rightarrow$ FUNCTION).

MAX KISTLER

SELECTED BIBLIOGRAPHY

Berthoz, A. (2000). *The brain's sense of movement* (G. Weiss, Trans.). Cambridge, MA: Harvard University Press. (Original work published 1997.)

Cover, T., & Thomas, J. (1991). *Elements of information theory*. New York: Wiley.

Dretske, F. (1981). *Knowledge and the flow of information*. Cambridge, MA: MIT Press.

Dretske, F. (1988). *Explaining behavior: Reasons in a world of causes*. Cambridge, MA: MIT Press.

Fodor, J. (1983). *The modularity of mind*. Cambridge, MA: MIT Press.

Fodor, J. (2000). *The mind doesn't work that way: The scope and limits of computational psychology*. Cambridge, MA: MIT Press.

Shannon, C. E., & Weaver, W. (1949). *The mathematical theory of communication*. Urbana, IL: University of Illinois Press, 1949.

INHERITANCE

Artificial intelligence. — The notion of *inheritance* in knowledge representation first began to develop in the field of semantic networks, where it was used for organizing information into inheritance hierarchies of the type *sort-of* or *kind-of* ($\rightarrow$ INFORMATION, REPRESENTATION, SEMANTIC NETWORK). Since then, inheritance has become a fundamental part of object representation and object-oriented programming ($\rightarrow$ OBJECT). In an inheritance-based system, concepts are classified hierarchically: the most general concepts dominate the more specialized ones ($\rightarrow$ CATEGORIZATION, CONCEPT). For example [*vehicle*] can be seen as a more general concept than [*automobile*] and as a more specialized concept than [*physical object*]. This type of classification is found in all large-scale knowledge-representation systems (such as Douglas Lenat and Ramanathan Guha's CYC systems or Thomas Gruber's Ontolingua) ($\rightarrow$ KNOWLEDGE BASE).

Inheritance is a form of inference that can be formulated as follows: if *A* is a kind of *B* and *B* has property *P*, then *A* also has property *P*. Thus if [*nurses-its-young*] is a property of [*mammal*], then [*rodent*], a kind of [*mammal*], also possesses this property (→ LOGIC, REASONING AND RATIONALITY). The reasoning process is obviously transitive, so the [*nurses-its-young*] property will be assigned to the concept [*mouse*] because it is a kind of [*rodent*]. But inheritance is not limited to this type of systematic reasoning. It can also be used to express a form of reasoning by default, like that often associated with typicality, which can be stated as follows: if concept *A* is a kind of *B* and if *B* typically has property *P*, then *A* will also have property *P* unless explicitly stated otherwise. For instance, one can say that *birds typically fly*. This means that the property [*ability-to-fly*] is a property assigned to [*bird*]. Although canaries normally inherit this feature, the same is not true of ostriches, which do not fly. All it takes to stop the inheritance process is to state that ostriches are unable to fly. This type of reasoning is prevalent in commonsense knowledge, where most properties are in fact typical but not true in all cases (another example is a table, which typically has four legs, unless it is a pedestal table or a three-legged table).

When a concept inherits directly from one concept at a time, the inheritance is called *simple*. In this case, the set of concepts forms a tree: the most general concept is located at the root and the most specialized concepts are the tree's "leaves." This is how plants and animals are organized in Carolus Linnaeus's classification. But simple inheritance is often too restrictive to describe complex or poorly structured domains (→ DOMAIN SPECIFICITY). *Multiple inheritance* overcomes this drawback by allowing a concept to inherit from several others. A set of concepts is then described in a noncyclical graph, as in most large knowledge-representation systems.

Some investigators have attempted to formalize the idea of inheritance by defining what is called a *subsumption* relation (William Woods and James Schmolze). Starting from a formal language, term *A* in that language is said to subsume term *B* if the set it denotes includes the set denoted by *B*. For example, the concept [*mouse*] subsumes all more specific concepts such as [*mouse whose color = black*]. In this framework, inheritance corresponds to the process that determines the set of conditions enabling one to know whether a given term subsumes a given other term.

Despite its utility in knowledge representation, inheritance cannot be used to account for all forms of reasoning, whether the task is to describe relationships between properties other than by means of classification, or to describe complex inferences. In addition, even though the idea of classifying things seems very natural, classifications prove to be quite difficult when the number of concepts is high, due to the inconsistencies that inevitably arise. In this case, other representation techniques must be used to organize the knowledge.

JACQUES FERBER

SELECTED BIBLIOGRAPHY

Gruber, T. R. (1993). A translation approach to portable ontology specifications. *Knowledge Acquisition, 5*, 199–220.

Lenat, D., & Guha, R. V. (1989). *Building large knowledge-based systems: Reference and inference in the Cyc project*. Reading, MA: Addison-Wesley.

Lenzerini, M., Nardi, D., & Simi, M. (Eds.). (1991). *Inheritance hierarchies in knowledge representation and programming languages*. New York: Wiley.

Woods, W. A., & Schmolze, J. G. (1992). The KL-ONE family. In F. Lehmann (Ed.), *Semantic networks in artificial intelligence*. Oxford, England: Pergamon Press.

INTENTIONALITY

Philosophy. — This medieval term was reintroduced into contemporary philosophy by Franz Brentano to refer to the "aboutness" property of mental states—the fact that they are about objects and states of affairs. *Intentionality* can thus be regarded as a property of mental states, the property of representing states of affairs in the world, whether already realized (as in beliefs, whose content is about the state of the represented world) or to-be-realized (such as desires, whose content is about a state the world would ideally attain) (→ BELIEF, DESIRE, REPRESENTATION). However, the states represented are not necessarily ones that actually exist in the world, nor are they necessarily even possible. One might wish to meet Santa Clause, or even believe that 4 + 3 = 9. In other words, one can misrepresent a state of affairs. Paradigmatic cases of intentional states are propositional attitudes (→ PROPOSITIONAL ATTITUDE). The most widespread forms of intentionality in the animal world are certainly those related to perception and action (→ ACTION, ANIMAL COGNITION, PERCEPTION), whose intentional content might be nonpropositional, that is, imagistic or preconceptual (→ MENTAL IMAGERY, PROPOSITIONAL FORMAT). Contrary to classical views like Edmund Husserl's, which see intentionality as a property of conscious acts of representation, today's understanding of intentionality generally holds it to be independent of any awareness of the content of thought (→ CONSCIOUSNESS).

While Brentano regarded intentionality as a feature that differentiates the physical world from the mental world (and the sciences of nature from the sciences of the mind), a number of contemporary philosophers are striving to *naturalize* it, that is, give it a causal explanation that is acceptable in the sciences of nature (→ NATURALIZATION). *Teleosemanticists* such as Fred Dretske and Ruth Millikan have made the most radical attempts to naturalize mental contents. They explain the *representational capacity* of certain states of the brain as a special *function* those states have acquired through the relationships they allow to be established with external states of affairs (→ FUNCTION).

According to Dretske, a mental state has a certain representational function (for instance, it represents the presence of food) by virtue of the fact that it has been selected (by operant conditioning, for example; → LEARNING) to control a behavior that is driven by the information it naturally carries (→ CONTROL, INFORMATION). Information is seen as an omnipresent, natural relation that does not necessitate the presence of an interpreter: whenever a nomological correlation exists between two states of affairs, the later state indicates or conveys information about the earlier state. This theory runs up against several obstacles, only the most obvious of which will be mentioned here. First, its distinction between the causal role supposedly played by the historically acquired representational content of mental states and the causal role of the neurophysiological states that control behavior is problematic (→ CAUSALITY AND MENTAL CAUSATION). Second, recourse to operant conditioning runs the risk of circularity if it requires the use of a representational capacity.

Millikan proposes understanding our representational capacity in terms of the concept of biological function, for which she offers an etiological analysis. What she calls an *intentional icon* is a device whose biological function is to map to the world. This articulate device acts as a mediator between a producer that does the mapping, and a consumer-interpreter that utilizes the icon to meet the organism's needs (→ INTERPRETATION). One advantage of this analysis is that it explains misrepresentation as a case of dysfunction; the normative character of representations is derived from the etiological character of function acquisition (→ NORMATIVITY). The main shortcoming of this view is that it does not tell us what the representational capacity consists of, because it lacks (and rejects as irrelevant) a causal analysis of the dispositions upon which functions are based.

The term *intentionality* in the technical sense (meaning representational capacity) must not be confused with the terms *intention, intension,* and *intensionality.* An intention, say the intention to work, is a particular representational state aimed at guiding action. *Intension* refers to a term's conceptual content, as opposed to its *extension,* that is, the individuals it subsumes (→ CATEGORIZATION, CONCEPT). Intensionality is a property of languages (called *intensional languages*) by virtue of which coreferential terms cannot be substituted for each other without modifying the truth value of the sentence in which they occur; it is opposed to the property of *extensional languages*, where this type of *salva veritate* substitution is always possible (→ LANGUAGE, LOGIC).

JOËLLE PROUST

SELECTED BIBLIOGRAPHY

Brentano, F. (1995). *Psychology from an empirical standpoint* (L. McAlister, Ed; A. Rancurello, D. B. Terrell, & L. McAlister, Trans.). London; New York: Routledge. (Original work published 1924.)

Dretske, F. (1998). *Explaining behavior: Reasons in a world of causes*. Cambridge, MA: MIT Press.

Jacob, P. (1997). *What minds can do: Intentionality in a non-intentional world*. New York: Cambridge University Press.

Lyons, W. (1995). *Approaches to intentionality*. New York: Oxford University Press.

Millikan, R. (1984). *Language, thought, and other biological categories*. Cambridge, MA: MIT Press.

INTERACTION

Linguistics. — Verbal or nonverbal *interaction* between individuals (conversation, dialogue, discussion, controversy, but also exchanging looks or gestures) can be regarded as either the locus of the actualization and manifestation of preexisting human organization principles or as a privileged place where social, cognitive, and linguistic forms are constructed, where they emerge (→ COMMUNICATION, CONSTRUCTIVISM, EMERGENCE, LANGUAGE, SOCIAL COGNITION). This second, interactional or interactionist view has interested philosophers as varied as Francis Jacques and Jürgen Habermas, and has been studied empirically in several disciplines of the human sciences. It has led to conceptions of language and cognition that do not focus on the representation of references and hence on the relationship between words and things (→ SENSE/REFERENCE), but rather on the establishment of intersubjective relationships and hence on the construction of public versions of the world linked to actions in context (→ ACTION, CONTEXT AND SITUATION). This approach reformulates a number of questions about social relations and social order, child socialization and learning, and the emergence of grammar (→ GRAMMAR, LEARNING).

Interaction, particularly face-to-face interaction, can be regarded as the primary place where social relations are formed, ratified, and transformed. Social order is not achieved through the straightforward sharing of values, norms, knowledge, or beliefs; rather, it is constructed through constant renegotiation (→ BELIEF, NORMATIVITY). Interaction is an elementary form of sociability, but its underlying processes contribute to structuring more complex forms of social organization. According to George Herbert Mead and *symbolic interactionism* (→ SYMBOL), the social world is not a factual given; it is formed, in interaction, by the local production of sensible actions. In *ethnomethodology*, social order depends on how the mutual intelligibility of actions and the objectivation of the social world are accomplished interactively in real situations.

Children interacting with their mother and/or father, and then with other children or adults, initiate and pursue their socialization and learning, in particular of language. At a very general level, interaction constitutes a place and a means for learning (→ COGNITIVE DEVELOPMENT): through coordination and exchange with more competent individuals in the course of socially situated activities, the child, the learner, or the novice is able to exhibit capacities and knowledge that surpass his or her individual possibilities. This is what Lev Vygotsky called the *zone of proximal development* (see also studies by Jerome Bruner). In this view, learning cannot be reduced to the internalization of preexisting knowledge, but is instead achieved through participatory production processes that, being linked to a singular context of practice, generate objects of knowledge that are flexible, contingent, and new. As such, these processes are more like collective improvisation than like the passive recording of knowledge on the part of an isolated subject (→ DISTRIBUTED INTELLIGENCE).

Interaction is the prototypical place for putting language to use: a language is not simply actualized as a system of preexisting potentialities; it is configured, reworked, and transformed by the elaborations of speakers as they adjust to each other and adapt their activity to the context (→ PRAGMATICS). In other words, the resources made available by the grammar are not merely exploited in different ways that depend on current goals and contexts: grammar takes shape within interactive processes and is thus organized socially, since it is formed in and by the contributions of participants during linguistic exchange.

Thus, whether with respect to cognition, socialization, or language, the interactionist approach is not limited to regarding interaction as a place for the observation of certain phenomena; it argues that the interactional dimension contributes to determining how those phenomena are organized. Hence the importance of describing the principles governing interaction, seen as a collective, ordered activity based on alternating speech turns, local handling of sequentiality, and coordinated production-interpretation by the participants, whose resources are elaborated and utilized in an indexical way (→ INTERPRETATION, ORAL).

Interactions are organized around *turn-taking* (a process also found in areas unrelated to speech, such as lines at the bank or post office, board games, cars crossing an intersection without traffic lights): the ordered nature of conversation is based on the fact that the conversers speak one at a time and each in turn, that is, according to a system of synchronization and coordination. The way this turn-taking system operates, as described by Harvey Sacks, Emmanuel Schegloff, and Gail Jefferson, is defined by two features: (1) the fact that speaking turns are structured to contain potential completion points where another speaker can take the floor, and (2) techniques for transferring the speaking turn to the other person. Procedures aimed at locating the moment when the next turn can begin, and determining who the next speaker will be, are devised by the participants using verbal devices; for example, a speaker may employ a syntactic structure that accepts additional phrases on the right in order to prolong his speaking turn ($\rightarrow$ SYNTAX) as well as nonverbal indicators such as looks or gestures.

The participants in a conversation organize the pathway of the interaction in situ, one turn at a time. Their respective speaking turns have both a prospective and a retrospective impact on the developing conversation, due to the constraints they impose on the upcoming sequence and the interpretations of preceding turns they manifest. The speakers modify the sequentiality of the conversation in an after-the-fact way by making references to earlier statements, or by backtracking to points in the conversation where a misunderstanding, a difficulty, or a mistake is sensed. "Repair" techniques allow them to identify the problem and offer a solution.

The most spectacular manifestations of coordination and collaboration in action are found in phenomena such as unison replies, listener-oriented planning with projections and anticipations, and the coproduction of a single utterance in two successive parts by different speakers. The actors work continuously to produce and interpret the observable forms toward which they are aiming, and which they analyze as the development of reciprocities. This work is contextual: the paths are not fully defined in advance by rules or conventions, nor are they entirely shared by the participants. On the contrary, they are built in a flexible and local way, with ongoing tuning in to the context and to the perspectives of others, while leaving room for repairs as the action unfolds. Thus, an interaction can be said to *coconstruct* its progression, its objects, and its resources, which are not predetermined and do not pertain to the intentionality of any one speaker. In this way, the contributions of each participant define the overall route of the interaction: through retakes and transformations achieved by chaining or contesting, the topics of the current conversation take shape through contrasts; through negotiations about the form of an expression, the right word to use, or the meaning of a term, the language itself is remolded.

With the interactional approach, then, one can show that the forms, objects, relationships, and categories ($\rightarrow$ CATEGORIZATION) that enter into any interaction are constantly undergoing a process of elaboration, reformulation, repetition, or subversion. Their sedimentation into seemingly autonomous entities is the fruit of iterations and changes that ratify and reinforce, but that also shift social structures, cognitive schemas, and the language system.

LORENZA MONDADA

SELECTED BIBLIOGRAPHY

Bruner, J. S. (1983). *Child's talk: Learning to use language*. New York: W. W. Norton.

Bruner, J. (1990). *Acts of meaning*. Cambridge, MA: Harvard University Press.

Knapp, M., & Daly, J. (Eds.) (2002). *Handbook of interpersonal communication* (3rd ed.). London; Thousand Oaks, CA: Sage.

Knapp, M., & Hall, J. (2001). *Nonverbal communication in human interaction* (5th ed.). Australia; US: Wadsworth/Thomson Learning.

Ochs, E., Schegloff, E. A., & Thompson, S. A. (Eds.). *Interaction and grammar*. Cambridge, England: Cambridge University Press, 1997.

Van Dijk, T. A. (1997). *Discourse as social interaction*. London: Sage.

Vygotsky, L. (1986). *Thought and language* (Rev. ed.; A. Kozalin, Trans. and Ed.). Cambridge, MA: MIT Press.

INTERPRETATION

Linguistics. — The term *interpretation* is employed in cognitive science to refer to very different concepts, depending on the discipline and the paradigm. In artificial intelligence (AI) and philosophy, the predominant acceptation comes from logical semantics (→ SEMANTICS), where a crucial distinction is made between *semantic interpretation* and *syntactic interpretation* (→ SYNTAX). Semantic interpretation maps a truth value to each proposition in a formal system (→ LOGIC). A proposition is said to be valid in a formal system if it receives the value *true* in all interpretations. Syntactic interpretation makes the meaning of a proposition be the result of a transcoding process. This obviously implies that the syntactic and semantic levels are separate, but also that the interpreted language and the transcoding language are compatible (→ LANGUAGE).

In linguistics, the syntactic view leads us to define interpretation as the transcoding of the "natural" language into an artificial language, a process that poses a number of unresolved theoretical problems. It is not surprising, then, that for an author like Richard Montague, (intensional) semantics is a carbon copy of syntax.

Quite often (e.g., in knowledge representation), the concept of interpretation takes on a broader meaning: the formulas in the language of representation become meaningful when related to a domain of objectivity or ontology (→ DOMAIN SPECIFICITY, REPRESENTATION). In this case, interpretation is the assignment of a *referent* (→ SENSE/REFERENCE).

In pragmatics, especially cognitive pragmatics, interpretation is the transition from the literal sense of an utterance to its derived sense (→ PRAGMATICS, SENSE). The transition is achieved by a series of inferences that, according to Dan Sperber and Deirdre Wilson, are driven by a principle of *relevance* whereby any ostensive act of communication transmits the presumption of its own optimal relevance (→ COMMUNICATION, RELEVANCE). Like any irenic principle, the principle of relevance establishes a regime of clarity. The more processing effort an utterance requires, the less relevant it is judged to be. At the word level, pragmatics ensure lexical uni-vocity (→ LEXICON). The modified version of Occam's razor principle, which we owe to Paul Grice, stipulates that one should avoid assigning multiple meanings to an expression (→ MEANING AND SIGNIFICATION). Accordingly, words have a single meaning but several senses, which are derived by pragmatic principles in keeping with usage, and the context is not determined on the basis of the situation, but depends on how consistent it is with the principle of relevance posited a priori (→ CONTEXT AND SITUATION).

In cognitive semantics, interpretation is understood to mean compre-hension, and consists mainly in specifying the relationships between *types* and *tokens* (→ TYPE/TOKEN). The problem of interpretation is posed in two main ways. At the word level, the idea is to match the lexical sense to a prototype: the prototype does not necessarily subsume it because the token may be a "deviant" (→ CATEGORIZATION). At the sentence or text level, the idea is to match the to-be-interpreted element to a relevant schema or con-ceptual framework: this is what in cognitive semantics is called the *frame problem* (→ FRAME PROBLEM, TEXT). In both cases, there is pattern match-ing much like that found in AI. But one difficulty arises: if all interpreta-tions are recognitions, then how can one account for the fact that people can interpret words and utterances for which the prototype and conceptual framework are unknown?

The problem of interpretation is posed in very different ways, depend-ing on whether comprehension is defined as the recognition of old knowl-edge or the elaboration of new knowledge (→ CREATIVITY). In the latter case, interpretation can be redefined in terms of how and in what ways the tokens are different from the types, or even in terms of how the types are generated or reconfigured by the tokens.

Opposed to the logical understanding of interpretation is a rhetorical-hermeneutic conception that is based not on logic but on the human and social sciences of psychology, sociology, and anthropology. Fundamen-tally, interpretation is seen as a pathway through a text or a semiotic per-formance (→ SEMIOTICS). This involves four factors that are lacking in the syntactic and logicosemantic views of interpretation: a situated subject-interpreter, a social practice, and hence, an action and a temporality (→ ACTION, TIME AND TENSE).

Since about the mid-1980s, following studies like those by Hubert Dreyfus and then Terry Winograd and Fernando Flores, the topic of inter-pretation has been reconsidered and developed in totally different terms borrowed from contemporary philosophical hermeneutics (Edmund Husserl, Martin Heidegger). This line of inquiry has not become an estab-lished trend, but the general ideas of *phenomenology* have been taken up by various authors who claim allegiance to constructivism or situated cog-nition (→ CONSTRUCTIVISM). In place of the definition of interpretation as the matching of concepts to objects (→ CONCEPT), these authors substitute the idea that sense emerges from the subject's flow of consciousness and of bodily experience (on this point, references to Maurice Merleau-Ponty's existential phenomenology have proliferated) (→ CONSCIOUSNESS, EMERGENCE). In linguistic semantics, one can link this line of inquiry to the appearance of phenomenological issues in work by authors as varied as Ray Jackendoff and Mark Johnson. Much remains to be accomplished, however, before a phenomenology of language is devised that satisfies the needs of linguistic description.

FRANÇOIS RASTIER

Philosophy. — In the philosophy of mind, the problem of interpretation amounts to knowing how to identify the content of the mental states of others: on the basis of what criteria are mental states attributed (→ REASONING AND RATIONALITY, SOCIAL COGNITION, THEORY OF MIND)? Accordingly, any theory of interpretation should both state the attribution criteria and assess whether such an attribution is theoretically justified, that is, if it correctly identifies the contents of others' thoughts. A number of philosophers, such as Donald Davidson and Dan Dennett, argue that the very idea of arriving at a single correct interpretation does not make sense, due to the fact that a mental state is nothing more than the product of an interpretation (*interpretivist theory*). Others, such as David Lewis and Jerry Fodor, argue that subjects possess an at-least-partially innate folk psychological theory, through which they interpret the beliefs and desires of others (*theory-theory*) (→ BELIEF, DESIRE). Still others, such as Alvin Goldman, contend that subjects do not have an internal representation of an ordinary (or folk) psychological theory, but predict the behavior of others by modeling internally—as if it were their own—the situation as experienced by the to-be-interpreted subject. This is how they are able to simulate the decisions of others (*projectivist theory*).

Interpretivism follows from adherence to Willard Quine's conception of *radical translation*, extended in the present case to radical interpretation, that is, the attribution of mental states to a subject by an observer. (Thus, for example, linguistic anthropologists are in a radical translation situation when they have to write a translation manual of an unknown language spoken by a linguistically isolated community.) As Quine showed, all possible observations of verbal and nonverbal behavior are compatible with systems of mutually incompatible analytic hypotheses (proposals for translation that give the intentional content of those behaviors). It follows from this, as Davidson and Dennett stressed, that, in reality, there are no objective facts about what someone means; such facts are always relative to an interpreter. Davidson also argues that the indeterminacy of interpretation is limited by the application of a normative principle called the *principle of charity*, by virtue of which one must agree that most beliefs of the subject being interpreted have to be true and consistent for interpretation to be possible (→ NORMATIVITY, TRUTH).

JOËLLE PROUST

SELECTED BIBLIOGRAPHY

Davidson, D. (1984). *Inquiries into truth and interpretation*. New York: Oxford University Press.
Dennett, D. (1987). *The intentional stance*. Cambridge, MA: MIT Press.
Dreyfus, H. (1979). *What computers can't do: The limits of artificial intelligence* (Rev. ed.). New York: Harper & Row.
Dreyfus, H. (1992). *What computers still can't do: A critique of artificial reason*. Cambridge, MA: MIT Press.
Dreyfus, H., & Dreyfus, S. (with Athanasiou, T.). (1986). *Mind over machine: The power of human intuition and expertise in the era of the computer*. New York: Free Press.
Quine, W. (1960). *Word and object*. Cambridge, MA: MIT Press.
Winograd, T., & Flores, F. (1986). *Understanding computers and cognition: A new foundation for design*. Norwood, NJ: Ablex.

INTROSPECTION

Philosophy. — People seem to know "immediately" much of what they are thinking and feeling at any particular time: they seem to be able to "see within" or *introspect* their own minds (→ MIND). However, neither the nature nor the extent of this ability is well understood. Many philosophers (for example, René Descartes) have claimed that there is some sort of "logical" connection between a mental state and a person's ability to introspect it. But others (for example, Gottfried Leibniz) have thought there were many reasons to believe that there were "unconscious" mental processes not accessible to introspection (→ CONSCIOUSNESS). This latter hypothesis was made scientifically plausible in the work of Sigmund Freud and has become something of a commonplace in contemporary linguistics and cognitive psychology. The latter discipline presumes that most of the cognitive processes responsible for people's intelligent behavior are not introspectible.

Fairly direct evidence of discrepancies between introspections and the mental processes supposedly introspected was reviewed by Richard Nisbett and Timothy Wilson. People have been shown to be susceptible to a wide range of cognitive factors that they are not only unable to introspect, but whose presence they will often introspectively deny. For example, asked to choose among an array of socks, 75 percent of subjects will choose the rightmost pair, even though all the pairs are in fact identical. When asked why they chose as they did, the subjects report a variety of considerations, all of which can be shown to be irrelevant, and, when asked about the effect of position, will emphatically deny that it was relevant at all. Nisbett and Wilson argue that what people take to be a special process of introspection is no more than an effort to make sense of themselves in much the same way as they might of anyone else (see Wilfred Sellars for a similar hypothesis).

Nisbett and Wilson's article stimulated a great deal of reaction, the most systematic of which is the work of Lars Ericsson and Herbert Simon, who try to develop a detailed computational theory of the mechanisms of introspection ($\rightarrow$ COMPUTATIONAL ANALYSIS), distinguishing, for example, material that is in fact immediately available in short-term memory for report ($\rightarrow$ MEMORY) from material that must be retrieved from long-term memory, and from speculative hypotheses about mental function ($\rightarrow$ FUNCTION).

What all such research underscores is a logical point: even if some things can be known by introspection, it does not follow that we can know introspectively just which things those are. Knowing what we can know introspectively may itself be knowable only by developing a nonintrospected theory of the structure of the mind.

GEORGES REY

SELECTED BIBLIOGRAPHY

Ericsson, L., & Simon, H. (1993). *Protocol analysis: Verbal reports as data*. Cambridge, MA: MIT Press.

Freud, S. (1915/1984). The unconscious. *On metapsychology: The theory of psychoanalysis*. London: Penguin.

Hurlburt, R. & Heavey, C. (2001). Telling what we know: Describing inner experience. *Trends in Cognitive Sciences, 5*, 400–403.

Nisbett, R., & Wilson, T. (1977). On telling more than we can know. *Psychological Review, 84*, 231–259.

Sellars, W. (1956). Empiricism and the philosophy of mind. In P. Feyerabend & G. Maxwell (Eds.), *Minnesota studies in the philosophy of science* (Vol. 1) (pp. 253–329). Minneapolis, MN: University of Minnesota Press.

Varela, F., & Shear, J. (Eds.). (1999). *The view from within: First-person approaches to the study of consciousness*. Thorverton, England; Bowling Green, OH: Imprint Academic.

K

KNOWLEDGE ACQUISITION

Artificial intelligence. — Knowledge acquisition is studied in several disciplines of the cognitive sciences, particularly in psychology, where the topic is addressed in research on learning and cognitive development (→ COGNITIVE DEVELOPMENT, LEARNING) using a symbolic and/or connectionist approach (→ COGNITIVISM, CONNECTIONISM, SYMBOL). In artificial intelligence, the utility of a *knowledge-based system*, or KBS (→ KNOWLEDGE BASE), depends for a large part on the richness and quality of the knowledge it contains. The construction of a KBS thus necessitates acquiring knowledge specific to a given *domain of application* (→ DOMAIN SPECIFICITY). However, it is not easy to elicit knowledge from experts in the field, precisely because they are usually completely unaware of most of the mechanisms underlying their expertise (→ CONSCIOUSNESS, INTROSPECTION). It is therefore important to have methodologies and tools to assist in acquiring this knowledge.

Approaches to knowledge acquisition have evolved considerably. The process was first seen as a knowledge extraction task whose goal was to transfer the real knowledge of experts into a knowledge base in the form of *production rules* of the type: *IF the situation exhibits a certain characteristic, THEN execute a certain action* (→ ACTION). Knowledge was acquired by means of interviews of experts and data collection.

The difficulties encountered using this method gradually converted the task into a *modeling* process that produced a conceptual model of the application (→ MODEL). The model acts as a formal intermediary, a sort of common ground shared and understood by all individuals working on the application, including the expert in the domain, the cognitive scientist, and the computer programmer. With this new perspective, the objectives and methods of knowledge acquisition changed: the focus was now on the nature of the knowledge gathered, its specificity relative to the problem-solving process (→ PROBLEM SOLVING), and its organization using modeling primitives. Different generic methods for problem solving were identified and modeled, along with their links to the major types of tasks (diagnosis, design, etc.) and the role played by domain knowledge in their implementation.

Once the methods and tasks shared by different applications are determined and abstract descriptions of domain knowledge and reasoning processes are produced (→ REASONING AND RATIONALITY), existing models can be reused. A complementary approach consists in giving the KBS the ability to acquire new knowledge automatically. This is done by applying *automatic learning algorithms* capable of taking examples (and counterexamples) and producing new rules or new concepts (→ AUTOMATISM, CONCEPT). The integration of modeling and automatic learning techniques is a promising route toward achieving incremental and global knowledge acquisition in the future.

MARIE-CHRISTINE ROUSSET

SELECTED BIBLIOGRAPHY

Debenham, J. (1998). *Knowledge engineering: Unifying knowledge base and database design.* Berlin, Germany; New York: Springer-Verlag.

KNOWLEDGE BASE

Artificial intelligence. — In artificial intelligence, a *knowledge base* is not a piece of software, but a body of compiled information to be used by a computer program, the *inference engine*. Together, they form what is called a *knowledge-based system* (KBS).

A KBS is designed to accomplish a particular task (for example, diagnosis, design) in a given *domain of application* (for example, automobile mechanics, medicine) (→ DOMAIN SPECIFICITY). The essential characteristic of a KBS is that it manipulates domain-specific knowledge represented in a knowledge base separately from the procedures developed to utilize it, which are assembled in the inference engine.

The main assumption underlying the construction of a KBS is that knowledge plays a major role in problem solving (→ PROBLEM SOLVING). In fact, it turns out that the performance and competence of a KBS stem more from the size and quality of its knowledge base than from the powerfulness of the general problem-solving techniques installed in its inference engine.

Building a knowledge base involves *modeling* and *representing* knowledge (→ MODEL, REPRESENTATION) in view of its utilization by the reasoning

mechanisms located in the inference engine (→ REASONING AND RATIONAL-
ITY). Knowledge modeling requires identifying and characterizing the various kinds of knowledge at play and the different properties in each case.
The medium used for such a model is a notation system whose most essential feature is readability and understandability by the different human
users involved in developing the KBS.

Representing this knowledge requires translating it into a *formal system*
suited for processing by a computer. This step is called *symbolic encoding*
because the coding process is achieved using symbols (→ SYMBOL) and the
reasoning done on the coded knowledge can be mechanized in the form of
symbol-manipulating algorithms. There are many formalisms for representing knowledge. They vary in the syntax used to define what statements
are legal, and in the semantics or interpretations given to those statements
(→ INTERPRETATION, SEMANTICS, SYNTAX). A property generally required of
any formal knowledge-representation system is that it must be *declarative*:
it must permit the expression of statements that represent pieces of knowledge, without specifying how those statements are to be utilized. Most
formalisms are based on logic (→ LOGIC): the statements are formulas to
which one can associate a formal semantics, and the reasoning performed
on those formulas corresponds to the *inference rules* of a deductive system.
The inference algorithms, which produce new statements from existing
ones, are implemented in the inference engine.

Difficulty going from the model of a body of knowledge to its representation is rooted in the problem of striking a balance between the expressive
power of the formal system (→ EXPRESSIVENESS), the validity of the associated inferences, and the fit between the representation and the model.

Knowledge bases generally bring together large quantities of piece-
meal knowledge. For each particular problem, the inference engine must
retrieve the relevant information for the problem at hand and organize it in
view of finding a solution. Precompilation of the knowledge base is done
before executing the KBS in order to convert the data into a format the inference engine can process. For example, one might index the knowledge
base to make useful data items easier to identify during execution. One
might also draw a dependency graph that brings out certain sequential relationships among elements stored in the knowledge base. Such partial orders can be exploited during KBS execution in order to optimize the
process that generates the deductive chains needed to solve the problem.

In the first KBSs, called *expert systems,* all knowledge was represented
in the same way, namely, as *production rules* that express useful associations between the properties of a problem and the elements of its solution.
It was believed that such knowledge could easily be acquired by merely
asking experts in the domain. This simple but powerful idea gave rise to
many operational systems in the early 1980s. But at the same time, it raised

new questions related to problems acquiring knowledge ($\rightarrow$ KNOWLEDGE ACQUISITION) and producing explanations ($\rightarrow$ EXPLANATION), and system robustness. This led to extensive research on second-generation expert systems, which led to a more sophisticated kind of KBS. Instead of the uniformity that characterized both the knowledge and the representations in the early expert systems, the problem-solving knowledge compiled in these new systems could be heterogeneous, and so could the formalisms employed to represent it. Today's KBSs are becoming increasingly rich in terms of the knowledge modeled, and increasingly complex in terms of the formal representation systems utilized and the reasoning mechanisms associated with them.

MARIE-CHRISTINE ROUSSET

SELECTED BIBLIOGRAPHY

Debenham, J. (1998). *Knowledge engineering: Unifying knowledge base and database design*. Berlin, Germany; New York: Springer-Verlag.

Levesque, H., & Lakemeyer, G. (2000). *The logic of knowledge bases*. Cambridge, MA: MIT Press.

L

LANGUAGE

Psychology. — In its initial stages, research on *language processing* in experimental psychology (see also → ORAL, READING, TEXT, WRITING) was largely inspired by the development of formal linguistic theories such as Noam Chomsky's *generative-transformational grammar* (→ GRAMMAR). Despite the immediate impact of this theory on the first research conducted in psycholinguistics, it quickly became clear that the formal description proposed in linguistics could not be envisaged as a relevant characterization of the mental representations and cognitive operations at play during language processing (→ REPRESENTATION).

It is important to note, however, that the doubt cast on approaches aimed at integrating a particular linguistic model into psycholinguistic models of language processing does not imply that psycholinguistic research can disregard descriptive linguistics (see *linguistics* below). In fact, taking linguistic descriptions into account is a prerequisite to any serious attempt to devise a model. Note simply on this point that numerous studies, both on language perception and language production, have shown that the way subjects process language is highly constrained by the structural properties of the language they speak.

To address the issue of language processing, it is useful first to describe the essential properties of this type of processing. Two basic although apparently contradictory functional properties have been brought to bear: *automaticity* and *flexibility* (→ AUTOMATISM). The automatic nature of language processing is manifested principally by the fact that the underlying operations are generally very rapid, irrepressible, and inaccessible to conscious inspection (→ CONSCIOUSNESS, INTROSPECTION). For example, when a sequence of letters that form a word is presented visually, quasiimmediate and irrepressible access to the word's meaning occurs (→ MEANING, PERCEPTION). The same holds true for a sequence of words that form a sentence: the meaning of the whole sentence comes directly to mind. Flexibility of processing refers mainly to the fact that the interpretation of a word or a statement is closely tied to its context of utterance (→ CONTEXT AND SITUATION).

The existence of these two properties, automaticity and flexibility, has given rise to two separate approaches in psycholinguistics, an *autonomous* or *modular* approach proposed in particular by Kenneth Forster and Merrill Garrett mainly to account for processing automaticity (→ MODULARITY), and an *interactionist* approach, first defended by William Marslen-Wilson and aimed more at accounting for processing flexibility. According to the modular view, distinct language processing components are associated with the different *levels* of structural description proposed by linguists: phonological, lexical, syntactic, semantic, and pragmatic (→ LEXICON, PRAGMATICS, SEMANTICS, SYNTAX). This approach postulates the psychological relevance of the notion of level in language representations and hence language processing. However, contrary to a widespread idea, it does not assume a serial organization for processing at the different levels. The interactionist approach, on the other hand, posits that various kinds of information at different levels interact more or less freely during processing. This means that decisions made at a given level can be affected by information coming from any other level (→ INFORMATION). An extreme version of this approach completely denies the relevance of the concept of processing level.

Variations on these two positions coexist today in some domains. However, it is probably in the area of *sentence processing* that the two perspectives have triggered the greatest number of studies. In the sentence-processing research, the modularity hypothesis leads to the postulate that the syntactic organization of a sentence is calculated solely on the basis of its structural properties, whereas the interactionist hypothesis suggests that other kinds of information of a lexical, semantic, and/or pragmatic nature also enter into the calculation. This sharp opposition was clearly a major driving force in the development of this line of research, but it is no longer debated today. It now seems well established that information of various kinds can have a bearing on sentence processing. This does not mean, though, that all types of information act freely and without constraints.

A current empirical endeavor is to determine exactly when and how phonological, lexical, syntactic, semantic, and pragmatic sources of information contribute to language perception, comprehension, and production. To answer this question, psycholinguists have devised experimental procedures with more or less indirect, real-time measures capable of informing us about the nature of these language processes as they are actually taking place. It is clear that relying on introspection is no help at all in this do-main, since most of the mental operations and representations at play are not accessible to conscious inspection. Only the final outcome can be so.

As the language-processing research evolved, hybrid models ranging from more modular ones to more interactive ones emerged. Some of these theories assume an initial stage of sentence processing where all potential structural patterns are generated in parallel. Then one of the candidates is selected on the basis of lexical, semantic, and pragmatic information (→ ACTIVATION/INHIBITION). In this case, the model is autonomous only during the pattern-generation phase. More generally, the earlier an opera-tion takes place and hence the closer it is to the signal, the greater its chances of being automatic, irrepressible, and so on. This idea is often ex-pressed by saying that linguistic identification processes are modular whereas interpretation processes are *nonencapsulated* (→ INTERPRETATION).

Regarding the semantic interpretation of sentences, a variety of proposals have been made, some derived from theories of prototypes or semantic net-works, others from postulates revolving around the concept of sense (→ CAT-EGORIZATION, SEMANTIC NETWORK, SENSE). Only the componential approach, which sees the meaning of words as being determined by a set of semantic features, has given rise to a relatively large body of research. Theories of meaning have been applied the most in the area of sentence verification.

However, the study of language processing cannot be reduced to sen-tences alone. *Text processing* is an important branch of contemporary psy-cholinguistics. This issue has mainly been addressed in the framework of Philip Johnson-Laird's theory of *mental models* (→ REASONING AND RATIO-NALITY). According to this theory, the interpretation of a sentence depends first of all on a propositional representation that is calculated automatically (→ PROPOSITIONAL FORMAT). Then procedural semantics comes into play to derive a mental model of the situation from the representation.

Text comprehension is regarded as a dual process in which the subject integrates the information found in the various constituents of the text and then builds a text model based on his or her general knowledge. Compre-hension thus depends to a large extent both on how coherent the text is, that is, on the nature of the links that connect the different parts to each other, and on its plausibility relative to the subject's prior knowledge. Plau-sibility in this sense is based on a representation of the text's content that is not a linguistic semantic one but a representation of a state of the world.

Finally, let us stress that language processing under ordinary communi-cation conditions (→ COMMUNICATION) requires the consistent and effective use by the subject of many kinds of knowledge (linguistic, encyclopedic, pragmatic, situational, etc.). It can be studied only by relying on a funda-mentally multidisciplinary approach, and in this respect, this research field undeniably poses a major challenge for the cognitive sciences. Despite some interesting attempts to model discourse processing (→ DISCOURSE) and the conditions of language usage, these areas remain largely unexplored from an experimental standpoint.

JUAN SEGUI

Neuroscience. — The ability to master language, a faculty specific to the human species, is an extremely complex process that necessitates the participation of a large number of *functional subsystems* (→ COMPUTATIONAL ANALYSIS). We shall look here at the contribution of cognitive neuroscience to the study of language production and comprehension (→ ORAL, READING, WRITING). Current research into brain-language relationships is showing more and more often that these two aspects of language mastery are tightly intertwined.

The wide variety of language disorders observed after an acquired brain lesion, called *aphasias*, reveals the complexity of this faculty and the large number of cerebral regions it involves (→ LOCALIZATION OF FUNCTION, NEUROPHYSCHOLOGY). The two major forms of aphasia traditionally distinguished in neuropsychology are (Paul) *Broca's aphasia*, an articulation disorder manifested by nonfluent speech (→ DISCOURSE) but no comprehension problems (damage to the posterior-inferior part of the third frontal convolution of the left hemisphere, or *Broca's area*), and (Carl) *Wernicke's aphasia*, the opposite disorder involving a comprehension deficit and no articulatory problems, with fluent, sometimes logorrheic speech often accompanied by paraphasia or even jargon aphasia (lesion of the posterior part of the first left temporal convolution, or *Wernicke's area*). Broca's and Wernicke's areas—the latter being connected to the former, which it controls (→ CONTROL)—are considered respectively to be the seats of the motor and auditory images of words. Damage to both areas causes global aphasia. Other types of aphasia are *conduction aphasia* (alteration of the connection between the two areas, characterized by fluent discourse, phonemic paraphasia, trouble repeating, but no articulatory or comprehension deficit) and aphasic forms caused by damaged connections to other parts of the brain, particularly to the hypothetical "idea or concept center" (*transcortical motor aphasia, transcortical sensory aphasia, mixed transcortical aphasia*) or to the motor effector system (*pure anarthria*) or auditory receptor system (verbal deafness). Finally, there are *subcortical aphasias* (left hemispheric lesions affecting the thalamus, central gray nuclei, or certain parts of the white matter) and *amnesic aphasias* (difficulty naming, inability to find the right word or anomia → MEMORY). This wide range of dysfunctions attests to the complexity of the speech faculty. Moreover, some studies go against the classical dogma of exclusive dominance of the left cerebral hemisphere for language and suggest that the right hemisphere may be involved in functions like understanding and producing prosody, lexicosemantic aspects of language, communication pragmatics (→ COMMUNICATION, LEXICON, PRAGMATICS, SEMANTICS), and even mood processing.

It is agreed today that caution must be exercised in classifying patients into the major categories of aphasia. The extreme complexity of the many language disorders that can appear following brain damage cannot be perfectly captured by the set of symptoms characterizing a given syndrome. One of the consequences of this complexity for research in cognitive neuropsychology is that grouping patients together on the basis of these main categories and then taking averages of their performance is highly risky. The most suitable method appears to be a case-study approach.

For a number of years now, work in brain imaging has been contributing substantially to identifying and locating the subsystems of language production (→ FUNCTIONAL NEUROIMAGING). In the very first brain imaging studies conducted in the late 1980s, subjects were asked simply to look at words on a computer screen or to read the words aloud. The brain activity observed in the silent reading condition was subtracted from that observed in the reading aloud condition, revealing several regions specific to language production (including Broca's area): the primary motor cortex (M1) of the left hemisphere (in the area corresponding to the mouth), the left sylvian cortex and premotor cortex, the primary motor cortex and lateral sylvian cortex of the right hemisphere, and the supplementary motor area. The same findings were obtained when the stimuli were presented in auditory form. Additional research has shown that certain regions (including the sylvian cortex) are also activated when subjects are asked only to move their tongue and mouth without speaking, which means that these regions are involved in motor programming or motor control of the phonatory organs, not in speech production as such. What stands out from these studies is that certain regions are involved in the planning of language production, whereas others serve actually to accomplish the movements that generate the sounds.

But language production is not confined to areas located in the anterior part of the brain. It has been shown using silent verb-generation tasks (by comparison to measures of activation at rest) that several posterior regions are involved in addition to the left inferior frontal regions (such as Broca's area) and the supplementary motor area; these include the inferior medial temporal and parietal regions, which exhibit greater activation in the left hemisphere. Activity in these temporal and parietal areas is probably indicative of the involvement of a vast network responsible for lexicosemantic processing.

Although the temporal and parietal areas are indeed involved in language production, it is now known that areas supposedly specific to production, such as Broca's area, are involved as well in linguistic processing that does not explicitly concern production. For example, activation of Broca's area has been observed in tasks like lexical decision making, phoneme detection in nonwords, and detection of rhyming letters (for example, deciding whether letters such as *B*, *T*, *R*, or *H* end in the sound /ē/). Such frontal activation is most likely associated with the phonological-articulatory transcoding required by these tasks.

Language production must therefore be regarded as an extremely complicated cognitive activity involving a large number of functional subsystems, each in charge of a specific facet of the task. Any model that involves only the frontal areas is definitively outdated.

Language comprehension is also a complex faculty that offers a wide variety of possibilities for analysis. Humans are not only able to understand isolated words, no matter who the speaker is and despite considerable differences in pronunciation or accent, but can also understand combinations of words in sentences and go beyond the literal meaning of a sentence to make sense out of a metaphor. The sound waves that convey this information contain a wealth of other information, such as cues that indicate the speaker's emotional state, or even his or her age or sex (→ EMOTION). These behaviors are made possible by the interplay of an entire series of subsystems, each in charge of a particular aspect of the comprehension mechanism.

It is generally agreed that in the simplest case—understanding an isolated word pronounced correctly—auditory patterns associated with all the words a listener knows are stored in memory and the (stored) pattern that best fits the pattern generated by the perceptual stimulus is activated (→ ACTIVATION/INHIBITION, PERCEPTION). Some authors call this information store the *auditory input lexicon*. However, before the lexical entry itself is activated, the listener probably identifies the more elementary units or phonemes the word contains. Accordingly, the lexical representation (→ REPRESENTATION) would not be activated until a certain number of phonemes have been detected. The first processing phase, where individual phonemes are identified, is thought to be carried out by an auditory analysis subsystem that preprocesses the complex sound wave. Because of the many possible sources of variation in speech signals, this mandatory preprocessing stage is needed to extract fixed patterns from the signal that are insensitive to variations in pronunciation and can thereby activate the lexical units stored in memory. It is well known, for instance, that consonants like *b* and *p* in *ba* and *pa* are perceived in terms of discrete categories (→ CATEGORIZATION). Depending on the time lapse between two critical parameters, the burst of air and the beginning of vocal cord vibrations (voice onset time), either *ba* or *pa* will be perceived. There is a very fine line between these two perceptions of the sound: if the time lapse is less than 25 ms, the sound *ba* is perceived; if it is longer than that, the sound *pa* is perceived. On the other hand, temporal variations within each category (*ba* or *pa*) do not change what is perceived, which is why this critical phenomenon in speech preprocessing is called *categorical perception.*

Neuroimaging studies have provided some interesting new data on the mechanisms of language comprehension. It has been shown that at least six brain regions (including Wernicke's area) are activated when subjects simply listen to words. Four of them are in the left hemisphere: the superior posterior temporal cortex, the superior anterior temporal cortex, the temporoparietal cortex, and the anterior inferior cingulate cortex. The other two are in the temporal cortex of the right hemisphere. Note that none of these regions is activated when words are presented in the form of visual stimuli, which means that these areas are in fact specialized in the auditory processing of stimuli. Note also that when nonlinguistic stimuli are perceived, the same regions are activated (except for the temporoparietal and superior anterior temporal areas). It thus seems that preprocessing is carried out by a specific set of brain regions (probably) specialized in performing different elementary operations on the complex sound wave. One of these operations is thought to be the extraction of prosodic information.

When a lexical representation is activated in the auditory input lexicon, it may in turn activate a representation stored in a semantic system called *associative memory*, which retrieves the meaning of the word heard. Brain imaging studies have shown that the semantic processing of words necessitates the participation of various regions located in the prefrontal and temporal cortices.

OLIVIER KOENIG

Linguistics. — The following uses of the term *language* must be distinguished: (1) languages (at least 3,000 languages still exist today); (2) language as a system, as in Ferdinand de Saussure's definition, which opposes the system per se (*langue*) to its usage (*parole*); (3) language as both a general faculty of the species, in the sense of "language organ," and as an abstraction that linguists construct from natural languages to describe their general or even universal characteristics; and (4) languages or artificial symbolic systems, the best known being programming languages (see *artificial intelligence* below) (→ LOGIC).

The most fundamental of these distinctions is the one that opposes *natural* and *formal* languages, although this is still a controversial issue. Certain influential authors such as Richard Montague have contended that there is no essential difference between the two. According to Dan Sperber and Deirdre Wilson, a language is a set of well-formed formulas with a *semantic interpretation* (→ INTERPRETATION, SEMANTICS). The formulas of a language have a semantic interpretation if they are all systematically associated with other objects, say, the formulas of another language, the internal states of the language user, or real or possible states of affairs. A language is a representation system governed by a grammar (→ GRAMMAR, REPRESENTATION). In this respect, natural and formal languages cannot be differentiated; linguistic signs are not distinguishable from the symbols of formal languages (→ SIGN, SYMBOL) and therefore become meaningful only through their interpretation, that is, a term-to-term matching with nonlinguistic realities such as mental states or states of affairs.

The analogy between formal and natural languages is based essentially on a shared theoretical framework: the semiotics of logical positivism and the ensuing tripartite division into syntax, semantics, and pragmatics (→ PRAGMATICS, SEMIOTICS, SYNTAX).

According to Ronald Langacker (in 1986), the main points of agreement in contemporary linguistic theory include the following: (a) language is a self-contained system that can be characterized using algorithms and is sufficiently autonomous to be studied on its own, independently of any broader cognitive considerations; (b) grammar (syntax in particular) is an independent aspect of linguistic structure, distinct from its lexicon and its semantics (→ LEXICON); and finally, (c) its meaning is subject to linguistic analysis and is correctly described by a sort of formal logic founded on truth conditions. Langacker opposes to this the fact that grammatical structures do not constitute an autonomous formal system or level of representation: on the contrary, they are symbolic by nature and permit the structuring and conventional symbolization of conceptual content (→ CONCEPT). Lexicon, morphology (→ MORPHOLOGY), and syntax form a continuum of symbolic units that cannot be arbitrarily divided into separate components. This way of contesting the tripartite division proposed by Charles Morris and Rudolf Carnap allows for a redefinition of the economy of linguistics, and in particular the place of semantics therein.

While Langacker's contentions are generally acknowledged by researchers in cognitive linguistics (except those who are closer to the orthodox cognitivism of Chomsky or Jerry Fodor; → COGNITIVISM), cognitive linguists are in no sense unified. Those who set out to psychologize a semantics derived from formal semantics (for example, Ray Jackendoff) must be distinguished from those who, like Langacker, further widen the gap between their view and the logical conception.

While many disciplines study language, linguistics is the only one to treat languages in all their diversity. But just what do linguists study about languages? Many contemporary linguists consider the language system to be their sole object of study and argue that the diversities observed in language usage do not fall within their scope. In fact, two important simplifications follow from this. (1) The concept of a language is already a linguist's abstraction, insofar as it (legitimately) encompasses all kinds of diversity (regional, social, etc.). When one chooses to study the standardized written form of a language, in the ordinary way, one is making a normative decision fraught with consequences: descriptive linguistics is founded on an implicit norm, which is reflected by the corpus or language level chosen as the object of study (→ NORMATIVITY). Even then, the resulting uniformity masks a substantial amount of diversity. Written language indeed remains very heterogeneous, due to the highly varied kinds of writing systems used. These differences affect not only the lexicon, but also the syntax and the semantic structure of text (→ TEXT). They are an irreducible factor of diversity, even in the most standardized languages. (2) A language is not composed of one and only one system, but of several regulatory levels that are constantly interacting and evolving in different time frames. Between the rules of the language and the regularities prescribed by other norms, such as genres, there is only a difference in degree, not in nature.

In cognitive linguistics, language is an integral part of human cognition (Langacker) or is considered a "product of cognitive processes" (Catherine Harris). The etiological value given here to mental processes presupposes two theses: language is a product of thought, and language is an instrument of thought. Only a functional approach is useful here: if language is a conceptual tool of humans, then it cannot be studied in an autonomous way but must be considered relative to its cognitive functions (→ FUNCTION): interpreting, ordering, fixing, and expressing human experience (Dirk Geeraerts) (→ EXPERIENCE).

The cognitive approach to languages is driven by the postulate that language is "an open window onto cognition" (Jackendoff). Several hypotheses are explored: either languages represent a formal language, the language of thought (Fodor) (→ LANGUAGE OF THOUGHT), or languages represent an abstract space in which the cognitive operations carried out define a sort of grammar of representations (Langacker), or yet again, the invariant properties of languages provide access to the categories of the human mind (→ MIND). These invariants are described as universal structures (like predication) or as categories (accordingly, some argue that grammatical categories attest to the existence of a sort of "alphabet of thought") (→ CATEGORIZATION). In any case, universalism in language is an ongoing preoccupation.

FRANÇOIS RASTIER

Artificial intelligence. — Since the 1960s it has been possible in AI to use natural language to query databases of facts and there are systems that can solve word problems of the kind found in schoolbooks (→ PROBLEM SOLV-ING). In 1970 Terry Winograd wrote a program capable of executing complex orders expressed in English, within a simple universe, the "world of blocks." Since then, oral or written dialogue systems have been developed that make use of various kinds of knowledge about language and about the world (→ COMMUNICATION). Although we are still far from having a machine capable of truly understanding, some systems can be accredited with a basic level of comprehension.

Most of these systems break down the comprehension process into *modules*, a choice probably based on the desire to model human cognition (see *psychology* above) or perhaps simply on computer-related constraints (→ MODULARITY). When the input is in vocal format, the initial modules process the speech signal, segment it, and propose an ordered list of possible phonemes for each segment. These segments are then connected in order to make words in the lexicon (→ LEXICON). Certain systems, especially those derived from Gestalt theory and/or connectionism (→ CONNECTIONISM, PERCEPTION), perform global recognition. If the input is a text, a morphological-lexical module identifies the words by applying, for example, the inflection and conjugation rules of the language under consideration.

Given that these kinds of data are *noisy* (imperfect recognition of phonemes, spelling mistakes, typographical errors, etc.) and that languages contain homophones and homographs, these analyses generally retain several hypotheses. At this point, a syntactic model of the language is necessary (→ SYNTAX), both for choosing among the hypotheses retained and for assigning a structure to the statement to be understood. The models proposed have evolved considerably, primarily through the impact of the computer. Starting from Zellig Harris's *string grammars* and Chomsky's transformational grammars, both popular in the 1960s, the next decade moved on to William Woods's *augmented transition networks* and Alain Colmerauer's *metamorphosis grammars*, and then in the early 1980s, to *unification grammars*, the most widely used today (→ GRAMMAR). For content processing, the task is often split between a semantic module and a pragmatic module (→ PRAGMATICS, SEMANTICS), with the former generating a logical form that expresses the *truth conditions* of the utterance, that is, what must occur in the universe for the statement to be true (→ INTERPRETATION, LOGIC), and the latter modifying the result obtained by taking the context of utterance into account (→ CONTEXT AND SITUATION).

The concept of truth condition poses a number of problems. For instance, it is not easily applicable to questions. A more difficult issue is the problem of *performatives:* although stating *p* does not make *p* true, statements like *I promise p* or *I order that p* become true by the sheer fact that they are uttered. The truth conditions depend on the situation in which the utterance is made, for example, whether the utterance contains a deictic (*here*, *I*, etc.). The output of the semantic processing step is a *logical form*. Various logical forms exist. The feature of natural language that allows propositions to be reified ad infinitum (while *p* is a proposition, *the fact that p* is a term) requires us to rely on higher-order logic systems: the grammatical future and past necessitate a temporal logic ($\rightarrow$ TIME AND TENSE); the conditional imposes reference to an unrealized universe, which calls for a modal logic (possible worlds $\rightarrow$ MODALITY); intensifiers (*very*, *little*, etc.) are more readily represented in a multivalued logic, and so on. Gottlob Frege pointed out relatively early that the confusion between *sense* and *reference* leads to errors: *John thinks that the capital of Sweden is Oslo* is not deemed to have the same meaning as *John thinks that Stockholm is Oslo* ($\rightarrow$ MEANING AND SIGNIFICATION, SENSE/REFERENCE). Richard Montague proposed an *intensional logic* for overcoming this difficulty, and designed a (very partial) system that could produce an intensional-logic form for any statement. His program has since been completed, in particular by David Dowty, Barbara Partee, and others; this work is noted for its *compositionality* hypothesis, according to which the logical form of a given structure is systematically built up from the logical forms associated with its constituents. This very strong hypothesis apparently fails when the semantic structure of the sentence does not correspond exactly to its syntactic structure. For example, a sentence beginning with *Every man who owns a donkey . . .* is easy to analyze if the suspension points stand for a unary property $P(x)$ (e.g., *lives on a farm*); the first-order expression for its logical form is: $(\forall x)((MAN(x) \wedge (\exists y)(DONKEY(y) \wedge OWN(x, y))) \supset P(x))$. But if the suspension points are replaced by *beats it*, the translation is quite different: $(\forall x, y)((MAN(x) \wedge DONKEY(y) \wedge OWN(x, y)) \supset BEAT(x, y))$, which defies the principle of compositionality. The *discourse-representation structures* proposed by Hans Kamp restore this principle by postulating an intermediate level between the syntactic structure and the logical form ($\rightarrow$ DISCOURSE, REPRESENTATION). These structures also resolve certain *coreferences*, that is, they can identify the same object designated in different ways, for example, when pronouns are used.

Semantics addresses other questions, such as handling priorities between quantifiers (*many books have few readers* does not have the same truth conditions as *few readers read many books*), negation (which in language has neither the same value nor the same scope as in logic), temporal and spatial expression processing ($\rightarrow$ SPACE), plurals, and so forth. Assuming that these questions are resolved, we know how to construct a logical form from predicates that presumably express the meanings of words ($\rightarrow$ MEANING), but we do not attempt to analyze the link between the word and its predicative representation: this is a job for lexical semanticists. Around 1970 Roger Schank (for verbs) and Yorick Wilks attempted to break down the meaning of all words into semantic primitives; others took up this endeavor in different forms. Another task is deciding whether a word is polysemous, that is, whether it has more than one representation. The complexities and nuances of this issue led investigators like Alan Cruse to speak of "semidistinct" acceptations, and Robert Martin to distinguish between polysemy of sense and polysemy of acceptation.

When a word has a variety of interpretations, it is difficult to determine what comes from the word itself and what is rooted in the word's context; for the time being, the boundary line between semantics and pragmatics remains blurred. Several studies by James Pustejovsky, Geoffrey Nunberg, and others have looked at systematic variations in the meaning of a word according to the construction in which it is employed. Recourse to so-called encyclopedic knowledge to solve this problem and many others is considered to fall within the realm of pragmatics, and in spite of the work by Schank and his collaborators on scripts and MOP (*memory organization packet*), the importance of this kind of knowledge is still largely underestimated.

Pragmatics looks especially at the conventions that dictate linguistic exchanges. For instance, Paul Grice's maxims bring out the role of indirectly communicated content, or *implicatures*. Sperber and Wilson attempted to reduce these maxims to a single principle, relevance ($\to$ RELEVANCE). Finally, pragmatics accounts for the intentions of interlocutors ($\to$ THEORY OF MIND) and examines the argumentative effects of certain lexical and stylistic choices.

This overview may make it seem like language comprehension is broken up into a multitude of specific types of processing, each with its own difficulties and obstacles. In reality, the main contribution of computer scientists is to integrate all of these kinds of processing. In doing so, they necessarily run into the question of the validity of the boundaries and the partiality of the objectives they set. We have noted the cross-permeability of semantics and pragmatics; analogous observations could be made at every level, particularly between syntax and semantics.

In addition to the question of natural-language understanding, the notion of language is introduced at another level in computer science, that of programming languages. Let V be a vocabulary (a set of words). V^* is usually used to denote the (infinite) set of all sequences one can construct using elements of V. A language on V is a subset of V^*. Consider for example $V = \{child, and, cries, laughs, a\}$: V itself is a language on V, as are the empty set, the infinite set V^*, and a set made up of the two sequences $\{a$ *and child*, *laughs and and*$\}$.

As the above example shows, such a definition supplies a view of language that is much too basic to be usable. This is why an auxiliary set must be added—a "nonterminal" vocabulary for Chomsky, a set of types in other theories. The auxiliary set is used to express the constraints imposed on the sequences that belong to the language in question. Accordingly, one can assign to the elements of *V* the respective types *noun, conjunction, verb*, and *determiner*, and then introduce the type *elementary sentence* by specifying that an element of this type is a sequence formed by a *determiner*, a *noun*, and a *verb*. Finally, the type *sentence* can be (recursively) defined as consisting of sequences of the type *elementary sentence*, along with sequences made up of two elements of the type *sentence*, separated by a *conjunction*. The type *sentence* now contains an infinite number of elements (for example, *a child laughs, a child cries and a child cries and a child laughs*, etc.). A language is defined as the set of sequences that belongs to a particular type, called an *axiom* by analogy to deductive systems; here, the axiom would be the type *sentence*.

There are many formalisms that enable one to both refine the constraints a sequence must obey in order to belong to a language, and assign a structure to the legal sequences. Depending on the type of constraint, there are problems of *membership* (does a given sequence satisfy the constraints?); *vacuity* (is there at least one sequence that satisfies the constraints?); *equivalence* (do two sets of constraints determine the same language?); and *ambiguity* (are there any sequences that are mapped to two distinct structures?), which may or may not be decidable.

This formal definition is a good one for artificial languages like mathematical or logical notation. It is indispensable for programming languages. Computers execute instructions expressed as strings in the binary alphabet {0, 1}. However, writing a program made up of such instructions is tedious and inevitably error-ridden. For this reason, right from the beginning of computer science languages that could be translated into computer instructions by specialized software (interpreters and compilers) were developed. They were designed to take into account (1) human ways of thinking (user-friendly programming environments have vastly improved the productivity of programmers), (2) the type of application (users do not express themselves in the same way to query a database, assess a company's production level, or calculate upcoming changes in the weather, yet all of these modes of expression are translated into the same instructions in the end), and (3) the type of computer hardware (for example, some languages contain instructions applicable to parallel machines only). In all cases, the syntax of the languages (what character strings are legal) and their semantics (what the computer is supposed to do) must be rigorously defined.

The adequacy of this type of definition for describing natural languages is much less clear, however. In natural languages, vocabulary *V* is more difficult to delineate, and more important, it is far from evident that a language defines a partition on set *V**, that is, that an ideal "informant" can always decide whether or not a sequence of elements from *V* is acceptable in his or her language. This requirement is sometimes made more lenient by speaking of degrees of acceptability, although the procedure for measuring this degree is rarely specified. Whatever the case may be, at the present time, no one claims to have devised a formal system that can furnish a correct and complete description of any language.

DANIEL KAYSER

SELECTED BIBLIOGRAPHY

Allen, J. (1995). *Natural language understanding* (2nd ed.). Redwood City, CA: Benjamin Cummings.

Damon, W. (Ed.) (1998). *Handbook of child psychology: Vol. 2. Cognition, perception, and language* (5th ed.). New York: Wiley.

Dupoux, E. (Ed.). (2001). *Language, brain, and cognitive development.* Cambridge, MA: MIT Press.

Gazzaniga, M. (Ed.) (2000). *The new cognitive neurosciences* (Section VII, *Language*). Cambridge, MA: MIT Press.

Hauser, M. D., Chomsky, N., & Fitch, W. T. (2002). The faculty of language: What is it, who has it, and how did it evolve? *Science, 298,* 1569–1579.

Jackendoff, R. (2002). *Foundations of language: Brain, meaning, grammar, evolution.* New York: Oxford University Press.

Langacker, R. (1987–1991). *Foundations of cognitive grammar* (Vols. 1–2). Stanford, CA: Stanford University Press.

Pinker, S. (1994). *The language instinct: How the mind creates language.* New York: William Morrow.

Scovel, T. (1998). *Psycholinguistics.* Oxford, England; New York: Oxford University Press.

Winograd, T., & Flores, F. (1986). *Understanding computers and cognition: A new foundation for design.* Norwood, NJ: Ablex.

LANGUAGE OF THOUGHT

Philosophy. — The *language of thought* (LOT) is a special language (→ LANGUAGE) that has been postulated by a number of writers (Wilfrid Sellars, Gilbert Harman, Jerry Fodor) to explain how humans and many animals represent and think about the world (→ ANIMAL COGNITION, COGNITIVISM, INTENTIONALITY, REPRESENTATION). It is claimed to be coded into their brains in the way certain formal languages are coded into the circuitry of a computer. There are different theories of how these symbols possess meaning, but most of them appeal to causal relations among the symbols (which might mirror a process of inference) and/or to causal relations the individual symbols bear to phenomena in the world (for example, a symbol *S* might causally covary with snow) (→ CAUSALITY AND MENTAL CAUSATION, SYMBOL). The LOT need not be a natural language (that people use for speaking); indeed, given that the relevant sorts of intelligent behavior are displayed by many creatures that lack a natural language, such as infants and chimpanzees (→ INFANT COGNITION), its postulation need not be confined to natural language users. What makes it a language is that it possesses semantically valuable, causally efficacious logicosyntactic structure; that is, it consists, for example, of names, predicates, variables, quantifiers (*all, some*), and logical connectives (*not, and, only if*) that are combined to form complex sentences that can be true or false (→ LOGIC, PROPOSITIONAL FORMAT, SEMANTICS, SYNTAX). In this way, the LOT is superior in its expressive power to systems of pure images, for instance (→ MENTAL IMAGERY), which seem incapable of expressing logically complex thoughts (e.g., that someone doesn't love everyone).

Fodor has argued that the main reasons for believing in an LOT is that it would explain three interesting phenomena associated with the mind (→ MIND): (1) the *productivity* of thought, for people can in principle understand a potentially infinite number of different thoughts that can be formed by logical combinations of simpler ones (for example, we can go on endlessly understanding claims about the louse that lived on the mouse that had a spouse . . . that lived in the house that Jack built); (2) the *systematicity* of thought: if a person can think some thought, *p*, then he can also think all logical permutations of *p* (for example, he can think that not everyone loves someone if and only if they can think that someone doesn't love everyone); (3) the *intensionality* of thought: people can think of things in one way without thinking of them in another (for example, they can think that the morning star is Venus without thinking that the evening star is), and sometimes they can think about nonexistent things (such as the fountain of youth). According to the LOT hypothesis, these phenomena are possible because thought consists in people bearing relations to linguistic symbols that can be caused to combine and recombine in all logically permissible ways in their brains, some of which may form different representations of the same thing, others which may form representations of nothing whatsoever.

GEORGES REY

SELECTED BIBLIOGRAPHY

Fodor, J. (1975). *The language of thought*. New York: Crowell.

Fodor, J. (1987). *Psychosemantics: The problem of meaning in the philosophy of mind*. Cambridge, MA: MIT Press.

Fodor, J. (2000). *The mind doesn't work that way: The scope and limits of computational psychology*. Cambridge, MA: MIT Press.

Harman, G. (1972). *Thought*. Princeton, NJ: Princeton University Press.

Sellars, W. (1956). Empiricism and the philosophy of mind. In M. Scriven, P. Feyerabend, & G. Maxwell (Eds.), *Minnesota studies in the philosophy of science* (Vol. 1) (pp. 253–329). Minneapolis, MN: University of Minnesota Press.

LEARNING

Psychology. — *Learning* refers to a modification in the ability to accomplish a task, brought about by an interaction with the environment. It differs from a behavioral change that occurs through *maturation* (internal evolution of the organism following a developmental program characteristic of the species). The concept of learning is invoked both at the most elementary level of life (for example, behavioral plasticity of certain one-celled animals) and in sophisticated artificial systems (for example, back-propagation algorithms in connectionist networks) (→ CONNECTIONISM, NEURAL NETWORK). Obviously, it is also brought to bear in the study of human cognitive development (→ COGNITIVE DEVELOPMENT).

Two major types of learning are generally distinguished, depending on the level at which the psychological processes are integrated into the cognitive system: *elementary, stimulus-driven learning* (imprinting, habituation, classical conditioning, operant or instrumental conditioning) and *complex, representation-mediated learning* (→ REPRESENTATION, SYMBOL). The former is largely determined by the physical characteristics of the environmental stimulus and is contingent upon such factors as contiguity, repetition, intensity, and predictive value. The latter is dependent upon the meaning the subject attributes to the stimulus (→ MEANING AND SIGNIFICATION): it brings symbolic representations into play and leads to stable modifications of representations stored in memory (→ MEMORY). This is reminiscent of the theoretical opposition between *behaviorism* (elementary, stimulus-driven learning) and *cognitivism* (complex, representation-mediated learning; → COGNITIVISM). Added to this classic dichotomy is the partially redundant distinction between the *symbolic* and *connectionist* approaches to knowledge acquisition. The symbolic approach corresponds to the second type of learning described above. The connectionist approach is unique because of its ability to do without the concept of symbol. It retains the idea of a representation, that is, the meaning attributed to a stimulus, but redefines it in terms of digital patterns of activation (subsymbolic activation of elementary processors or formal neurons; → ACTIVATION/INHIBITION). Learning algorithms bring these patterns into play and cause stable modifications in the activation patterns stored in memory (memory is the very structure of the system).

In the case of elementary learning controlled by environmental stimuli, the two main mechanisms studied in animals and humans are *classical conditioning* and *operant* or *instrumental conditioning*. In classical conditioning, which we owe to Ivan Pavlov, a pair of stimuli is presented repeatedly. One of the stimuli (*conditioned stimulus* or CS) is initially neutral, in that it does not trigger a specific reaction; the other (*unconditioned stimulus* or US) triggers a characteristic reaction called the *unconditioned reaction* (UR). After repetition of the pairs a variable number of times, the first stimulus starts to trigger the same or a similar reaction to the second, called the *conditioned reaction* (CR). In operant conditioning, invented by Burrhus Skinner, a pleasant or unpleasant stimulus is presented following a specific action performed by the experimental subject. The action is called the *instrumental response* in that it determines the consecutive stimulus. Repeated pairing of the instrumental response and the consecutive stimulus, in a device specially designed for this purpose (a Skinner box), increases the probability that the subject will produce the response if the consecutive stimulus (feedback) is pleasant (reinforcement) and decreases that probability if it is unpleasant (punishment). Whenever the same action causes different effects depending on the situation, contextual stimuli that precede or are concurrent with the response, called *discriminative stimuli*, allow subjects to discern what type of situation they are in (→ CONTEXT AND SITUATION). Whether the conditioning is classical or operant, the fundamental factors of conditioned learning are *contiguity* (between the CS and the US for the former, between the instrumental response and the consecutive stimulus for the latter), *repetition* of the pairs (two stimuli, or a response and a stimulus), and *intensity* (of the US, or of the reinforcing or punishing stimulus). Another important factor is the *predictive value*, also called the *informational value* (→ INFORMATION), which, in the case of classical conditioning, is the predictive value of CS relative to US (a factor that is not to be confounded with repetition of the stimulus pair).

In the case of complex learning mediated by symbolic representations, the characteristics of the learning environment are not studied as much as are the learner, his or her prior knowledge, and the cognitive information processes implemented. Research on learning-by-doing or *learning through action* is a good example (→ ACTION). This type of learning takes place whenever knowledge acquisition can be ascribed to actions, the sources of new information. Operant conditioning is thus an example of learning through action, but according to the behaviorist view, the change it triggers is strictly limited to behavior. The cognitive approach to action-based learning looks at *problem-solving* situations (→ PROBLEM SOLVING) in which subjects have to learn artificial rules (rules of a game, sorting criteria, etc.) or natural rules (physical laws, etc.). This approach goes beyond behavior and focuses on mental strategies for action planning and the operations performed on the information taken in. When subjects base their activity on a hypothesis, they can ascribe their success or failure to that hypothesis. This same approach, centered on the organization and reorganization of memory representations, is applied to *text-based* or *picture-based learning* (→ TEXT). Studies on the mental processes carried out during this kind of learning have pointed out a number of important cognitive mechanisms: analogy, hypothesis making and testing, induction, knowledge generalization, mapping to a known case, and so forth. Note also that these mechanisms (and hence learning) are constrained by the subject's working memory capacity and selective attention resources ($\rightarrow$ ATTENTION). Research also deals with *explicit* and *implicit* learning and its metacognitive dimension ($\rightarrow$ METACOGNITION). In addition to these individual forms of learning, there are various kinds of *sociocognitive learning*, such as learning by observation, by model imitation, and by coconstruction ($\rightarrow$ INTERACTION, SOCIAL COGNITION).

Running counter to the cognitive approach to learning based on symbolic representations, the connectionist approach began to develop. In this framework, learning is described as a subsymbolic adjustment of weights assigned to arcs in a network (connections between elementary processors or formal neurons) in view of "capturing" the regularities contained in a series of examples of external input-output associations. This learning mode is implicit, inseparable from the processing machinery itself, and inaccessible to introspection or verbalization ($\rightarrow$ INTROSPECTION). Several *learning algorithms* have been proposed. Here is a simple one, the *Widrow-Hoff algorithm*, which has five steps: (1) consider the first situation and set the corresponding input units and output units; (2) add D to the weight of all connections whose input and output units are both active; (3) set the input units only; (4) evaluate the output units based on the network's initial weights; and (5) add D to the weight of all connections whose input and output units are both active. If on Step 4, the output units evaluated are the expected ones (the ones set on Step 1), then Step 5 resets that part of the network; if not, the network is modified. This is when the network learns. Other, more complex algorithms have been designed, such as the backpropagation learning procedure for multilayer networks.

Although connectionism seems to have renewed its ties with the classical view of learning in which contiguities generate connections (behaviorism), this idea is applied here with an unprecedented degree of sophistication. In addition, formal neural networks supply a new tool for modeling the relationships between maturation and learning ($\rightarrow$ MODEL). The characteristics of the networks that define the basic architecture correspond to maturation, and the changes resulting from the interaction between a network with a given architecture and its environment constitute learning. An objective of future research will be to account for the complex relationships between learning and cognition at the symbolic and subsymbolic levels.

OLIVIER HOUDÉ

Neuroscience. — In cognitive neuroscience, it is conventional to distinguish between two types of learning, according to whether implicit or explicit memory is involved ($\rightarrow$ MEMORY). Each type calls upon different brain structures.

Skill learning involves an adaptive modification of behavior achieved through task repetition. It occurs in situations such as learning to ski or mirror drawing (a common experimental task). This type of learning is considered to fall into the implicit memory category, in that it is manifested through behavior (improved performance across training sessions) and occurs without the subject's being able consciously to recollect the learning episodes. An example of implicit learning is found in amnesic patients who cannot remember learning episodes they have experienced. This type of learning probably involves the central gray nuclei, since it appears to be altered in patients suffering from Parkinson's disease or in patients with a dopamine deficiency leading to dysfunction of the striatum.

The learning that takes place in intentional memorization situations, such as memorizing a list of words, a shopping list, or a poem, is of a different nature. This kind of learning, called *intentional learning,* is considered to depend on explicit memory since it can be expressed via language (→ LANGUAGE) rather than solely through behavior, and the learner can state when and where the learning episodes took place (→ SPACE, TIME AND TENSE). Intentional learning is disrupted in amnesia, a syndrome observed in patients with brain lesions in the mediotemporal regions (particularly the hippocampus) or in the diencephalon (thalamus and mammilary body). It therefore seems to involve these brain structures, which are critical for encoding new information in memory (→ INFORMATION). It is well known today, though, that these structures are not used for information storage.

JEAN DECÉTY AND OLIVIER KOENIG

Artificial intelligence. — In 1950, even before the term *artificial intelligence* (AI) was coined, Alan Turing had already pointed out the importance of learning in the design of "intelligent" machines. According to Turing, a machine that boasts of intelligence must appear insightful in most situations it faces, even the most disconcerting ones. Yet to appear insightful, it must have at its disposal knowledge that enables it to act in an appropriate way. It must therefore possess extensive knowledge for coping with the unexpected. This means either that one must tell it everything, which is likely to be highly time-consuming, or that it must be able to learn on its own, which would be preferable. Daily experience has confirmed this: a machine that reacts in strictly the same way to every request it receives cannot be deemed intelligent.

The crux of AI is the study of the mechanisms likely to enable a machine to make good use of its experience, that is, to learn (→ EXPERIENCE). This line of research is aimed first and foremost at building machines capable of adapting and acting more efficiently, but that is not all. Another AI task is simulating certain aspects of human or animal learning; such simulations improve our understanding of the learning process (see *psychology* above). Note that designing machines to help humans learn does not fall directly under what is conventionally called learning in AI; it is preferable in this case to refer to *computer-assisted teaching*.

Despite their common goal to acquire knowledge (→ KNOWLEDGE ACQUISITION), the functions and mechanisms of learning are multiple and varied. For simplicity's sake, let us begin by distinguishing four major learning functions. (1) Learning involves *memory storage and organization* such that memories can be retrieved at the opportune time (→ MEMORY). (2) Learning involves the *acquisition of concepts*: when given different examples and counterexamples of a category (for example, *table, scalpel, carburetor*), a very general function is launched to differentiate between the examples and the counterexamples in each category (→ CATEGORIZATION, CONCEPT). (3) Learning is based on the *compilation of know-how*. A task executed several times is accomplished faster, since the same errors are not made and the same hesitations are no longer needed. Accordingly, once it has executed a task, a machine should be in a position to draw from its experience in order to work more quickly. (4) Finally, like human beings, a machine should be capable of *inventing* new theories to explain or summarize a body of facts or a series of events. This is the most difficult operation of the mind to figure out, and the most exciting objective that can be set.

Attempts to simulate these four major functions rests on a number of fundamental mechanisms, which can be implemented on a computer. The crucial operation common to all learning mechanisms is *generalization*, a process that takes examples (points in a representation space; → REPRESENTATION) and generates a function (→ FUNCTION) that in turn partitions the representation space on the basis of a given criterion. Generalization techniques vary: first, according to the structure of the representation space, for example, Boolean, discrete, continuous, or first-order logic (→ LOGIC); second, according to whether the examples are input all at once or one by one (the latter property of learning systems is called *incrementality*); and finally, according to the potential metaphors employed to describe them, such as neural networks, genetic algorithms, and so forth (→ ARTIFICIAL LIFE, CONNECTIONISM, NEURAL NETWORK).

Symbolic learning utilizes examples described in either *extended propositional logic* or *first-order predicate calculus*. In the first case, the learning process proceeds by constructing decision trees or sets of production rules and calling upon procedures like those used in data analysis. The general principle is to eliminate specific features and save common features. For example, the two descriptions *Color-Flower-Yellow & Narcissus* and *Color-Flower-White & Narcissus* are generalized as *Narcissus*. In this framework, the originality of symbolic learning, as compared to data analysis, lies not only in its use of formal knowledge-representation systems, which are more than just simple data tables, but also in its introduction of knowledge that is implicit in the descriptions. Continuing with the above example, if the system knows that a daffodil is a yellow narcissus, it will be able to generalize the descriptions *Daffodil* and *Color-Flower-White & Narcissus* to *Narcissus*.

When the examples are described in first-order logic, the generalization process not only eliminates specific features but also performs a *matching* operation that pairs similar elements. To grasp the role of matching, imagine two bouquets of flowers, one containing white narcissus and yellow roses and the other containing white roses and daffodils. Two generalizations are permitted here: the bouquets can be characterized in terms of their color, white or yellow, or in terms of the type of flowers in them, roses or narcissus. Each of these generalizations corresponds to a particular matching: the white narcissus are matched with the white roses and the yellow roses with the daffodils in the first bouquet, and the white roses are matched with the yellow roses and the white narcissus with the daffodils in the second.

The generalization of structured objects represented in first-order logic or in some other more or less equivalent formalism is specific to symbolic learning only. This type of generalization has given rise to many formalizations in recent years. However, symbolic learning does not address questions of incrementality from the practical standpoint; most of the time, the examples are given all at once. A totally different situation exists for the *gradient-backpropagation technique,* which adjusts the synaptic weights of multilayer formal neural networks by taking into account the discrepancy between the actual response obtained and the desired response. The success of these learning techniques is responsible for the renewed interest in the connectionist approach, initially derived from the cybernetic trend, that began in the 1980s.

Also worth mentioning are techniques called *adaptive learning,* particularly those customarily called *genetic algorithms* (in artificial life), first developed by John Holland in the early 1970s. To begin, a population of individuals in charge of accomplishing various tasks in response to stimuli is simulated. Every individual in the population is endowed with a "genetic makeup" that defines its particular character. A procedure tests the adaptiveness of each individual by evaluating the relevance of its responses. Following a series of experiences, those least-adapted disappear and the best-adapted reproduce by giving birth to individuals whose genetic makeup results from cross-breeding or mutation of the genetic makeup of their ancestors (see also → NEURAL DARWINISM). After a few generations, the population must be adapted to the tasks it was assigned.

In the end, though, not everything can be learned. First, for a machine to learn, it must have examples described in a language (→ LANGUAGE), which is always heavily loaded with implicit meanings. In this same vein, all learning algorithms make use of additional knowledge one might call *learning biases*, which must be learned but are not specifically taught. Some of this knowledge is explicit (for example, the fact that a daffodil is a yellow narcissus); some is implicit and results from the parameter configurations or settings of the learning system. Finally, there are formal limitations on machine learning, due to the algorithmic complexity of the procedures. These theoretical limitations are being studied by specialists of formal learning theories (or *learnability*).

JEAN-GABRIEL GANASCIA

SELECTED BIBLIOGRAPHY

Bechtel, W., & Abrahamsen, A. (2002). *Connectionism and the mind: Parallel processing dynamics and evolution* (2nd ed.). Oxford, England: Blackwell.

Byrnes, J. (2001). *Cognitive development and learning in instructional contexts* (2nd ed.). Boston: Allyn & Bacon.

Goldberg, D. (1989). *Genetic algorithms in search, optimization and machine learning*. Reading, MA: Addison-Wesley.

Kandel, E., Schwartz, J., & Jessell, T. (Eds.) (2000). *Principles of neural science* (Section IX, *Language, thought, mood, learning, and memory*) (4th ed.). New York: McGraw-Hill/Appleton & Lange.

Kayser, D., & Vosniadou, S. (Eds.) (1999). *Modelling changes in understanding* Amsterdam; New York: Pergamon Press.

Marcus, G. (2001). *The algebraic mind: Integrating connectionism and cognitive science*. Cambridge, MA: MIT Press.

Mitchell, T. (1997). *Machine learning*. New York: McGraw-Hill.

Schunk, D. (1999). *Learning theories: An educational perspective* (3rd ed.). Upper Saddle River, NJ: Prentice Hall.

LEXICON

Linguistics. — The lexicon is an important object of study, not only in linguistics but also in the philosophy of language, cognitive psychology ($\rightarrow$ LANGUAGE), anthropology, and the communication sciences ($\rightarrow$ COMMUNICATION). The common ground in these disciplines is that they all treat words as signs and examine the relationships between them ($\rightarrow$ SIGN). Although acknowledged as important, the lexicon is nonetheless a vague concept, even for linguists. It ranges from being a set of partially regular forms to a set of representations of content structured by ill-defined laws that differ across authors ($\rightarrow$ REPRESENTATION).

Etymologically speaking, the term *lexicon* means "list of words," that is, a glossary or vocabulary. The oldest views of the lexicon see it as a nomenclature or list of words, mostly nouns. The characteristic feature of nomenclatures is the one-to-one correspondence they establish between the things being referred to and the names used to refer to them: each thing possesses one and only one name, and each name corresponds to one and only one thing. The methods used today in dictionary making are still strongly marked by this tradition. A second, more recent understanding of the lexicon sees it as a set of items organized into a system. This postulate is found in Ferdinand de Saussure's work, but it in fact goes back to the Aristotelian tradition with its taxonomic understanding of the lexicon (→ CATEGORIZATION). This view was taken up in particular by Carolus Linnaeus in his famous zoological taxonomy. Debates revolving around this conception generally concern how the lexicon is organized: Are words organized into strict hierarchies (as in Porphyry's tree) or into trellis-like structures? If one agrees that the lexicon is an arboreal or circular system, it follows that it is structured by, and reducible to, a finite set of distinctive features and relationships between the elements of the system. This approach raises the additional question of degree of membership (→ INHERITANCE). Terminologists, for example, prefer a taxonomic model with absolute membership only.

In the third conception, any lexicon is a reconstruction in which both text and context are disregarded (→ CONTEXT AND SITUATION, TEXT). This view draws from the functional models developed in phonology and grammar (→ FUNCTION, GRAMMAR). The difficulty of achieving such a reconstruction is evident: the phonological and grammatical systems of English contain forty or so phonemes and a hundred or so grammatical categories, respectively; these figures are nothing next to the number of words (simple and complex) in the lexicon, which easily exceeds a half a million if we include only the most common technical terms. However, if we give up on the idea that the lexicon is one large system that forms a unit and search instead for small local systems, some structural principles show up. Each local system is made up of reciprocally related words, in such a way that the sense of each one is dependent upon that of the others and a change in one engenders a change in all the others (→ DOMAIN SPECIFICITY, MEANING AND SIGNIFICATION, SEMANTICS). These microsystems are called *lexical fields* or *semantic fields*. The commonly used example is the lexical field pertaining to kinship. Starting from the linguistic formants *grand, great*, and *in-law*, and the basic terms *father, mother, son*, and *daughter*, one can define the semantic field of kinship using three criteria: generation, not-blood-relative, and sex. In a sociolinguistic study, one can then compare the lexical fields of kinship across languages.

Lexical fields are organized on the basis of morphological (→ MORPHOLOGY), semantic, and social criteria, among others (some examples of lexical fields are the names of colors, military ranks, means of transportation, varieties of seats, etc.). To define such an organization, the lexical senses of words are broken down into primitive elements or *semes*, and each item in a given lexical field is defined in terms of whether these semes are present or absent. For example, the lexical field relating to seats can be defined using the semes */back/, /arm(s)/, /feet/, /designed for one (or more)* *persons/*, and so on. The word *stool* is thus defined as a seat without a back or arms that has feet and is designed for one person. This *differential* analysis must not be confused with *componential* models, in which signified concepts are defined independently of each other in terms of referential features (Jerrold Katz and Jerry Fodor).

Although it is agreed that *lexicology* is the science of the lexicon, that is, the scientific study of lexical structures, and that *lexicography* is the technique of making dictionaries, the debate about what constitutes a *word*, the basic linguistic unit to be considered by the lexicographer, is not fully resolved. A word is defined as a meaningful unit that is always identifiable as such and can be used in commutation tests. The term *lexeme* is also readily employed here. This definition goes against the more common one in which a word is a unit coded graphically by a space to the right and to the left. Some authors make the distinction between *full* or *content* words (nouns, verbs, adjectives, adverbs, etc.) and *empty* or *function* words (prepositions, articles, etc.). The former are said to pertain to *lexical semantics*, and the latter, to *grammatical semantics*. Only full words are represented in semantic networks, for example (→ SEMANTIC NETWORK). A remaining question concerns the boundary between the lexical unit coded graphically and the lexical unit defined semantically; for example, lexical units that are larger than one word (like *floating-point arithmetic*) or smaller than one word (*proto-* in *protoplasma, -tic* in *phonetic*). Lexemes can be simple (for example, *program*), compound (*character-recognition program*), or complex (*execute a program*). In this context, a *morpheme* is the smallest meaningful unit uttered, that is, the immediate constituents of a word (for example, *cats* is composed of two morphemes, *cat-* and *-s;* the first is a lexical morpheme and the second is a grammatical morpheme).

All lexical units can be described by at least three sets of features: phonological, syntactic (→ SYNTAX), and semantic. The last set is traditionally presented in the form of a dictionary definition, and some linguists have even contended that it is the only complete form in semantic analysis; in any case, it is certainly the most common.

Lexicology is currently exploring some new lines of research dealing with *lexicon-grammars* and the use of computer tools and electronic lexica. The notion of lexicon-grammar is founded on the idea that the smallest meaningful unit is not the word but rather the elementary sentence (subject-verb-essential complements). The data in lexicon-grammars are mainly destined for use in automatic text analysis. As for the computer, while it plays an undeniably positive role in the preparation phases of traditional dictionaries (automatic searching, sorting, knowledge representation, etc.) and in developing tools for their use (CD-Roms, Internet, remote querying, on-line dictionaries), its contribution is not so clear cut when it comes to automated tools for lexicon processing and text generation, as attested by the problems encountered in machine translation.

GABRIEL OTMAN

SELECTED BIBLIOGRAPHY

Altmann, G. (Ed.) (1998). *Cognitive models of speech processing: Psycholinguistic & computational perspectives on the lexicon.* New York: Taylor and Francis.

Greimas, A. (1983). *Structural semantics* (D. McDowell, R. Schleifer, & A. Velie, Trans.). Lincoln: University of Nebraska Press. (Original work published 1966.)

LOCALIZATION OF FUNCTION

Neuroscience.— *Localization of brain function* refers to the assignment of functions to particular regions of the brain (→ FUNCTION). The question of cerebral localization partially overlaps with the more fundamental problem of the relationship between body and mind (→ DUALISM/MONISM, MIND). Historically, the first step was the discovery of the brain's role in controlling the organism (ancient Egypt) (→ CONTROL) and in intelligence (ancient Greece). Already by the Galenic era, investigators were trying to distribute the different aspects of mental activity across the regions of the brain. But methods were lacking. It was not until the Renaissance, with studies on anatomy, and the classical era, with the anatomical-clinical correlations observed in brain-damaged patients, that reliable evidence began to surface.

In the seventeenth century, Thomas Willis was the first to make the connection between intelligence and wrinkles on the cerebral cortex. The notion of brain area finally emerged in the nineteenth century. After Franz Gall's unsuccessful attempts (with his *phrenology*, or study of the "bumps of the skull"), experimental studies on animals and clinical studies on humans began to lay the groundwork for localizing the functions of the brain. Paul Broca, who related a speech impairment to a restricted part of the left hemisphere (→ LANGUAGE), was responsible for a radical change in the localization research by being the first to accurately apply this approach to a specifically human function (→ NEUROPSYCHOLOGY). By the end of the nineteenth century, two opposing views had developed: the first, prolocalization, attempts to define the link between an elementary unit of anatomy (a brain area or structure) and an element of mental activity (a function); the second, antilocalization, tries to bring these elements back together in order to reestablish the (lost) unity of the brain and behavior.

Today, the use of functional brain imaging techniques—especially positron emission tomography (PET) and functional magnetic resonance imaging (fMRI)—is renewing the issue of localization of function with unprecedented technical precision (→ FUNCTIONAL NEUROIMAGING). Most of the results have partially confirmed the validity, for normal subjects, of the localization data established earlier in clinical neuropsychology for brain-damaged patients (for example, *Broca's area* for word production), while nonetheless suggesting that there are networks or neural circuits spanning several brain regions for each function studied.

ÉRIC SIÉROFF

SELECTED BIBLIOGRAPHY

Clarke, E., & Dewhurst, K. (1996). *An illustrated history of brain function: Imaging the brain from antiquity to the present* (2nd ed. rev. and enl.). San Francisco, CA: Norman Publishing.
Frackowiak, R., Friston, K., Dolan, R., Mazziotta, J., & Frith, C. (Eds.). (1997). *Human brain function*. San Diego, CA: Academic Press.
Kertesz, A. (Ed.) (1994). *Localization and neuroimaging in neuropsychology*. New York: Academic Press.
Kosik, K. (2003). Beyond phrenology, at last. *Nature Reviews Neuroscience, 4*, 234–239.
Posner, M. L., & Raichle, M. E. (1994/1997). *Images of mind*. New York: Freeman.
Shallice, T. (1988). *From neuropsychology to mental structure*. New York: Cambridge University Press.

LOGIC

Artificial intelligence. — The adjective *logical* applies intuitively to reasoning that conforms to good common sense (→ REASONING AND RATIONALITY), whereas the noun *logic* (examined here) refers to a science that has only a tenuous relationship to commonsense reasoning. Technically speaking, a logic is defined by an (artificial) *language* (→ LANGUAGE), a *deductive system*, and a *truth-value calculus* (→ TRUTH). Logic is an essential tool not only in artificial intelligence (AI), but also in other cognitive sciences (in particular, psychology, linguistics, and philosophy) (→ LOGICISM/PSYCHOLOGISM).

The most elementary language of logic, the language of *propositions*, is based on an alphabet made of letters denoting propositions (p, q, r, etc.), the symbols ¬ (negation) and ∧ (conjunction), and parentheses. A *formula* in the language is a letter, a negated formula, or the conjunction of two formulas, with parentheses serving to delineate the formulas. For example, p, $q \wedge \neg r$, and $\neg (p \wedge \neg r) \wedge q$ are three formulas in the language. Abbreviation conventions extend the language. For example, if f and g are formulas, the formula $\neg (f \wedge \neg g)$ is abbreviated as $f \supset g$ (read: f implies g).

A deductive system S is defined by formulas of the language, axioms, and operations (called *inference rules*) that take formulas as their input and produce formulas as their output. For example, the operation called *substitution*, which replaces all occurrences of a given letter by a given formula, is an inference rule in many deductive systems. Another common rule is *modus ponens:* given two formulas, one stating $f \supset g$ and the other being f itself, the *modus ponens* operation outputs the formula g.

The *proof* of a formula f in a deductive system S is a sequence of formulas whose last formula is f. Each formula in the sequence is either an axiom of S or the result of an inference rule of S applied to some of the formulas that precede it in the sequence. Accordingly, in any deductive system S that has the formula $p \supset (q \supset p)$ as one of its axioms and the above operations (substitution and *modus ponens*) as inference rules, the sequence

(1) $p \supset (q \supset p)$
(2) $(q \supset (p \supset q)) \supset (p \supset (q \supset (p \supset q)))$
(3) $q \supset (p \supset q)$
(4) $p \supset (q \supset (p \supset q))$

is a proof of $p \supset (q \supset (p \supset q))$.

Indeed, Step 1 is an axiom of S; Step 2 is obtained from Step 1 by substituting $q \supset (p \supset q)$ for p and p for q; Step 3 is obtained from Step 1 by substituting q for p and p for q; Step 4, which is the formula to prove, is obtained by *modus ponens* from Step 2, which has the form $f \supset g$ (if we take f to be $q \supset (p \supset q)$ and g to be the formula to prove), and from Step 3, which is indeed f. A formula for which a proof exists in S is called a *theorem* of S.

In the same way as abbreviations make formulas in the language easier to read, proofs are made simpler by using *derived inference rules*, also called *metatheorems*. For example, in many deductive systems, one can demonstrate that for any pair of formulas f and g, if f and g are theorems, then $(f \wedge g)$ is also a theorem.

A deductive system S is said to be *consistent* if there is no formula f such that both f and $\neg f$ are theorems of S. It is said to be *decidable* if there exists an algorithm which determines, for any formula f, whether f is a theorem of S in a finite amount of time ($\rightarrow$ COMPLEXITY).

Calculating the truth value of a formula f requires an interpretive framework ($\rightarrow$ INTERPRETATION). In the case of propositional logic, an interpretive framework I is merely a mapping from the alphabet of letters into the set $\{true, false\}$. According to the definition of the language, there are three cases to consider: (a) f is a proposition letter; in this case, the truth value of f is $I(f)$; (b) f is the negation of formula g; then the value of f is *true* if and only if the value of g is *false;* (c) f is the conjunction of two formulas g and h; f has the value *true* if and only if the values of g and h are *true*.

A formula f is called *valid*, denoted $\models f$, if and only if it takes on the value *true* in all interpretations. This is the case of $\neg (p \wedge \neg p)$. Indeed, if $I(p) = true$ by (a), the formula p will have the value *true;* by (b), $\neg p$ will have the value *false;* and by (c) $p \land \neg p$ will have the value *false*, so applying (b) again will give *f* the value *true;* but if $I(p) = false$, a similar reasoning process can be used to show that *f* will also have the value *true*.

A formula *f* is a *consequence* of a set of formulas *E*, denoted $E \mid = f$, if any interpretation that makes all formulas in *E* true also makes *f* true. In particular, if *E* contains two opposing formulas *g* and $\neg g$, every formula *f* is a consequence of *E*.

A deductive system *S* is *correct* if every theorem of *S* is a valid formula. One can easily verify that this holds in the example above. A deductive system *S* is *complete* if the reciprocal of this property is true, that is, if every valid formula is a theorem of *S*. (Note that the word *complete* has another meaning in logic, which will not be used here: a set of formulas *E* is called complete if for any formula *f* in the language, either *f* is in *E*, or $\neg f$ is in *E*.) The above system is not complete.

Since 1910, when Bertrand Russell and Alfred Whitehead published their *Principia mathematica*, many correct and complete deductive systems have been developed for propositional calculus. These systems are decidable insofar as a formula is a theorem in these systems if and only if it is valid, and the validity of a formula can be tested in a finite amount of time. More stringent systems of proofs have since been designed, such as Luitzen Brouwer's *intuitionist proofs*, where it is illegal to conclude *f* if one can only show that $\neg f$ is false, and Alan Anderson and Nuel Belnap's *relevance proofs*, in which all premises must actually be "used," and so forth ($\rightarrow$ RELEVANCE).

Propositional logic is far from being capable of expressing all types of commonsense reasoning, for it cannot examine the content of the propositions it manipulates. For example, *Paul is a man*, *Pierre is a man*, and *Easter falls on a Sunday* are three different propositions, but nothing in this logic allows us to consider the first two closer to each other than the last. One way to "get inside" and see the content of propositions is to change logics.

The language of *first-order logic* is richer: its alphabet contains symbols for *functions*, *predicates* (also called *relation symbols*), *variables*, and a *quantifier* $\forall$ ($\rightarrow$ FUNCTION). Each function symbol or relation symbol is assigned a nonnegative integer, called its *arity*, which indicates how many arguments it has (for example, equality is a binary relation, so its arity is 2). A function with an arity of 0 is a constant. A term is either a variable symbol or a function symbol of arity *n* accompanied by *n* terms. A formula can be a relation symbol of arity *n* accompanied by *n* terms, a negated formula, the conjunction of two formulas, or an expression of the form $(\forall x) f$ where *x* is a variable symbol and *f* is a formula.

To interpret this language, a universe of objects, *U*, must be specified. The interpretation assigns an application $I\phi$ of U^n into *U* to each function symbol ϕ of arity *n*, and a subset I_R of U^n to each relation symbol R of arity n. Finally, each variable is assigned an element of U. Term t is interpreted by the element $I(t)$ of U, calculated as follows: if t is a variable, $I(t)$ is given by assignment; if t is a function, ϕ, accompanied by the terms $t_1, \ldots, t_n$, $I(t)$ is the result of the application I_ϕ, given arguments $I(t_1), \ldots, I(t_n)$.

The truth value $v(f)$ of a formula f is obtained in the following manner: if f is a relation R accompanied by $t_1, \ldots, t_n$, $v(f)$ is *true* if and only if element $I(t_1), \ldots, I(t_n)$ of U^n belongs to the subset I_R. Negation and conjunction are treated as in propositional logic. Finally, $v((\forall x) f)$ is *true* if and only if $v(f)$ is *true* no matter what element of U is assigned to x.

Like propositional logic, first-order logic has correct and complete deductive systems (Kurt Gödel in 1930). However, these systems are only *semidecidable*, that is, there exist algorithms that, when given formula f as input, conclude in a finite amount of time that f is a theorem of the system, if indeed it is; but for certain formulas that are not theorems, the execution of the algorithm never finishes.

If one wishes to specify not only the properties of objects, but also the properties of relations between objects, a higher-order logic must be defined. Gödel showed that there could not exist deductive systems that are both correct and complete in these higher-order logic systems.

Other interesting extensions have been introduced at various times. Classical logic recognizes only the modalities *true* and *false* for qualifying propositions, whereas some kinds of reasoning require a much wider range of modalities ($\rightarrow$ MODALITY). The most useful distinctions are the *alethic* modalities (*necessary, possible*), the *deontic* modalities (*obligatory, permissible*), the *temporal* modalities (*past,* single or multiple *future*; $\rightarrow$ TIME AND TENSE), and the *epistemic* modalities (*known* or *assumed to be true* by one or more agents; $\rightarrow$ EPISTEMIC), and possibly to varying degrees (fuzzy logic; $\rightarrow$ FUZZY). At first (with Clarence Lewis in 1918–1932), a modal logic was a simple language equipped with a deductive system but devoid of truth calculations. It was not until 1960 that Jaako Hintikka and Saul Kripke proposed a suitable calculus based on "possible worlds." This concept, together with λ-calculus, was taken up by Richard Montague to devise his *intensional logic*, often used to study natural language semantics.

Jean-Yves Girard's work in 1987 led to the definition of a logic called *linear logic* in which propositions act as "consumable" resources. This opened new doors for modeling cognitive processes such as planning, syntactic analysis, and so forth ($\rightarrow$ MODEL, SYNTAX).

However, an obstacle to using logic in the cognitive sciences is the problem of proofs. Any proof of f in a deductive system S that takes a set A of formulas as axioms is, ipso facto, a proof of f in any deductive system S' whose set of axioms includes A. This property of a logic is called *monotonicity.* Yet it often happens that formula f is seen as a consequence of set E

but is no longer so for set E' that includes E. For example, from E = {John took the train at 9:47 from the downtown station to go to Chicago, Pierre took the train at 9:47 from the downtown station to go to Chicago}, one will conclude f = John and Pierre travelled in the same train. But from E' = $E \cup$ {there are two trains that leave the downtown station at 9:47 in the direction of Chicago}, one will not draw the same conclusion. One might refuse to use the term *logic* to refer to this notion of consequence, but it remains nonetheless necessary to model the very widespread form of reasoning it describes.

This was the very task the designers of *nonmonotonic logic* set out to accomplish in the late 1970s. In 1980 Raymond Reiter proposed a logic of reasoning by default, in which consequences were calculated using a fixed-point equation; at the same time, John McCarthy, who relied on the idea of "preferred model," arrived at quite a different way of calculating the "extension" of a theory. Many other systems were developed during the 1980s. In 1990 Sarit Kraus, Daniel Lehmann, and Menachem Magidor proposed that nonmonotonic deducibility be studied in its own right, independently of the system employed to calculate consequences.

Logic was initially aimed at expressing only atemporal truths. Several ideas were then proposed that enabled logicians to overcome this limitation. In first-order logic, for example, nothing prevents one from introducing a temporal variable t. If a relation between a and b can evolve over time, a ternary relation symbol R is chosen to represent it, and the formula $(\forall t)\,(t_1 \leq t \leq t_2 \supset R(a, b, t))$ means that a and b are related during time interval $[t_1, t_2]$. As we have seen, with modal logic one can express more qualitative notions like the future and the past, which are often easier to manipulate. More specific logics have focused on the notion of *action*, defined as a process (instantaneous or durable) that changes the truth value of certain propositions ($\rightarrow$ ACTION). However, determining these changes ($\rightarrow$ FRAME PROBLEM) is a delicate task that has recently inspired many theoretical studies on revision. By generalizing the techniques introduced to handle temporality, some authors have proposed a logic of spatial reasoning ($\rightarrow$ SPACE).

Finally, inputting formula f into deductive system S can initiate a process to determine whether or not f is a theorem of S. We can therefore draw an analogy between expressions in a logic language and expressions in a programming language, both aimed at triggering algorithms. This idea gave birth to logic programming and the well-known language PROLOG created in 1972 by Alain Colmerauer. The logic used is a subset of first-order logic, but with certain allowances that deviate from classical logic (for example, *NOT f* is considered to be true, not if f is false but if all attempts to prove f fail). This type of language is often used in cognitive science and nicely resolves the problem of the tradeoff between expressing the inference principles in a declarative way and achieving algorithmic efficiency.

DANIEL KAYSER

SELECTED BIBLIOGRAPHY

Gabbay, D., & Guenther, F. (Eds.) (2001). *Handbook of philosophical logic* (2nd ed.). Boston: Kluwer.

Gabbay, D., Hogger, C. J., & Robinson, J. A. (Eds.). (1993–1998). *Handbook of logic in artificial intelligence and logic programming.* 5 vols. New York: Oxford University Press.

Kraus, S., Lehmann, D., & Magidor, M. (1990). Non-monotonic reasoning, preferential models, and cumulative logics. *Artificial Intelligence, 44,* 167–207.

Mendelson, E. (1997). *Introduction to mathematical logic* (4th ed.). London: Chapman & Hall.

Priest, G. (2001). *An introduction to non-classical logic.* New York: Cambridge University Press.

Whitehead, A., & Russell, B. (2002). *Principia mathematica to *56* (2nd ed.). New York: Cambridge University Press.

LOGICISM/PSYCHOLOGISM

Psychology. — Logicomathematical *formalization* is a heuristic tool for psychologists; it helps them "manage things" and put their thoughts in order. This pragmatic fit between psychology and logic exposes the logician to the temptation of *psychologism* (viewing the task of logic as that of describing human thought processes) (→ LOGIC) and the psychologist to the temptation of *logicism* (the view that whatever works in a formal system will work in psychology too). Formalization also raises the question of *realism* and *constructivism* (→ CONSTRUCTIVISM, REALISM): Do logicomathematical objects exist outside the human brain as an ideal representation of the universe (hence their relevance to psychology as well as to physics, biology, economics, and the like), or are they precisely the product of a symbolic neural construction of the human brain and mind (→ MIND, NUMBER)?

Dictionaries define mathematical logic as "a science of developing and representing logical principles by means of a formalized system consisting of primitive symbols, combinations of these symbols, axioms, and rules of inference" (*Webster's New Collegiate Dictionary*) (→ SYMBOL). This type of definition excludes all psychological processes and therefore corresponds to antipsychologism. However, we know that this idea has not always been the prevailing one, particularly in the nineteenth century, when mathematical logic took its first steps. Indeed, one of the fundamental books in the field, written by George Boole, was entitled *An investigation of the laws of thought*. More radically, John Stuart Mill's view states that the laws of logic are entirely derived from acts determined by the human mental makeup. The law of noncontradiction, for example, is said to be rooted in the subjective feeling that a given belief and its opposite are mutually exclusive (→ BELIEF). Opposed to this view is Gottlob Frege and Edmund Husserl's no-less-radical antipsychologism. Frege argued along two lines: because of their objectivity and public character, the laws of logic cannot derive from subjective, private representations (→ REPRESENTATION); because of their necessity, they cannot derive from representations that vary across individuals (→ DIFFERENTIATION). This analysis sees logicomathematical objects as a world independent of the mind, that of "the laws of being-true" (→ TRUTH). Antipsychologism rubs shoulders here with realism. Like Frege, Husserl rejected psychologism—with naturalism reducing logic to approximate generalities (→ NATURALIZATION)—contending that the laws of logic have an ideal, objective content that excludes all anthropological relativity, and that these laws are submitted, as they are, to consciousness (→ CONSCIOUSNESS).

Although today's mathematical logic by definition disregards both the matter to which its applies and all psychological processes, the antipsychologism advocated by Frege and Husserl is no longer in circulation today, for progress in psychology during the twentieth century has changed the problem data. As the philosopher Pascal Engel showed, novel forms of anthropological relativity have come into the picture and have defined new relationships between logic and psychology (and more broadly, between logic and the cognitive sciences). Whether it be in Piagetian theory or in *cognitivism* (→ COGNITIVE DEVELOPMENT, COGNITIVISM), introspection is outdated (→ INTROSPECTION). Without giving in to the unobservable (which behaviorism does out of rigor), the object of study is no longer confined to the subjective representations discredited by antipsychologism. Jean Piaget thus postulated the existence of endogenous processes that are common to all subjects and that, during ontogenesis, attain the different states of *logicomathematical construction* (operatory logic: operation grouping, combinatorial systems, and formal grouping structures). These processes correspond to increasingly abstract ways of structuring the predefined properties of the world. Following the same path, the classical cognitivist scheme presupposes objective representations (symbols) of a predetermined outside world, and an inference system (calculus) that transforms them. The question here is determining the extent to which the rules of this system are like those of logic (and what logic?), in the same way that, in Piagetian theory, the problem is determining the relevance of the isomorphism established between the states of the child's or adolescent's abstract constructions and the postulated logicomathematical structures. These questions, raised by the threat of logicism, have recently come into the foreground in the philosophy of mind, cognitive psychology, and cognitive neuroscience, where, as far as possible, they must be treated in accordance with the stipulations of the experimental method (→ REA-SONING AND RATIONALITY).

In its most common acceptation, the term *logicism* refers to the planned reduction of mathematics to logic. That project was defended by Frege and by Bertrand Russell but disparaged by Henri Poincaré, Léon Brunschvicg, and others, and its utopianism became apparent with Kurt Gödel's work on the intrinsic limitations of formalization. The logicism that still holds today is of another kind. It reduces the sciences of the mind to logic, or, more precisely, it interprets psychological data in reference to a fragment of logic identified as (the one and only) "logic," forgetting that it is impossible to give an unequivocal answer to the question: What is logic? Thus, as the philosopher and logician Gilbert Hottois stated, it all depends on what period is at stake, and often within that period, on what logician is under consideration.

Piaget's genetic psychology is often said to be the study of child and adolescent logic. It is in fact the study of the acquisition of a certain number of scientific concepts and of Boolean algebra, a formal system just one of whose interpretations is used in Piagetian theory: *class logic* (associated with an interpretation of propositional logic founded on the class-inclusion relation) (→ CATEGORIZATION). Logicism in this case is not as much a matter of reducing psychology to logic—which was never Piaget's goal—as it is a matter of choosing a single normative framework representing one particular way of understanding logic, and hence psychology (→ NORMA-TIVITY). As he said himself, Piaget nevertheless set out to "clean up his operatory logic," particularly by making his extensional logic evolve into an intensional logical or "logic of meanings" (→ RELEVANCE).

Concerning cognitivism, a radical logicism dominated the scene during the initial years of the cybernetic period (Alan Turing, Warren McCulloch and Walter Pitts, John von Neumann, etc.). It was a kind of logicism that is neatly summarized by the title of the original 1943 article by McCulloch and Pitts: "A logical calculus of the ideas immanent in nervous activity." This article suggests that logic is the appropriate discipline for analyzing the functioning of the brain, conceived of as a deductive machine whose constituents (neurons) embody logical principles. For instance, one can interconnect three neurons—automata whose activation status (active or inactive) indicates the logical value (true or false)—to perform the logical operation *OR*. From these theoretical analyses it was a short step to the invention of the computer, and that step was taken by von Neumann: replace the neurons with vacuum tubes or, today, with silicon chips. Mathematical logic thus asserted itself as the key formalism of cognitivism. Its instrumental accomplishments in artificial intelligence (IA) over the past few decades have supported the development of high-level programming languages such as PROLOG (PROgramming in LOGic) based on first-order predicate logic. In psychology, with the impetus of the computer metaphor, the logicomathematical roots of cognitivism led to the postulate that there exists a mental logic whose formal rules subtend reasoning processes. Raising the issue of logicism here amounts to finding out whether all valid reasoning requires the alleged mental logic. It is the task of AI research to determine whether programs based on classical predicate logic suffice for "capturing" the operations performed by the human intelligence.

OLIVIER HOUDÉ

SELECTED BIBLIOGRAPHY

Boole, G. (1854). *An investigation of the laws of thought, on which are founded the mathematical theories of logic and probabilities.* London: Macmillan.

Changeux, J.-P., & Connes, A. (1995). *Conversations on mind, matter, and mathematics* (M. B. DeBeveoise, Ed. & Trans.). Princeton, NJ: Princeton University Press. (Original work published 1989.)

Engel, P. (1991). *The norm of truth: An introduction to the philosophy of logic* (M. Kochan & P. Engel, Trans.). Toronto, Ontario; Buffalo, NY: University of Toronto Press.

Fischer, K., & Kaplan, U. (2003). Piaget, Jean. In L. Nadel (Ed.), *The encyclopedia of cognitive science* (Vol. 1, pp. 679–682). London: Nature Publishing Group, Macmillan.

McCulloch, W. S., & Pitts, W. (1943). A logical calculus of the ideas immanent in nervous activity. *Bulletin of Mathematical Biophysics, 5*, 115–133

M

MEANING AND SIGNIFICATION

Linguistics. — Like many terms in semantics (→ SEMANTICS), the word *signification* originated in Scholasticism (William of Sherwood). Its sense in modern French usage dates back to the eighteenth century, when Nicolas Beauzée declared that every word had its own primitive and fundamental signification, which was then divided into an objective signification (a fundamental idea that was the individual object of the word's signification or meaning) and a formal signification (equivalent to the Scholastic "mode of signifying"). This view made the signification of a word its primitive and fundamental sense, with the figurative senses falling among its various acceptations, all of which depended upon the fundamental sense (→ SENSE). This distinction is still considered valid by many authors today.

Most contemporary French linguists make the distinction between signification and *sense*, but it is usually applied only to lexical words: the signification of a word is rooted in the language (*langue*, in French) whereas its sense is discourse-dependent (*parole*, in the Saussurian sense of the term) (→ DISCOURSE, LANGUAGE, LEXICON, ORAL). In other words, the meaning of a word is a *type*, and the senses that it takes on during speech are *tokens* of that type (→ TYPE/TOKEN).

In English linguistics, the distinction between sense and meaning is not clear cut, especially since the word *meaning* refers to various forms of intentionality (→ INTENTIONALITY). In addition, the word *sense* is often employed to refer to the conceptual meaning or core meaning of a word (→ CONCEPT), which makes it the translation of the French word *signification*. In all cases, though, the signification or meaning of a word is a stable form that is independent of the context, whereas the sense varies with the context and is no longer defined relative to an isolated sign (→ CONTEXT AND SITUATION, SIGN).

In logic, meaning is often akin to the comprehension (or *intension*) of the concept signified by a word, in opposition to its *extension* (→ CATEGORIZATION, LOGIC). Gottlob Frege's view, according to which meaning or sense determines *denotation*, is a testimony to this:

> It is natural, now, to think of there being connected with a sign (name, combination of words, letter), besides that to which the sign refers, which may be called the reference of the sign [*Bedeutung*], also what I should like to call the sense of the sign [*Sinn*], wherein the mode of presentation is contained.

Contemporary intensional semantics studies meaning under this definition.

The link between meaning and denotation was specified by Charles Morris and Rudolf Carnap in their theory of *necessary and sufficient conditions* (NSC): to each element of meaning corresponds a condition of denotation. Cognitive semantics gave up on the issue of denotation and turned instead to the question of the relationships between concepts within the same category (or class). Drawing from Eleanor Rosch's work in psychology, cognitive semantics adopted the concept of *prototype*, which is sometimes defined as a privileged exemplar or paragon (for example, *canary* is the prototype of the bird category) and sometimes as an abstract type, with the various members of the class being either central or peripheral occurrences of it (*canary* is a central exemplar of the bird category, while *ostrich* is a peripheral exemplar).

Three questions arise in determining the status of meaning: Is meaning rooted in language or mental contents (→ MIND, LANGUAGE)? Is it attached to the linguistic expression of concepts or is it independent of that expression? How does it become linked to sense in the first hypothesis, and to denotation in the second? As a general rule, for authors who claim to be cognitive semanticists, meaning is mental content that is universal in nature, either by virtue of the primitives that comprise it (as suggested by Roger Schank and Anna Wierzbicka in artificial intelligence and linguistics, respectively) or by the operations that constitute it.

Finally, one can distinguish the various theories of meaning by the relationships they emphasize. Logical theories place priority on reference (→ SENSE/REFERENCE), pragmatic theories, on inference (→ PRAGMATICS). Linguistic semantics, with its structural tradition, focuses on differences: it is oppositions within and between semantic classes that define lexical content. Cognitive semantics has reassessed the issue of differences by introducing or recognizing quantitative inequalities between members of categories (or lexical classes) and introducing forms of graduality into the organization of categories.

FRANÇOIS RASTIER

SELECTED BIBLIOGRAPHY

Allwood, J., & Gärdenfors, P. (Eds.). (1999). *Cognitive semantics: Meaning and cognition.* Amsterdam; Philadelphia: J. Benjamins.

Cruse, D. A. (2000). *Meaning in language: An introduction to semantics and pragmatics.* Oxford, England; New York: Oxford University Press.

Grice, H. P. (1989). *Studies in the way of words.* Cambridge, MA: Harvard University Press.

Jackendoff, R. (2002). *Foundations of language: Brain, meaning, grammar, evolution.* Oxford, England; New York: Oxford University Press.

Kintsch, W. (1974). *The representation of meaning in memory.* Hillsdale, NJ: Erlbaum.

Rastier, F. (1997). *Meaning and textuality* (F. Collins & P. Perron, Trans.). Toronto, Ontario; Buffalo, NY: University of Toronto Press. (Original work published 1989.)

Shore, B. (with Bruner, J.). (1996). *Culture in mind: Cognition, culture, and the problem of meaning.* New York: Oxford University Press.

MEMORY

Psychology. — In cognitive psychology, the concept of *memory* pertains to mental states that carry information, whereas *learning* refers to the transition from one mental state to another (→ LEARNING, INFORMATION). In everyday usage, the term *memory* seems to evoke a single information storage mechanism, yet in psychology research on memory has found evidence of a wide variety of mental representations and processes (→ REPRESENTATION). Several distinctions are generally made in memory research, although recent theoretical advances relating to brain-activation phenomena argue in favor of a structural unity that overarches this functional variety.

The first distinction concerns the temporary (*short-term memory*) or permanent (*long-term memory*) nature of mental states. Short-term memory handles a limited amount of information (span) and is particularly sensitive to any kind of interfering activity. This distinction resulted in the introduction of the concept of *working memory*, a transient kind of memory that accomplishes cognitive activities and whose role is contingent upon the temporal dimension of those activities and hence upon the necessary establishment of relationships between different pieces of information spread over time. The most common view, developed by Alan Baddeley, postulates the existence of autonomous modules corresponding to the different modalities in which information is represented (phonological-articulatory, visuospatial), all controlled by a "central executive" whose function is primarily attentional (→ ATTENTION, CONTROL, MODULARITY). The limited capacity of working memory concerns both the amount of information stored in memory and the cognitive cost of the processes involved in its functioning. In neostructuralist theories of cognitive development, the functional capacities of working memory are hypothesized to increase as development progresses (→ COGNITIVE DEVELOPMENT).

Conceptions of long-term memory are also based on a number of distinctions. Endel Tulving proposed the now-classical opposition between *episodic memory*, or information that can be situated in time and space and whose retrieval is context-dependent (→ CONTEXT AND SITUATION, SPACE, TIME AND TENSE), and *semantic memory*, or general knowledge of the world that is independent of the time and place where it was acquired, and whose retrieval is closely tied to its internal organization (→ SEMANTIC NETWORK, SEMANTICS). Both of these forms of memory fall under the heading of *declarative memory:* knowledge that can be represented in natural language or in the form of mental images, and is therefore theoretically accessible to conscious awareness (→ CONSCIOUSNESS, MENTAL IMAGERY, LANGUAGE). In line with John Anderson's view, declarative memory is opposed here to *procedural memory*, which is involved in the accomplishment of perceptuomotor or cognitive processes and whose content remains essentially inaccessible (→ ACTION, PERCEPTION). Still another, more recent opposition distinguishes *explicit memory* and *implicit memory*. Explicit memory relies on intentional information-searching strategies, whereas implicit memory does not involve conscious access to information but shows up in mental activities that use information incidentally encountered at an earlier time. Perceptual and conceptual processes and lexical access are examples of some of the cognitive activities studied from this angle (→ CATEGORIZATION, CONCEPT, LEXICON).

Long-term memory has been the topic of many studies aimed both at demonstrating its organized character (assumed to be necessary due to the large quantity of information memorized) and at analyzing the most critical types of organization. Many concepts have been developed to account for these structures, including conceptual and propositional networks (→ PROPOSITIONAL FORMAT), typicality, frames, schemas, and scripts. The way these structures are constructed and evolve is a major issue in the developmental study of memory.

The emergence of *activation/inhibition* theories has led to conceptions that depart considerably from those based on the structural-architecture premise (→ ACTIVATION/INHIBITION). When the impact of the permanent properties of memorized information (for example, lexical frequency) on working-memory functions is taken into account, working memory can be seen as the activated part of long-term memory. The limited capacity of working memory in this case would act as a functional limitation on the number of elements that can be simultaneously activated, or even on the degree or duration of activation of each one. These conceptions support models that attempt to articulate memory theory and attention theory, such as that of Nelson Cowan.

DANIEL GAONAC'H

Neuroscience. — In cognitive neuroscience, it is nearly impossible to address the question of memory without also considering the mechanisms of perception (→ PERCEPTION). All feelings of familiarity, and all activities involving the recognition or identification of a perceived object, necessarily activate representations in memory (→ ACTIVATION/INHIBITION, REPRESENTATION). The nature of these representations and the mechanisms through which they are constructed and modified are important topics of study today.

As has been done with other cognitive systems, memory can be divided into many *functional subsystems* (→ COMPUTATIONAL ANALYSIS, FUNCTION). However, given the ever-present nature of memory and its tight links to perception, it is not surprising to find that it shares many neural and cognitive subsystems with the functional architectures of perception. Accordingly, the subsystems that store perceptual or semantic representations (→ SEMANTICS) are also part of the functional subsystems of memory, supplementing the more specific subsystems. It is now widely acknowledged that human memory can be separated into different components, each of which can be selectively deteriorated by brain lesions (→ LOCALIZATION OF FUNCTION, NEUROPSYCHOLOGY).

However, these components, often called *memory subsystems*, should be regarded as different in kind from those found in a functional architecture. The term *memory subsystem* originated in studies of human memory conducted by different authors at different periods, and according to different levels of analysis (see *psychology* above). One of these levels is the temporal level. Analyses at this level look at how long memory traces are sustained in sensory memory (a few hundred milliseconds), short-term memory (20 or 30 seconds), and long-term memory (more than 30 seconds). Other temporal analyses attempt to account for the transformation of episodic information into semantic information (→ INFORMATION). Still other, clinical analyses oppose *retrograde memory* to *anterograde memory*, the former corresponding to a loss of information acquired before the appearance of a brain lesion, and the latter, to a loss of the ability to store new information in long-term memory following brain damage. Another level of analysis hinges on the evaluation of the knowledge stored in long-term memory, where explicit memory is opposed to implicit memory. In implicit memory, two distinct processes are defined: *priming*, or the unconscious influence of the prior presentation of a stimulus on the current processing of that same stimulus or another one associated with it (→ CONSCIOUSNESS), and *procedure learning* (→ LEARNING).

All of the facets of human memory studied by psychologists are important, for each one corresponds to an anatomical or anatomofunctional reality. The validity of the distinction between short-term memory and long-term memory is supported by neuropsychological observations of patients with amnesia, whose short-term memory capacities are intact at the same time as their long-term memory capacities are deficient. Amnesic patients also exhibit a selective deficit in explicit memory processes while their implicit memory is spared. As stressed above, descriptions of the different memory subsystems are nevertheless the product of ways of breaking down mental processes that differ from those used to characterize the functional subsystems defined in computational analysis. Computational analysis works at a finer-grained level and deals precisely with the identification and study of the processing subsystems that implement the different facets of memory mentioned above. Cognitive neuroscience attempts, for example, to determine which subsystems are involved in the unconscious acquisition of new procedures or skills.

The neuropsychological dissociations observed in human memory pathology, along with the results of studies on experimentally lesioned animals, have proven to be of considerable theoretical utility for understanding normal mnesic mechanisms. It is now clear that some regions in the mediotemporal part of the brain (e.g., the hippocampus) and in the diencephalon (e.g., the thalamus) are critically involved in the mechanisms of explicit information storage in long-term memory. On the other hand, these regions do not appear to be the place where information is stored, since intact memories can be retrieved even when these areas are damaged. It is also agreed today that information storage takes place in the areas responsible for stimulus encoding or perceptual analysis. Neither the acquisition of new skills nor the effects of priming seem to depend on mediotemporal and diencephalic structures. Apparently, the sole condition for the occurrence of a priming effect is the integrity of the cortical zones responsible for perceptual information processing.

Neurophysiological research on extremely simple organisms like Aplysiidae—whose nervous system no longer holds many secrets for memory neurobiologists—has found evidence of learning mechanisms in these organisms, albeit elementary ones, but mechanisms that could be the basis of more advanced learning (→ ANIMAL COGNITION). Finally, simulation studies have been particularly useful for analyzing and testing the mechanisms underlying the formation of memory traces (→ CONNECTIONISM, NEURAL NETWORK) and for gaining insight into the nature of the representations stored in neural networks and how they evolve as new information arrives or old information is reactivated in new contexts.

OLIVIER KOENIG

Artificial intelligence. — In computer science, the term *memory* refers to a physical device that is a part of any computer. It can record a fixed quantity of information at specified addresses and recover that information after an undetermined amount of time (→ INFORMATION). One of the genuine feats accomplished by the pioneers of computer science was that of obtaining the elaborate behaviors they did, despite the lack of program intelligibility and the low memory capacities available at the time. Considerable progress in the memory capacity, reliability, access speed, and cost of computers has completely eliminated this state of affairs. Obviously, though, the limits of what can actually be computed are still determined by the spatial complexity of algorithms (→ COMPLEXITY).

DANIEL KAYSER

SELECTED BIBLIOGRAPHY

Anderson, J. R. (1983). *The architecture of cognition*. Cambridge, MA: Harvard University Press.

Baddeley, A. (1986). *Working memory*. Oxford, England; New York: Oxford University Press.

Baddeley, A., Aggleton, J. P., & Conway, M. A. (Eds.). (2002). *Episodic memory: New directions in research*. New York: Oxford University Press.

Cowan, N. (1985). *Attention and memory: An integrated framework*. Oxford, England; New York: Oxford University Press.

Fuster, J. (1995). *Memory in the cerebral cortex: An empirical approach to neural networks in the human and nonhuman primate*. Cambridge, MA: MIT Press.

Gazzaniga, M. (Ed.). (2000). *The new cognitive neurosciences* (Section VI, *Memory*) (2nd ed.). Cambridge, MA: MIT Press.

Kandel, E., Schwartz, J., & Jessell, T. (2000). *Principles of neural science* (Section IX, *Language, thought, mood, learning, and memory*) (4th ed.). New York: McGraw-Hill.

Schacter, D., & Tulving, E. (1994). *Memory systems*. Cambridge, MA: MIT Press.

Squire, L., & Schacter, D. (2002). *Neuropsychology of memory* (3rd ed.). New York: Guilford Press.

MENTAL IMAGERY

Psychology. — The human mind retains traces of the sensory events it perceives (→ MIND). It is capable of evoking them in the form of inner experiences. These cognitive events, which are figurative in nature, are called *mental images*. The term *mental imagery* refers to the mechanisms by means of which individuals construct internal representations that preserve the figurative aspects of objects, record them in memory, and then cognitively reinstate them in future situations (→ MEMORY, REPRESENTATION). All sensory domains are concerned with mental imagery, but most of the work done so far has dealt with visual imagery. The research is aimed first at providing evidence of the existence of image-based psychological events, and then at describing their internal organization, examining their role in cognitive functioning, and, especially, characterizing the specificity of this form of representation in the human cognitive system.

Proving the existence of private events is a major difficulty facing research in psychology. Beyond verbal or graphic testimonies, investigators have been seeking indicators of such events for quite some time. Visual images are accompanied by physiological events that vary with the properties of the image. For example, the dilation of the pupils during the formation of a visual image increases as the image becomes more difficult to evoke. However, pupil dilation also accompanies cognitive activities other than mental imagery, which severely limits its validity as a cue. There is growing interest today in another indicator: variations in the regional brain activity accompanying visual-image building and inspection. Evoked potential studies have revealed intense participation of the posterior cerebral regions in image generation. Brain imaging techniques ($\rightarrow$ FUNCTIONAL NEUROIMAGING) are also providing increasingly finer demonstrations of the involvement of the occipital regions in visual imagery tasks (see *neuroscience* below).

The idea that mental images have a structure and an internal organization that might be detected using experimental operations did not become fully recognized until recently. This idea led to various hypotheses about the processes underlying mental imagery (*generation, retention, exploration, transformation*). The use of a chronometric measure has been a preferential means of accessing certain aspects of the structure of images. Stephen Kosslyn showed that the time taken to mentally explore a visual image increases with the distance to cover. Similarly, Roger Shepard showed that the time taken to mentally rotate an object lengthens with the size of the rotation angle. These findings suggest not only that mental images have a structure that is an analogical reflection of the structure of the objects and scenes represented, but also that the transformation processes applied to images exhibit an analogy with those applied to objects actually perceived or manipulated ($\rightarrow$ PERCEPTION, SPACE). However, positing that the visual images we generate and manipulate are analogical says nothing about the degree of abstractness of the long-term representations that activate them ($\rightarrow$ PROPOSITIONAL FORMAT) (see *philosophy* below).

Images sometimes appear during thinking, even when no tasks revolving around cognitive performance are underway. But a more important issue in mental imagery concerns its contribution to cognitive functioning when an individual is solving problems or answering new questions. First, verbal-information storage is known to depend on the use of visual images ($\rightarrow$ LANGUAGE); by encoding verbal information in image format, individuals are able to record additional figurative aspects of the concepts being stored ($\rightarrow$ CONCEPT). Similarly, text understanding is facilitated by the construction of images that allow readers to visualize complex relationships in a text ($\rightarrow$ TEXT). Images also fulfill important functions in reasoning and in tasks that require the subject to visualize unfamiliar relations or features ($\rightarrow$ REASONING AND RATIONALITY). Images even offer the opportunity to simulate unperceived events and to anticipate novel states of reality. They thereby help to solve new problems and play a special role in creative activity ($\rightarrow$ CREATIVITY).

Finally, an important research objective is to account for the relationship between how images are structured and how they operate. The hypothesis here is that images owe a large part of their functionality to the structural properties they share in an exclusive manner with perceptual events. Unlike other, more abstract forms of representation, images contain information whose structure is analogous to that of perceptual information. This unique quality is a powerful tool for adaptation to the environment. Imagery supplies representations that enable individuals to reason and retrieve information, even when the objects it evokes are not visible ($\rightarrow$ INFORMATION), and thus to process remote objects cognitively. The fact that image processes have features in common with perceptual processes clearly facilitates cognitive operations. On the whole, imagery is not disconnected from other cognitive functions. In particular, it is tightly intertwined with perception, from which it receives its initial content and structure, and for which it acts as a functional substitute in many circumstances of cognitive life.

MICHEL DENIS

Neuroscience. — Among the various types of mental imagery (visual, motor, etc.), visual imagery is the most highly studied in cognitive neuroscience, as in psychology (see *psychology* above). It has benefited from a new surge of interest in the past few years with the advent of brain imaging techniques ($\rightarrow$ FUNCTIONAL NEUROIMAGING).

Visual mental imagery is not a single process. It is subtended by various subsystems, each specialized in specific cognitive operations. Identifying these subsystems has been a goal of many studies of brain-damaged patient ($\rightarrow$ LOCALIZATION OF FUNCTION, NEUROPSYCHOLOGY) and tomography-based studies. As a whole, the findings support the view that visual mental imagery and visual perception share many functional subsystems ($\rightarrow$ PERCEPTION). In particular, several tomography studies have been conducted to determine whether the primary visual area (V1) is activated during visual image processing. With this goal in mind, Kosslyn and his collaborators measured the brain activity of subjects performing a mental imagery task and a perception task. In the imagery task, the subjects were given a lowercase letter; they had to imagine the corresponding uppercase letter drawn on a grid and decide whether the imagined letter covered a given square of the grid (marked with a *X*). In the perception task, the uppercase letter was actually shown on the grid. The activation patterns observed in the imagery and perception conditions were similar. This study offers an interesting demonstration of the overlapping of the brain areas involved in mental imagery and visual perception.

Another way to demonstrate the overlapping of imagery and perception processes is to look in imagery for the functional principles known to dictate vision. Using this approach, Kosslyn showed that the topographic organization of the visual cortex can also be mapped using an imagery task. Subjects with their eyes closed had to listen to names of letters, build a mental image of the uppercase letter just heard, and then say, for example, whether the letter contained a curved line. The originality of this study lies in the fact that the subjects were asked to imagine letters that were as small as possible or as large as possible. The slides obtained showed activation of the primary visual area V1 during imagery, with more marked activation of the posterior part of V1 (corresponding to the fovea) for small letters, and of the anterior part of V1 (corresponding to the parafoveal areas) for large letters. These findings are in line with current knowledge of the topographic organization of V1 and support the hypothesized sharing of mechanisms by vision and mental imagery.

The shared-mechanism hypothesis was further validated by Kosslyn in another study where subjects had to listen passively to the names of objects (control condition), or build different-sized mental images of an object described by its name (test condition). As in the previous study, residual activation in V1 was observed after subtraction of the two conditions. Activation was posterior for small images, anterior for large images, and in the middle for medium-sized images. Note, however, that some authors have not found V1 activation during visual imagery tasks. This issue is under debate today. The discrepancy could probably be eliminated through a precise comparison of the experimental protocols used.

Recent work on functional brain imaging has also confirmed that in visual mental imagery as in perception, there are two distinct neural circuits involved in the two essential aspects of object processing in space: *Where is it?* and *What is it?* ($\rightarrow$ SPACE). The "where" circuit is the pathway called *dorsal*, which includes the regions situated along an occipito-parietal axis extending into the superior parietal lobe. This pathway is responsible for locating objects and analyzing the spatial attributes of imagined (or perceived) scenes. The "what" circuit is the pathway called *ventral*, which is situated along an occipitotemporal axis extending into the inferior temporal gyrus. This pathway is specialized in shape processing, and more generally, in treating the figural characteristics of objects (identification operations).

OLIVIER KOENIG

Philosophy. — In ancient philosophy, the privileged medium of thought was iconic or pictorial; understanding language thus required the juxtaposition of images ($\rightarrow$ LANGUAGE). Two assumptions defined this view: Thesis A, in which mental images are pictorial representations ($\rightarrow$ REPRESENTATION), and Thesis B, which holds that imagination resembles perception carried out under deprived conditions (→ PERCEPTION). This tradition was taken up by modern philosophers: from René Descartes to John Locke and David Hume, thinking is manipulating simple ideas, seen as weakened images of the impressions of the senses that can be combined to form complex ideas.

George Berkeley was the first to criticize this view, arguing that images are always determinate (Thesis C). It followed from this, he contended, that general concepts could not be images (the image of a triangle always depicts a triangle with certain angles, whereas the general concept of triangle does not have to have any particular feature) (→ CONCEPT). Jerry Fodor derived support from a remark by Ludwig Wittgenstein (the image of a man walking up a hill can also be the image of that same man sliding down the hill backward) to pursue Berkeley's criticism and refute the capability of images to convey truth and falsity, and thus to have a definite propositional content (→ TRUTH). Indeed, images (mental ideas in this case, but also photographs) do not appear abstract enough to be the medium of conceptual representation.

Theses A, B, and C have repeatedly been discounted, both in philosophy and in psychology, for several reasons. The analogy with pictorial representations is weak, since images cannot be treated as physical objects; the perceptual model of imagination is problematic insofar as it is difficult to see where the alleged image scanning might take place; finally, images can be indeterminate, as illustrated by the mental image of a tiger with an unspecified number of stripes.

While considerably reducing the implication of images in the theory of thought, these criticisms are not applicable to the role of images in imagination. Even if we set aside data from introspection, whose theoretical validity is doubtful (→ INTROSPECTION), several empirical findings tend to show that at least part of the mental representation process is in fact based on an iconic structure and that visual perception and imagination share some processes (see *psychology* and *neuroscience* above). The classical experiments cited on this issue, conducted by Shepard and Kosslyn, respectively, concern mental rotation and *mental scanning:* (1) The time taken to determine whether two pictures represent the same object seen from two different angles is a linear function of the difference between the two angles (taken as a measure of rotation). Subjects thus seem to be able to mentally manipulate images at a fixed speed. (2) The time taken to mentally locate a landmark on an imagined map (a mental image of a map studied in advance) is a linear function of the distance on the real map between the landmark in question and the last landmark located by the subject. To explain experimental data of this kind, it is usually hypothesized that subjects mentally explore iconic entities. Images are seen as existing in a medium that can behave like space, and functional representations are thought to assign properties to positions in space (→ SPACE). Kosslyn's model suggests that there are three processes—image generation, scanning, and transformation—that are specific to imagination and distinct from other cognitive processes.

One objection to this view of images is that it is not conceptually clear and may be nothing more than a simple metaphor. This is particularly evident for those who propose a *propositional theory* to account for phenomena like Points 1 and 2 above (→ PROPOSITIONAL FORMAT). According to Zenon Pylyshyn, mental images are merely structural descriptions, that is, complex linguistic representations that use predicates like *object, part of object*, and *on the right* to describe the spatial structure of what they represent. Pylyshyn showed that (3) a subject's beliefs and linguistic competence (→ BELIEF) interfere with the speed of the operations supposedly carried out on images. For example, the difference between how fast a chess master and a novice memorize a chess layout decreases if a random combination of pieces is presented instead of an actual game position. In the iconic theory, where pattern scanning is a primitive, independent capacity, there should be no noticeable difference between the processing of linguistically structured and unstructured data.

Geoffrey Hinton proposed a variant of the propositional theory in which objects are associated with structural descriptions that rank the objects in a hierarchy of spatial relationships (for instance, we have a conceptual representation of the fact that the hand is connected to the arm, which in turn is connected to the shoulder). Image scanning would therefore be subject to the same distance effects as those present in the iconic theory, because it takes longer to activate the peripheral parts of the hierarchy than the central parts. Michael Tye proposed a compromise between iconic theory and linguistic theory wherein a spatial, iconic medium such as a grid is filled with symbolic propositional vectors that specify the property represented at each position in the grid.

ROBERTO CASATI

SELECTED BIBLIOGRAPHY

Denis, M., et al. (Eds.). (2001). *Imagery, language, and visuo-spatial thinking*. New York: Psychology Press.

Gazzaniga, M. (Ed.) (2000). *The new cognitive neurosciences* (Section VIII, *Higher cognitive functions*) (2nd ed.). Cambridge, MA: MIT Press.

Kosslyn, S. (1980). *Image and mind*. Cambridge, MA: Harvard University Press.

Kosslyn, S. (1994). *Image and brain*. Cambridge, MA: MIT Press.

Kosslyn, S., et al. (1993). Visual mental imagery activates topographically organized visual cortex: PET investigations. *Journal of Cognitive Neuroscience, 5*, 263–287.

Kosslyn, S., et al. (1995). Topographical representations of mental images in primary visual cortex. *Nature, 378*, 496–498.

Mazoyer, B., Mellet, E., & Tzourio, N. (2002). Visual and language area interactions during mental imagery. In A. Galaburda, S. Kosslyn, & Y. Christen (Eds.), *The languages of the brain* (pp. 207–214). Cambridge, MA: Harvard University Press.

Mellet, E., Petit, L., Denis, M., & Tzourio-Mazoyer, N. (1998). Reopening the mental imagery debate: Lessons from functional anatomy. *NeuroImage, 8,* 129–139.

Shepard, R., & Metzler, J. (1971). Mental rotation of three-dimensional objects. *Science, 171,* 701–703.

Tye, M. (1991). *The imagery debate.* Cambridge, MA: MIT Press.

METACOGNITION

Psychology. — *Metacognition* (cognition about cognition) encompasses the knowledge and cognitive processes whose object is cognition and whose task is to control and verify one's own cognitive functioning ($\rightarrow$ CONTROL). According to the psychologist John Flavell, whose work in the 1970s on intentional memorization in children made a powerful contribution to the development of research in this field ($\rightarrow$ MEMORY), two interdependent dimensions come into play: *metacognitive knowledge* and *metacognitive experiences*.

Metacognitive knowledge, or *metaknowledge*, is understood to be the set of knowledge and beliefs stored in long-term memory about factors likely to affect the progression and outcome of cognitive processes ($\rightarrow$ BELIEF). Metaknowledge pertains to *persons, tasks*, and *strategies*. The person category includes acquired knowledge and beliefs about human beings as information-processing systems. This knowledge concerns inter- and intraindividual differences ($\rightarrow$ DIFFERENTIATION), but also, and perhaps especially, the universal properties of human cognition. The task category includes metaknowledge about the nature of goals to be attained and information to be processed. The strategy category includes the knowledge and beliefs individuals have about cognitive strategies for progressing toward a goal, and about metacognitive strategies whose function is to control and check the unfolding of that process. Apart from the fact that metaknowledge is second-order knowledge (knowledge about knowledge), it does not differ qualitatively from other types of knowledge: it is acquired gradually, it can be activated automatically (via salient situational cues; $\rightarrow$ AUTOMATISM) or deliberately (during the conscious search for a solving strategy; $\rightarrow$ CONSCIOUSNESS), and it can be insufficient, inaccurate, incorrectly recalled, or misused.

Metacognitive experiences are understood to encompass all conscious cognitive or affective experiences ($\rightarrow$ EMOTION) linked to the solving of a particular problem. Such transient experiences occur especially when the subject is performing a relatively complex cognitive task—that is, complex for that particular subject's level of development or expertise ($\rightarrow$ COGNITIVE DEVELOPMENT)—that requires the implementation of control processes like planning, anticipation, and the assessment of strategies and/or outcomes. Metacognitive experiences fulfill various functions that are useful in regulating cognitive processes. For example, a reader who suddenly senses that he or she is not understanding what he or she reads may change his or her studying strategy, seek additional information elsewhere, break down his or her overall goal into subgoals, and so forth (→ READING).

Long-term metacognitive knowledge and transient metacognitive experiences are related to each other in a reciprocal way. Metaknowledge serves to interpret metacognitive experiences and respond in a more or less fitting manner (→ INTERPRETATION). In return, person-, task-, and strategy-related information acquired through metacognitive experiences enhances metacognitive knowledge by supplementing it with new metaknowledge, eliminating erroneous metaknowledge, generalizing, and so on.

Metacognition and its related concepts are also studied in disciplines other than psychology, such as artificial intelligence (see *artificial intelligence* below) and the education sciences. In the latter area, investigators such as Ann Brown, Michael Pressley, and Wolfgang Schneider have shown that it is possible to train subjects to use certain metacognitive skills in an effective way, particularly the capacity to reflect upon one's own functioning, which constitutes a fundamental aspect of human cognition (→ LEARNING).

In psychology, the study of metacognitive processes began by looking at memory mechanisms, but it now deals with many other cognitive activities, including communication, text comprehension, persuasion, problem solving, social cognition, and so forth (→ COMMUNICATION, SOCIAL COGNITION, TEXT). An important research trend in this vein, *naive psychology* or *theories of mind*, draws directly from metacognition research (→ THEORY OF MIND). The idea here is to study the development of children's representations of mental entities and phenomena (→ REPRESENTATION) while examining their ability to describe, predict, and interpret human behavior and emotions in reference to mental entities such as intention, desire (→ DESIRE), belief, ignorance, knowledge, and so on.

ANNE-MARIE MELOT

Artificial intelligence. — The prefix *meta-* means several things. In scientific neologisms, it often means that some object is applied to another object of the same kind; the noun after the prefix gives an idea of the type of object and the concerned application. This is often insufficient for defining both the object and the application, so it is better to clearly specify the sense of words prefixed with *meta-*.

Let us illustrate with two examples. Linguists are interested in *metadiscourse*, or discourse about discourse (→ DISCOURSE). Metadiscourse serves to organize a text (→ TEXT), clarify the meaning of certain words, correct what was said, and so forth. The first sentence in this paragraph is an example of metadiscourse: it adds no information about the subject. Notice its generality: it could be found in exactly the same form in a chemistry book. Any good text-generation system should be capable of generating metadiscourse in view of facilitating the reader's task (→ READING).

Psychologists study metacognition, that is, cognitive activities pertaining to human cognition (see *psychology* above). It would be useful for artificial intelligence (AI) systems to have metacognitive capabilities, such as knowing what they know and what they can do, or knowing the properties of the problem-solving methods they use (→ PROBLEM SOLVING). In a system where several robots have to work together, each robot must have an idea of its own aptitudes so as not to undertake a task it is incapable of executing (→ DISTRIBUTED INTELLIGENCE, ROBOTICS).

The major part of the AI research where a metaactivity is involved deals with two-level systems. At the *base level*, the system solves a problem; at the *metalevel* it observes the problem statement or what it did at the base level to solve the problem. It then changes its behavior in accordance with what it observed. Most chess programs settle for systematically developing all possible moves for as long as they can. In other words, they work solely at the base level. But some chess systems also examine the rules of the game and discover properties that allow the program to stop considering every legal move. For instance, a system could see that in a case of double check, it has to move the king. Noticing this makes is useless to contemplate any other moves and therefore speeds up the search. At the present time, it is the programmer who examines the rules of the game and finds such properties; but it is also the programmer who exhibits intelligence. This approach is satisfactory if the program plays only one game. To develop a system that can play any game, the programmer obviously cannot examine the rules of as-yet-unknown games. Without the possibility of examining the rules of every game to discover useful properties, the system will perform poorly on new games. On the other hand, a system can be both general and perform well if it can reason about the rules of any game (→ REASONING AND RATIONALITY).

To work at the metalevel, one needs a kind of knowledge that can manipulate base-level knowledge—that is, metaknowledge. An example of metaknowledge is: *If using a piece of knowledge often produces an undesirable result, then discard it.* This piece of metaknowledge is useful in systems capable of learning new knowledge, since they need to be able to delete knowledge that proves less useful than was hoped at the time it was generated (→ ACTIVATION/INHIBITION, LEARNING). When we express ourselves, we use metaknowledge to help us make the ideas we wish to transmit more understandable (→ COMMUNICATION). For instance, we can state that it is a good idea to give examples of the knowledge we are expressing.

Metaknowledge applies to itself. It is a particular type of knowledge. Its only particularity is its domain, which is knowledge per se rather than, say, mathematics or medicine (→ DOMAIN SPECIFICITY). Metaknowledge about discarding knowledge may very well be applied to itself: if using it often leads to the elimination of knowledge that would sometimes be very useful after all, it will satisfy its own conditions and will have every reason to "self-destruct." Note that we have just also applied the above metaknowledge about giving examples, by using it as an example.

The reflexivity of metaknowledge has several beneficial effects. First of all, it is not necessary to create "metametaknowledge" for processing metaknowledge; it is perfectly capable of self-processing. Another advantage is the possibility of *bootstrapping*, where a system uses itself to do its own setup. Metaknowledge about finding new knowledge, for instance, can find new metaknowledge about finding knowledge, and can therefore be self-enhancing. The history of technology has shown that bootstrapping is a widely used technique, as illustrated by the fact that today's computers are designed using computers. The bootstrapping capability has opened up a line of research where AI will be able to contribute to future developments in AI. Systems that utilize metaknowledge are difficult to design and test, which is why they are few and far between. But they implement an essential feature of intelligence: the ability to think about what we are doing. Hence our difficulty in understanding why we can make intelligent systems that cannot function at a metalevel.

JACQUES PITRAT

SELECTED BIBLIOGRAPHY

Brown, A. L. (1987). Metacognition, executive control, self-regulation, and other more mysterious mechanisms. In F. E. Weinert & R. H. Kluwe (Eds.), *Metacognition, motivation, and understanding*. Hillsdale, NJ: Erlbaum.

Carruthers, P., & Chamberlain, A. (2000). *Evolution and the human mind: Modularity, language, and meta-cognition*. New York: Cambridge University Press.

Flavell, J. H., Green, F. L., & Flavell, E. R. (Eds.). (1995). *Young children's knowledge about thinking*. Chicago: University of Chicago Press.

Flavell, J. H., & Wellman, H. M. (1977). Metamemory. In R. V. Kail & J. W. Hagen (Eds.), *Perspectives on the development of memory and cognition*. Hillsdale, NJ: Erlbaum.

Metcalfe, J., & Shimamura, A. (Eds.). (1994). *Metacognition: Knowing about knowing*. Cambridge, MA: MIT Press.

MIND

Philosophy. — Wondering what the mind is made of amounts to asking what criterion a state, process, or property must satisfy to be called *mental* (as opposed to a state, process, or property that is solely physical). Two criteria are generally proposed. One is the property of being *conscious* (→ CONSCIOUSNESS): a conscious state is a state that has the property of being sensed by its bearer. Referring to Thomas Nagel's definition, a conscious organism is an organism that senses that "there is something that it is like to be that organism." Having a mind is essentially being conscious or capable of consciousness. The other criterion is what Franz Brentano called the "intentionality of mental states" (→ INTENTIONALITY). The mental states in question are about states of affairs; they *represent* them (→ REPRESENTATION). Having a mind is being capable of building representations. However, the second criterion must be supplemented with the criterion that the representational content of mental states has to play a causal role in the behavior of the organism or system under consideration—otherwise, a photograph could be considered to be "mental" (→ CAUSALITY AND MENTAL CAUSATION, COGNITIVISM, FUNCTIONALISM).

While the first criterion grants a privileged role to sensations and qualia (→ QUALIA) and thereby denies a mind to any entity lacking conscious "phenomenology," the second contends that the most important class of mental states is the class of *propositional attitudes*, that is, the beliefs or desires that organisms form about their own environment or about themselves and that determine their behavior (→ BELIEF, DESIRE, PROPOSITIONAL ATTITUDE).

The choice of a criterion for being mental fully depends upon how the relationship between mind and body is understood (→ DUALISM/MONISM). *Mentalists* (George Berkeley) derive the physical world from the mind and its operations. *Materialists* (David Armstrong, Paul Churchland), on the contrary, strive to reduce the mind to the brain and body or to some of the brain's or body's properties (→ REDUCTIONISM). *Dualists* posit the existence of irreducible substances in the manner proposed by René Descartes, who opposed the mind, a thinking thing, to the body, an extended thing. By contrast, neutral *monists* (William James, Bertrand Russell) attempt to get rid of the opposition between the realms of physical and mental causality. *Functionalism* offers an interesting attempt to give a nonreductionist definition of mental states that nevertheless remains compatible with a materialistic ontology (in the "token physicalism" version; → PHYSICALISM).

JOËLLE PROUST

SELECTED BIBLIOGRAPHY

Armstrong, D. (1993). *A materialist theory of the mind*. London: Routledge.

Chalmers, D. (2002). *Philosophy of mind: Classical and contemporary readings*. New York: Oxford University Press.

Crumley, J. (1999). *Problems in mind: Readings in contemporary philosophy of mind*. New York: McGraw-Hill.

Gregory, R., & Zangwill, O. (Eds.). (1997). *The Oxford companion to the mind*. New York: Oxford University Press.

Nagel, T. (1979). *Mortal questions*. New York: Cambridge University Press.

Posner, M., & Raichle, M. (1994/1997). *Images of mind*. New York: Freeman.

Rey, G. (1996). *Contemporary philosophy of mind: A contentiously classical approach*. Oxford, England: Blackwell.

Thagard, P. (1996). *Mind: Introduction to cognitive science*. Cambridge, MA: MIT Press.

MODALITY

Philosophy. — One can evaluate a proposition not only as being true or false, but also as being so in a contingent or necessary way (→ LOGIC, TRUTH). A proposition can be defined as a set of "possible worlds," or as a function that assigns each world a truth value (→ FUNCTION). The *modality* of a proposition is its truth or falsity relative to the set of possible worlds. If it is true (or false) in all possible worlds, then it is necessarily true (or false); if it is true in some worlds, it is only possible. If it is true in this world, it is not only possible but real. When a modal term is applied to a statement that already contains one, as in *It is possible that it is necessary that P*, the modalities are said to be *nested*.

Classic problems in interpreting modality lie in understanding what a possible world is. "Possibilists" such as David Lewis contend that it is legitimate to assert the existence of worlds that are only possible, whereas "actualists" such as Robert Stalnaker limit their existence to the real world, a view that leads them to describe individuals that are only possible as a particular type of noninstantiated property (→ COUNTERFACTUAL).

JOËLLE PROUST

Linguistics. — Modality is the relation that links a proposition to an instance that grants it its validity (→ VALIDATION). According to this general definition, any stated proposition is therefore produced in a given modality (although a reductionist conception of the relationships between morphology and semantics has led a number of authors to see as modalized only those propositions containing a marker specifically and exclusively aimed at expressing modality; → MORPHOLOGY, SEMANTICS). In linguistics, the kind of modality to consider is the one that is displayed in a sentence. For example, in saying *It's raining*, the speaker is presenting a proposition as being objectively true at the moment the sentence is uttered—even if, based on nonlinguistic considerations, we also know that this assertion is grounded in a belief or perception of the speaking subject (→ BELIEF, PERCEPTION).

Two criteria are available for classifying linguistic modalities: the type of *validating instance* and the *force of the relation*. There are three types of validating instances. (1) The first is reality itself, in cases where the speaker does not state his or her own point of view; this type corresponds to the *alethic* or *ontic* modalities of the objective truth (→ TRUTH). (2) The second is when a subject expresses an opinion or belief; this type corresponds to the *epistemic* or *doxastic* modalities of the subjective truth (→ EPISTEMIC). The opinion or belief in question may be that of a particular person who is or is not participating in the conversation (*I, you, he*), or shared (*we, one*). (3) The third is an institutional authority (the law, moral standards, etc.) and corresponds to the *deontic* modalities of obligation and permission.

In the alethic and epistemic modalities, the "direction of fit" (in John Searle's sense of the term) goes from the statement to the world (the statement is supposed to conform to the objective world or to the world as it is perceived or understood by the subject), whereas in the deontic modalities the direction is reversed (the world must conform to the statement). This is why the deontic modalities pertain to obligation and not truth. The *volition* modalities (→ WILL), barely studied to date, are obtained by taking combinations of the reverse direction of fit and the subject's choice of validating instance.

The validating instance, which is the basis of modality, should not be confused with the source of information (→ INFORMATION), which is related to evidentiality, although these two phenomena are tightly linked and sometimes difficult to distinguish (consider statements like *According to Paul, Marie is the prettiest*).

The force of the relation ranges from maximal validation (which, for the alethic, epistemic, and deontic systems, gives the necessary, the certain, and the mandatory, respectively) to total invalidation (the impossible, the excluded, and the prohibited). Between these two poles—with variations, of course, that depend on the type of model adopted—we find intermediate modal values in each case: respectively, the possible and the contingent, the probable and the contestable, the permitted and the optional. From the standpoint of speech acts (→ PRAGMATICS), it is the modal value that determines the force of the obligations weighing on the speaker who is making an assertion or promise (compare: *I will come / I will surely come / I think I will come / Perhaps I will come*) or on the addressee receiving a directive *(You may leave / You should leave / You must leave)*.

While some linguists have borrowed from formal logic (→ LOGIC) a particular system (see Robert Martin's use of the logic of possible worlds) and use its formal operators to describe the values of linguistic markers (modal verbs, propositional attitude verbs, modal adverbs, mood, etc.; → PROPOSITIONAL ATTITUDE), this approach has its limitations due to the different aims of these two disciplines. While contemporary modal logics are essentially concerned with calculating implication relations between the outcomes of modalities, linguistics (which rarely has to deal with this type of situation) tries to reconcile the rigor of formalism with the description of often irregular, empirical phenomena. Logicians have proposed to organize and define modal values within the alethic, epistemic, and deontic systems by means of relations of opposition (in the form of a triangle, a square, or a hexagon). For example, the square (inspired by the Apuleius square) appears useful in accounting for the linguistic behavior of the French modal verbs *pouvoir* and *devoir* when employed to express the deontic modalities of permission and obligation, respectively. These modalities in English are expressed using the modal auxiliaries *may* and *must*, although their behavior is not exactly the same. The two-part marking of negation in French (*ne . . . pas*) is what makes this four-cornered opposition possible. In the case of *POUVOIR*: (1) *pouvoir* marks permission, *pouvoir ne pas* marks optionality (permitted that not *p*), *ne pas pouvoir* marks prohibition (not permitted that *p*), and *ne pas pouvoir ne pas* marks obligation (not permitted that not *p*). In the case of *DEVOIR*: (2) *devoir* marks obligation and *devoir ne pas* marks prohibition (obligatory that not *p*), but against all logical predictions (and this phenomenon is far from being rare), *ne pas devoir* in a sentence like *Vous ne devez pas fumer* (You must not smoke) marks prohibition, not optionality. (Note that these two notoriously polysemous markers can also express the alethic and epistemic modalities.)

Moreover, a fundamental difference in behavior specific to linguistics opposes alethic and deontic modality markers (or *root modalities*) to most (but not all) epistemic markers. According to Hans Kronning, the former express an act of "veridiction" (the modality itself being presented as true), whereas the latter merely "show" the modality. As such, only the former can be the object of a question or refutation: *Is it necessarily too late? It is not necessarily too late. *Is it probably too late? *It is not probably too late* (the asterisk indicates that the sentence is ungrammatical).

It is noteworthy that polysemous markers like *devoir* in French and *must* in English can be questioned, negated, or focalized only when they take on an alethic or deontic value. Accordingly, the epistemic interpretation (high probability) is ruled out and overridden by the deontic interpretation (obligation) in examples like *Must he be absent? He must*.

Finally, regarding the temporal modalities (alethic modalities defined with respect to time; → TIME AND TENSE), note that in the realm of language, it is no longer the present moment that draws the dividing line between the necessity of the past (its irreversibility) and the possibility of the future (its indeterminateness) but the moment in time used as the reference point in the utterance. This is why in the sentence *At that time, Luke was crossing the road*, the end of the process, which occurs after the temporal reference point, remains but a possibility (one cannot conclude that Luke reached the other side: something could have happened to prevent it). This principle lays the foundation for the inferential view of narrative text reading (→ TEXT): past events are seen as possible because they succeed the temporal reference point. Because of this, the reader will make forecasts about them, which the subsequent text will confirm or refute, according to Umberto Eco's analysis, proposed in possible-world semantics.

LAURENT GOSSELIN

SELECTED BIBLIOGRAPHY

Bybee, J. (1995). *Modality in grammar and discourse*. Philadelphia: J. Benjamins.
Eco, U. (1979). *The role of the reader: Explorations in the semiotics of texts* (Trans.). Bloomington, IN: Indiana University Press. (Original work published 1979.)
Kripke, S. (1972). *Naming and necessity*. Oxford, England: Blackwell.
Lewis, D. K. (1986). *On the plurality of worlds*. Oxford, England: Blackwell.
Martin, R. (1992). *Pour une logique du sens* [Toward a logic of meaning]. Paris: Presses Universitaires de France.
Stalnaker, R. (1979). Possible worlds. In M. J. Loux (Ed.), *The actual and the possible*. Ithaca, NY: Cornell University Press.

MODEL

Neuroscience. — Building a *model* of the normal cognitive system is the main goal of cognitive neuroscience. It is widely agreed today that cognitive activities like language and perception (→ LANGUAGE, PERCEPTION) are not global, undifferentiated activities but, on the contrary, are made possible through the operation of multiple *subsystems*, each performing an elementary process. To build a model of cognitive functioning, one must identify these processes and define how the appropriate subsystems are organized and interrelated in order to accomplish a given cognitive operation. The model thus describes a set of subsystems organized into a *functional architecture* (→ COMPUTATIONAL ANALYSIS, FUNCTION).

However, such a model must abide by two fundamental principles: biological plausibility and computational suitability. First, the model must be consistent with our knowledge of brain functioning. Second, the elementary processing steps taken by the different subsystems must be compatible with the results of a *computational analysis*, that is, a logical analysis that defines the processing steps any biological or artificial system must take to perform a given cognitive process (→ LOGIC). Only if the latter principle is obeyed will the description of the model be clear enough to be tested in a computerized simulation experiment.

OLIVIER KOENIG

Psychology. — Modeling in cognitive psychology now draws heavily from the approaches used in neuroscience, particularly in the area of computational analysis (see *neuroscience* above; → COMPUTATIONAL ANALYSIS, FUNCTION). In addition to reaping the benefits of models developed in connectionism and in the study of dynamic systems (→ CONNECTIONISM, DYNAMIC SYSTEM), cognitive modeling has taken on new directions that primarily result from the introduction in the 1990s of functional brain imaging techniques: positron emission tomography (PET), functional magnetic resonance imaging (fMRI), and electro- and magnetoencephalography (MEG) (→ FUNCTIONAL NEUROIMAGING).

The psychology of the 1970s and 1980s was strongly influenced by the ideas and technological accomplishments in artificial intelligence (AI). New ways of validating cognitive models appeared (→ VALIDATION), based on the careful articulation of experimental methodology and computer simulation, with physicalist and biological models being set aside (→ PHYSICALISM). In the 1990s, references to the brain were brought back into the foreground. Without knowing whether the history of science will dub functional brain imaging the "microscope of psychology," one can reasonably assume that within the next few years, it will no longer be possible for any major research laboratory to practice experimental psychology without relying on these techniques. The question now raised is: What new ways of testing cognitive models have been introduced by neurofunctional imaging? For neuroscientists, psychologists, and philosophers, this question is historically related to René Descartes's *dualism* between the mental world (cognitive functions) and the physical world (brain and body) (→ DUALISM/MONISM). Indeed, what is left (or will be left) of Cartesian dualism? The most radical materialists would answer, "Nothing!" But as the philosopher John Searle so rightly pointed out, the new materialists unknowingly accept the categories and the vocabulary of dualism. They are in some sense doomed to recognize the dichotomy of the physical and the mental by their very own claim that one of the terms of the dichotomy contains everything while the other is empty. Paradoxically, then, they do not refute Descartes's way of framing the debate.

The point of view that truly overthrows the Cartesian framework and the disciplinary breakdown that follows from it (neuroscience/psychology) is the claim that neurofunctional imaging techniques are able to delineate a radically new scientific object that falls outside the categories of dualism. Indeed, everything seems to suggest that images of the brain in operation—that is, as the subject executes an experimental task requiring a specific cognitive function—are pictures of an object that is neither matter alone nor mind alone. Nor is their union, in the Cartesian sense of a mysterious interaction between two components, one that can be subjected to mechanistic analysis and one that cannot (→ NATURALIZATION). But exactly what scientific object is this? Even if today we have a feeling of what it might be, coming up with a precise definition will remain a most ambitious and fascinating challenge in the years to come. A convincing example of this can be found in Stephen Kosslyn's brain images, which bring out the interrelationships between mental-image generating (mind) and topographic representations of the primary visual cortex (matter). It has even been demonstrated that this brain region changes topographically in accordance with whether the mental images generated by the subject correspond to small, medium-sized, or large objects (→ MENTAL IMAGERY).

However, this enterprise has only just begun, and many points remain obscure. As has been emphasized by contemporary philosophers of mind such as Daniel Pinkas, the unanimous antidualism that reigns in the cognitive sciences is more a reflection of agreement on the epistemologically hopeless nature of Cartesian dualism than it is a shared view of the paths that should be explored in order to clearly and accurately relate psychological functions to physical mechanisms.

In cognitive psychology as elsewhere, a model is defined by a *syntax* and a *semantics*. The syntax, derived from computer systems during the 1970s and 1980s, is now defined in cerebral terms: the physicochemical and neuroanatomical properties of the brain. The semantics correspond to the spatial and temporal projection of that syntax onto a psychologically meaningful reality (with resolution constraints that depend upon the imaging technique used). New theoretical and methodological debates are already attacking the issue of the various possible ways of achieving this projection and the validity of each one.

OLIVIER HOUDÉ

Artificial intelligence. — The logical sense of the term *model* deviates considerably from its everyday meaning. It is generally considered that a model of phenomenon A is a mathematical function (→ FUNCTION), an algorithm, or even another, more accessible phenomenon B. In logic, any model M has three constituents: (1) a *universe* (any set of objects), (2) an *interpretation*, in that universe, of predicate and function symbols (→ INTERPRETATION, LOGIC), and (3) an *assignment of free variables* to the elements of the universe. These constituents enable one to compute the *truth value* of any formula (→ TRUTH). M is said to be a model of theory T if the calculation of all formulas of T gives the value *true*.

We also speak in artificial intelligence (AI) of *cognitive modeling*. This less-developed branch of the discipline is aimed not only at obtaining results that exhibit an analogy with those produced by human intelligence, but also at acquiring them by means of methods that themselves exhibit an analogy with the mechanisms postulated in the psychology of reasoning (→ REASONING AND RATIONALITY). Another task in AI is *data modeling*, that is, specifying the attribute types of objects represented in a database and the dependency relations between those attributes (→ KNOWLEDGE BASE). Every state of the modeled database must meet the constraints dictated by the data model (→ CONSTRAINT). This supplies a convenient means of automatically detecting data-entry errors or updating errors when large quantities of data must be manipulated.

DANIEL KAYSER

Linguistics. — Although originating in the theory of mathematical models (Alfred Tarski), the notion of model is not really used in a technical way in linguistics: formal linguistics has not produced a formal calculus. The term *model* is employed in a general way to mean theory, stripped of any epistemological considerations.

Ordinarily, to model is to translate a natural language into a *language of representation* (→ LANGUAGE, REPRESENTATION). The languages used by the symbolic paradigm in cognitive research are logic languages. They are generally quite simple, as in first-order predicate calculus (→ COGNITIVISM, LOGIC, SYMBOL). A good example is the logical form, which in recent versions of Noam Chomsky's theory represents the semantic level of sentences (→ SEMANTICS). Cognitive models differ from the logical models of formal linguistics only by the (strong) hypothesis that they in fact correspond to mental representations. Jerry Fodor's *language of thought*, for example, is a psychological transposition of such a logical model (→ LANGUAGE OF THOUGHT). This hypothesis is rooted in rationalistic postulates and a formalist view of rationality (→ REASONING AND RATIONALITY). Although without breaking away from this general framework, cognitive grammars (in particular, Ronald Langacker's grammar) no longer use logical modeling languages, but replace them with various iconic representations lacking a precise topological base (→ GRAMMAR). They are semiotic forms that obey the principle of perceptual preeminence (particularly visual) and its associated localistic hypotheses, and more generally, are compatible with an iconicity whose pedagogical virtues override any theoretical justifications (→ PERCEPTION, SEMIOTICS).

FRANÇOIS RASTIER

SELECTED BIBLIOGRAPHY

Chomsky, N. (1988). *Language and problems of knowledge*. Cambridge, MA: MIT Press.

Fodor, J. (1975). *The language of thought*. New York: Crowell.

Fodor, J. (2000). *The mind doesn't work that way: The scope and limits of computational psychology*. Cambridge, MA: MIT Press.

Frackowiak, R., Friston,, K., Dolan, R., Mazziotta, J., & Frith, C. (Eds.). (1997). *Human brain function*. San Diego, CA: Academic Press.

Gaukroger, S. (2003). Descartes, René. In E. Nadel (Ed.), *The encyclopedia of cognitive science* (Vol. 1, pp. 947–950). London: Nature Publishing Group, Macmillan.

Hardcastle, V. (1996). *How to build a theory in cognitive science*. Albany, NY: State University of New York Press.

Hauser, M. D., Chomsky, N., & Fitch, W. T. (2002). The faculty of language: What is it, who has it, and how did it evolve? *Science, 298*, 1569–1579.

Kosslyn, S., & Koenig, O. (1992/1995). *Wet mind: The new cognitive neuroscience*. New York: Free Press.

Langacker, R. (1987–1991). *Foundations of cognitive grammar* (Vols. 1–2). Stanford, CA, Stanford University Press.

Pinkas, D. (1995). *La matérialité de l'esprit* [The materiality of the mind]. Paris: La Découverte.

Posner, M., & Raichle, M. (1994/1997). *Images of mind*. New York: Freeman.

Searle, J. (1992). *The rediscovery of the mind*. Cambridge, MA: MIT Press.

MODULARITY

Psychology. — The term *modularity* in psychology refers to a conception of the cognitive system whereby it is divided into functionally distinct *subsystems* (→ COMPUTATIONAL ANALYSIS, FUNCTION). This analytic approach becomes mandatory as soon as the psychologist tries to account for complex cognitive skills like reading (→ READING). The reading process is much easier to understand when broken down into separate parts, each achieved by specific components or *modules* of the reading system.

Conventional diagrams made up of boxes and arrows are used to show how the different components are connected to each other to form a system. They thus depict the *functional architecture* of the system under study. In such models, each component is characterized by the types of representations and procedures that are associated with it (→ MODEL, REPRESENTATION).

This standard view of modularity was updated and thoroughly revised by Jerry Fodor's proposals. Fodor laid down a set of criteria for distinguishing systems based on varying degrees of modularity. Among these criteria is the hard core of Fodor's theory, the idea of *informational encapsulation* (→ INFORMATION). A module is said to be informationally encapsulated when the input information it uses to make its computations is highly constrained and module-specific. This means that the module functions as if it were blind to information coming from other sources exogenous to the module itself. Several other functional properties of modules are closely tied to informational encapsulation. For instance, the more encapsulated a system is, the greater the likelihood that its calculations will be *automatic*—that is, fast, irrepressible, inaccessible to conscious inspection, and so on (→ AUTOMATISM, CONSCIOUSNESS, INTROSPECTION).

In applying his modularity criteria, Fodor was led to envisage modules as input systems that serve as interfaces between "low-level" sensory representations and the central processes that fix beliefs (→ BELIEF). According to Fodor, the latter processes cannot be regarded as modular. Among the input systems, he includes not only perceptual mechanisms but also language (→ LANGUAGE, PERCEPTION). This proposal is surprising if we think of language as a single system, but interesting if we accept that language processing can be broken down into more elementary components.

The language mechanisms to which Fodor refers (those involved in speech perception, syntactic processing, and lexical access) do indeed seem to satisfy the criteria for modularity (→ LEXICON, SYNTAX). Note on this point that Fodor dedicated his book *The Modularity of Mind* to Merrill Garrett, saying that his own ideas on modularity originated in Garrett's remark about the "nearly reflexive" character of sentence parsing.

JUAN SEGUI

Neuroscience. — The modular view of cognitive activities is a critical one in neuroscience. In this view, mental activities are described as sets of subsystems or modules, each executing a particular information processing step (→ COMPUTATIONAL ANALYSIS, INFORMATION, MODEL). One of the goals of cognitive neuroscience is precisely to identify these modules, define their activity, and understand how they are organized into a functional architecture (a set of processing modules that carries out a given cognitive task).

However, the modules described in cognitive neuroscience do not correspond exactly to those proposed by Fodor (see *psychology* above) in that they are not assumed to function totally independently of one another (as would encapsulated modules). This is why Stephen Kosslyn and Olivier Koenig qualify modularity in cognitive neuroscience as "weak." The idea of weak modularity implies that a module can be part of several processing systems. This argument is grounded on the fact that the same set of neurons can very well play a critical role in two different cognitive activities. For example, consider the neurons in visual area MT, which are activated in response to the perception of a movement (→ PERCEPTION): since perceiving a movement enables the observer both to extract an object from the background against which it is perceived (*figure-ground separation*) and to follow a moving object with the eyes, it can be inferred that the module formed by MT neurons is part of both an architecture responsible for the visual recognition of objects and an architecture involved in tracking moving objects. Clearly, then, this module is far from being independent and can be defined only in relation to the other modules with which it interacts.

The notion of weak modularity is not incompatible, though, with the fact that a brain lesion can selectively damage one or more modules (→ LOCALIZATION OF FUNCTION, NEUROPSYCHOLOGY). The *double dissociation technique*, an extremely powerful method in neuropsychology for deciding whether or not two cognitive activities call upon exactly the same processing modules, is based on the principle that modules can be selectively lesioned. However, there is no a priori reason for a brain lesion to follow the boundaries of the modules defined by computational analysis. A lesion can be diffuse and its size large enough to affect several modules. This restriction nevertheless seems insufficient to cast doubt on the double dissociation method and the conclusions drawn from it.

OLIVIER KOENIG

Philosophy. — The philosophy of mind is highly interested in a property of the cognitive system proposed by Fodor, the modularity of the mind ($\rightarrow$ MIND), considered to be well established by many investigators in the cognitive sciences. Over the past few decades, artificial intelligence, linguistics, neuroscience, and psychology have supplied many arguments in favor of a modular organization. However, the available empirical data do not support the strict dichotomy claimed by Fodor between peripheral systems (modular) and central systems (nonmodular), but suggest that gradual forms of modularity are found in certain central processes.

First, not all peripheral systems necessarily exhibit every characteristic Fodor assigns to modularity (see *psychology* above). It seems in particular that they are not informationally encapsulated in the strictest sense, but have limited access to information from other parts of the cognitive system ($\rightarrow$ INFORMATION). Moreover, evidence obtained in cognitive neuroscience does not fully support modularity. While suggesting that the sensory information-processing systems are largely localized in specialized brain regions ($\rightarrow$ LOCALIZATION OF FUNCTION), the findings also indicate that multiple cerebral areas can be simultaneously activated during a given cognitive process, such as visual perception ($\rightarrow$ PERCEPTION), and that numerous interconnections exist for exchanging information between different brain regions (see *neuroscience* above). Furthermore, certain central thought processes appear to exhibit a form of modularity. Recent work suggests, for example, that many conceptual thought processes are governed by domain-specific principles ($\rightarrow$ DOMAIN SPECIFICITY). All of these empirical findings provide philosophers and (neuro)psychologists with input for current debates on the modularity of the mind.

ÉLISABETH PACHERIE

SELECTED BIBLIOGRAPHY

Carruthers, P., & Chamberlain, A. (2000). *Evolution and the human mind: Modularity, language, and meta-cognition*. New York: Cambridge University Press.
Fodor, J. (1983). *The modularity of mind*. Cambridge, MA: MIT Press.
Fodor, J. (2000). *The mind doesn't work that way: The scope and limits of computational psychology*. Cambridge, MA: MIT Press.
Karmiloff-Smith, A. (1992). *Beyond modularity: A developmental perspective on cognitive science*. Cambridge, MA: MIT Press.
Kosslyn, S., & Koenig, O. (1992/1995). *Wet mind: The new cognitive neuroscience*. New York: Free Press.

MORPHOLOGY

Philosophy. — The *morphological* level is the level that qualitatively structures material substrates into sensible forms. According to the *morphodynamic* approach to cognition, this structuring process is objective, albeit qualitative, and results from the dynamic self-organization of physical substrates. To the extent that it accounts for the genesis of forms through the self-organization of material, physical, or neural substrates, morphodynamics makes the morphological level into a third term situated between the physical level and the symbolic structure level (→ DYNAMIC SYSTEM, EMERGENCE, PHYSICALISM, SYMBOL). It thus strives to establish both a physical theory of phenomenological properties and an ontology of structures, in an attempt to achieve a unitary conception of reality. Because of the importance it grants to the morphological level, this approach is reminiscent of Gestalt theory and phenomenology. Its originality lies in its choice of a naturalistic and monistic framework, and in its claim that the morphological level is an objective one (→ DUALISM/MONISM, NATURALIZATION). It also has much in common with connectionist models (→ CONNECTIONISM) of the subsymbolic paradigm, sharing with those models the view that relative to morphological infrastructures, the symbolic level is only a surface phenomenon.

ÉLISABETH PACHERIE

Linguistics. — Morphology is the part of grammar that deals with the makeup of complex lexical units (*derivational* or *lexical morphology*), and with variations in lexical forms (*inflectional morphology*) (→ GRAMMAR, LEXICON).

From the *syntagmatic* standpoint, a *lexical unit* is defined as the smallest linguistic segment whose semantic contribution remains the same in different sentences; it is a syntactic atom, that is, a unit that exhibits distributional independence and does not tolerate the insertion of linguistic material (Alan Cruse, Igor Mel'chuk) (→ CONTEXT AND SITUATION, SEMANTICS, SYNTAX).

From the *paradigmatic* standpoint, any lexical unit that, abstracted out of its variations in form, is prosodically autonomous and belongs to an open-ended list is a *lexeme*. In the sentence, *An acquaintance of his mother's friends saw a cat belonging to his mother-in-law's friend*, there are two occurrences of *mother*, but only the first one corresponds to the lexeme MOTHER. By contrast, *friend* and *friends* belong to the same lexeme FRIEND. The article *A* is also rendered by two occurrences, *a* and *an*, but it is not a lexeme (it is a grammatical word, also called a *function word*). According to a tradition reinforced by structuralism, the smallest constituents of lexical units are *morphemes* (or *monemes*, as André Martinet called them). The morpheme is generally defined as the smallest unit for which there is a fairly consistent correspondence between a phonic segment and a unit of meaning. For example, the word *selfish* can be broken down into SELF + ISH. Morphemes are realized in speech by *morphs* (here, /sĕlf + ĭsh/). When a morph has several variants, they are called *allomorphs:* in English / əz, s, z/ are allomorphs of the morph /Z/, which is the realization of the plurality morpheme PLU (for example, *boxes, cats, flowers,* respectively BOX + PLU, CAT + PLU, etc.). There is some disagreement about what to call the minimal units of meaning expressed in morphemes, as in "print + action-of." Classical morphology—where complex lexical units are combinations of morphemes—is at a loss whenever there is not a one-to-one correspondence between the phonic and semantic levels: a stretch of phonic material may correspond to several units of meaning (as in the French word *parla* [he/she/it spoke], where the *-a* ending marks the preterite, the third person, and the singular), and several different phonic sequences may correspond to a single unit of meaning (as found in two-part number marking in the past tense in Finnish: *e-*mme *puhu-nee-*t [we have not spoken], which is broken down into NEG-1PLU SPEAK-PPERF-PLU). The correspondence may even be multivocal (Stephen Anderson). This type of occurrence, added to the necessity of looking within the lexical unit to account for prosody-dependent phenomena (subtraction, reduplication, infixation as in Ulwa: *suulu* [dog], *suuka*lu [his/her dog]) led linguists to consider complex units to be the outcome of operations performed on a basic unit, the lexeme, with morphs simply being the phonic trace of those operations (Anderson, Robert Beard). Retaining the idea that the lexeme constitutes the privileged domain of morphological mechanisms, new approaches were developed that did not rely on sequential rules to describe these mechanisms, but instead used a declarative method (Robert Bird), based in particular on ranked and weighted constraints (optimality theory; see John McCarthy and Alan Prince).

Like syntax, morphology relates the phonic level to the semantic level. But unlike syntax, it is tightly linked to phonology, since phonetic realizations that depend on parameters that are not strictly phonological are overridden by morphophonological considerations (for example, the French word *asymmétrie* is pronounced /äsēmātrē/ rather than /äzēmātrē/, which violates French pronunciation rules in order to conform to the morphological composition of the word). The relationship between morphology and lexicon can be best understood by looking at how units are constructed and become lexicalized. In lexical morphology, complex lexical units are formed via specific mechanisms that differ from those found in syntax. These include derivation (by affixation, as in *management, unwrap, outweigh,* and *oversleep;* by apophony, as in *sing, song;* by reduplication, as in *helter-skelter,* etc.), compounding (as in *fly-fishing, thatch-roofed, long-legged, churchgoer*), and conversion (*brake, empty*). Of all possible units formed in this way, even attested ones, only some will become codified entities with a rule-based association between sound and sense that is socially recognized and employed as such. However, some phrases (e.g., *Middle Ages, cold room, line of sight, greatest common denominator*) and expressions (e.g., *cold shoulder, raining cats and dogs*) that exhibit normal syntax, or others that are formed in an irregular way (blends such as *Amerindian, brunch, guestimate, smog;* clipping: *lab, exam;* lax speech: *gotcha, gonna;* slang: *wannabee, druthers;* or backslang: *yob* for boy) may also become lexicalized.

Inflectional phenomena are nonexistent in certain languages (such as Vietnamese). But when they exist, they rely on mechanisms that only morphology can treat (for example, the role of perfect and present tense themes in the formation of Latin paradigms: see Mark Aronoff). Allomorphic phenomena (/flouər/ *flower* ⌢ /flôr/ *floral*) and suppletive phenomena (*good* ⌢ *better*), both very frequent in morphology, do not have clear-cut syntactic equivalents. The notions of frequency and variation of form make sense for lexical units, but they are meaningless for sentences. These features and many others are indicative of the irreducibility of morphology to syntax.

Two major cognition-related questions raised in morphology concern *marking* and *regularity*. One problem, for example, is finding out what conceptual categories are most often expressed by means of inflection (→ CATEGORIZATION, CONCEPT). Joan Bybee defends the (criticized) idea that conceptual categories are ones that are both the most general and the most relevant. Another claim is that the meanings expressed via morphological derivation reflect cognitive categories of the AGENT type, and so forth (see Irzy Szymanek, Beard) (→ MEANING). In the theory of natural morphology (Wolfgang Dressler and collaborators) *marker iconicity* is a key concept. According to this theory, for a given state of a language, morphological encoding becomes more transparent (diagrammatical) as the relationship between a unit of content (*signatum*) and its phonic expression (*signans*) approaches a one-to-one correspondence (thus, for example, affixation is more diagrammatical than apophony). Research tends to show that models of irregularity (e.g., irregular Spanish verbs) can be quite productive because they bring to bear factors related to frequency, autonomy, and centrality (of a form or a type of form) (Bybee). Analogy and paradigmatic regularization are also known to be instrumental in creating new lexical and inflectional forms (e.g., *-iamo* in present-day Italian, and the extension of the umlaut; Nigel Vincent, Carol Chapman, Jaap Van Marle). David Rumelhart and James McClelland proposed a connectionist model to describe the acquisition of verb inflections (→ CONNECTIONISM). Models of this type are developed to account for the emergence of new lexical items in text (→ TEXT).

BERNARD FRADIN

SELECTED BIBLIOGRAPHY

Anderson, S. (1992). *A-morphous morphology*. Cambridge, England: Cambridge University Press.

Dressler, W., Mayerthaler, W., Panagl, O., & Wurzel, W. U. (1987). *Leitmotives in natural morphology*. Amsterdam: J. Benjamins.

McCarthy, J., & Prince, A. (1993). Generalized alignment. *Yearbook of morphology* (pp. 79–153).

Payne, E. (1997). *Describing morphosyntax: A guide for field linguists*. Cambridge, England; New York: Cambridge University Press.

N

NATURALIZATION

Philosophy. — A philosophical theory is *naturalistic* when its goal is to use, in its analyses, only concepts and principles that are compatible with those of natural science. The project of *naturalizing* epistemology (→ EPIS-TEMOLOGY), defended by the philosopher and logician Willard Quine, is aimed at studying perception, learning, thought, language acquisition, and cultural transmissions in a scientific way, in an attempt to delineate the general conditions that justify our beliefs (→ BELIEF, LANGUAGE, LEARNING, PERCEPTION). This endeavor changes the goal of epistemology, taking it from grounding knowledge to exploring all factors (psychological, linguistic, etc.) that shape human knowledge, on the basis of what the sciences themselves teach us about it (this is also the approach used in Jean Piaget's genetic epistemology) (→ COGNITIVE DEVELOPMENT, CONSTRUC-TIVISM). This naturalization process is currently an important issue in the philosophy of mind, where concepts classically deemed to be foreign to the scientific approach, such as the premises of intentionality and con-sciousness (→ CONSCIOUSNESS, INTENTIONALITY), are submitted to natural-istic inquiry.

JOËLLE PROUST

SELECTED BIBLIOGRAPHY

Kornblith, H. (Ed.). (1994). *Naturalizing epistemology*. Cambridge, MA: MIT Press.
Piaget, J. (1970). *Genetic epistemology* (E. Duckworth, Trans.). New York: W. W. Norton. (Origi-nal work published 1970.)
Quine, W. (1969). *Ontological relativity, and other essays*. New York: Columbia University Press.

NEURAL DARWINISM

Psychology. — *Neural Darwinism* is mainly represented in France by Jean-Pierre Changeux and in the United States by Gerald Edelman. It is a speculative parallel of evolutionist thinking (Charles Darwin, etc.), proposed in cognitive neuroscience and psychology to answer questions about the construction of logicomathematical objects, aesthetic pleasure and emotion, perception, categorization, memory, consciousness, and so on (→ CATEGORIZATION, CONSCIOUSNESS, CONSTRUCTIVISM, EMOTION, LOGIC, MEMORY, PERCEPTION).

The underlying assumption of Changeux's neurobiological theory is that there are multiple *levels of functional organization* in the nervous system: the molecular and cellular level, the neural-circuit level (reflex arcs, local circuits), the understanding level (neuronal groups), and the reasoning level (ensemble of neuronal groups). In this mental architecture, which goes from molecular and cellular phenomena to mental objects, a given function (including cognitive ones) (→ FUNCTION) is assigned to a given organization level. But functions are not autonomous: they obey the laws of the level just below them but are also highly dependent upon (nested within) higher levels. To account for this two-way dependency of each pair of adjacent levels, Changeux proposes a Darwinian scheme of generalized *variation-selection*, with two components: a generator of diversity and a selection system (testing system). At the most elaborate levels of the architecture (understanding and reasoning, in Changeux's terms), the dynamics of variation-selection are as follows: (1) The generator of diversity produces spontaneous, transient activation in neuron assemblies, or *prerepresentations* (the neurocognitive equivalents of Darwin's variations) (→ ACTIVATION/INHIBITION, NEURAL NETWORK, REPRESENTATION). (2) The selection system then proceeds by combining these assemblies in a way that foresees upcoming interactions with the environment. Two cases are possible: either the internal state of the neural system can be *mapped* to the external state or it cannot, where mapping or a lack thereof is a function of the adaptive power of the neuron assembly(ies) or prerepresentations(s) generated. In the first case, there is stabilization and storage in memory; in the second, no memory storage takes place. Adequate mapping is challenged, in the case of sensory perception, through a resonance between perceptual prerepresentations, and in the case of motor action, through evaluation processes involving reward mechanisms.

We know that the variation-selection scheme is the classical one in the evolution of the species, and that it has been observed at work in the development of immunological responses, where variation (or diversity) results from genomic reorganization and gene expression, and selection is based on the survival of the fittest (including antigen-antibody adaptation). The same scheme can also account for the transition from one cell to multicellular organisms, and for the general morphogenesis of the brain. But Changeux goes one step further: he generalizes the Darwinian scheme to the interaction between the nervous system and the outside world, during postnatal development and throughout adulthood as higher cognitive functions are acquired (→ COGNITIVE DEVELOPMENT). The evolution nevertheless occurs here inside the brain, without there necessarily being a change of genetic material (contrary to Jean Piaget's biological views), and within the bounds of a short-term time scale: months, days, or even tenths of seconds (microgeneses) for the processing and reorganization of mental representations. It is thus assumed to involve autoevaluation mechanisms that mobilize higher-order reward processes.

One originality of this theory is its conceptual articulation of two time scales—*phylogeny* (the evolution of the species) and *ontogeny* (neurocognitive development, with its macrogenesis and microgeneses)—based on a generalized Darwin-like mechanism, variation-selection. Changeux stresses the involvement of the prefrontal cortex in this mechanism, and also of the limbic and mesencephalic reward system (→ CONTROL). For the most integrated cognitive functions, the theory is illustrated using logico-mathematical objects, both in the debate about constructivism and realism between Changeux and the mathematician Alain Connes, and in the neurofunctional models proposed by Changeux and Stanislas Dehaene in the domains of number and reasoning (→ NUMBER, REALISM, REASONING AND RATIONALITY). An attempt to generalize the theory to the relationship between reason and aesthetic pleasure has been undertaken, in the hope of solving part of the mystery of artistic creativity, especially pictorial, in neurofunctional terms (→ CREATIVITY). More recently, another generalization was proposed by Changeux on the question of truth (→ TRUTH).

Changeux's theory of neural Darwinism is consistent with current models of cognitive development, which accentuate not only the coordination-activation of structural units (as in neostructuralist theories inspired by Piaget), but also selection-inhibition. Moreover, it leads us to reject the classic cognitivist idea that the science of mental life is a particular kind of science, the science of the *language of thought* (Jerry Fodor; → COGNITIVISM, LANGUAGE OF THOUGHT). Against this programming-based idea and its associated hardware/software metaphor of the computer mind, Changeux discredits the radical proposal (of cognitivists like Philip Johnson-Laird) according to which the physical nature of the brain imposes no constraints on the structure of thought. Here, thought (understanding and reasoning), like neural circuits and cells, is a part of—and is constrained by—a multilevel neurofunctional architecture subjected to the Darwinian scheme of generalized variation-selection.

Another variant of neural Darwinism is Edelman's theory, whose *innatist-selectionist* approach is neatly summarized by the title of a chapter in his book, *A Biological Theory of Consciousness:* "Morphology and

Mind: Completing Darwin's Program" ($\rightarrow$ MIND). Here, the mind is a specific process that depends on particular ways of organizing matter, namely, the different forms of connectivity that link the brain's neuronal groups as they are assembled under the effects of genetic factors. As in Changeux's theory, Edelman proposes a generalized variation-selection scheme (based on connectivity between and within neuron groups) that is applied to cognitive functions such as perception, categorization, memory, and consciousness.

As tempting as neural Darwinism theories may be for cognitive neuroscience and psychology, they are only a metaphorical utilization of the theory of natural selection, as the physiologist Marc Jeannerod pointed out.

OLIVIER HOUDÉ

SELECTED BIBLIOGRAPHY

Changeux, J.-P. (1985). *Neuronal man: The biology of mind* (L. Garey, Trans.). New York: Pantheon. (Original work published 1983.)

Changeux, J.-P., & Connes, A. (1998). *Conversations on mind, matter, and mathematics* (M. B. DeBevoise, Ed. and Trans.). Princeton, NJ: Princeton University Press. (Original work published 1989)

Changeux, J.-P., & Dehaene, S. (1989). Neuronal models of cognitive functions. *Cognition, 33*, 63–109.

Changeux, J.-P., & Ricoeur, P. (2000). *What makes us think?: A neuroscientist and a philosopher argue about ethics, human nature, and the brain* (M. B. DeBevoise, Trans.). Princeton, NJ: Princeton University Press. (Original work published 1988.)

Edelman, G. (1987). *Neural Darwinism: The theory of neuronal group selection.* New York: Basic Books.

Edelman, G., & Changeux, J.-P. (Eds.). (2000). *The brain.* New Brunswick, NJ: Transaction Books.

Fodor, J. (1975). *The language of thought.* New York: Crowell.

Gazzaniga, M. (Ed.) (2000). *The new cognitive neurosciences* (Section X, *Evolution*) (2nd ed.). Cambridge, MA: MIT Press.

Johnson-Laird, P. (1988). *The computer and the mind: An introduction to cognitive science.* Oxford, England: Blackwell.

NEURAL NETWORK

Neuroscience. — The term *neural network* in cognitive neuroscience can be used to refer either to a computer simulation program in which interconnected units (or artificial neurons) work together to execute a particular calculation ($\rightarrow$ CONNECTIONISM), or to a group of real neurons situated in one or more parts of the brain where an elementary cognitive operation is performed ($\rightarrow$ COMPUTATIONAL ANALYSIS, FUNCTIONAL NEUROIMAGING, LOCALIZATION OF FUNCTION).

Networks of artificial neurons, often called *connectionist networks*, are very useful for testing models of cognitive functioning ($\rightarrow$ MODEL). They help us understand how a system (here, the network) manages to produce a particular response when given a particular stimulus. An artificial neural net is made up of units, each of which has its own activity level. The units are interconnected, and each connection is assigned a weight that modulates the way two units interact. A network of this type is capable of storing information and thus of learning (→ INFORMATION, LEARNING). The stored information is contained in the connection weights, and learning consists in modifying the weights in order to improve system performance.

Information is input into a network by adjusting the states of the units that form the network's *input layer*. The response the network puts out is expressed by the state of the units that form its *output layer*. The remaining units are called *hidden units*, which can be organized into one or more layers. During a learning process, the network adjusts the strength of the connections between the input layer units and the hidden units, and between the hidden units and the output units. However, learning is possible only if the network knows the correct response and can calculate an error signal to be used in adjusting the connection weights. This mechanism is called *error backpropagation*.

One of the most interesting capabilities of neural networks is their ability to generalize. When a network arrives at a suitable input-output match using a finite set of stimuli, it is capable of correctly processing (e.g., sorting) stimuli it has never seen before (→ CATEGORIZATION). This capability is valuable because it can be used to test the predictions of a particular processing theory and then compare the network's performance with human behavior. Such a model can also be effective for predicting the behavior of patients after brain damage (→ NEUROPSYCHOLOGY). The effects of a lesion are simulated by destroying units at different network levels or eliminating connections between them and then comparing the performance of the model and the patients.

Connectionist modeling has proven highly useful because it offers an explanation for empirical phenomena that, when approached in terms of other formalisms, seem counterintuitive. In some respects, the units in neural networks resemble real neurons, in that they too are interconnected and can be activated by signals received from a large number of other neurons. Real neural networks are infinitely more complex, however: a single neuron may have several thousands of connections, and no model of this size has ever been tested. In addition, the influence of one neuron on another may depend on the specific features of the receiving neuron, which further increases the complexity of real networks. Moreover, no evidence of a supervisory mechanism that enables error backpropagation (a key mechanism in artificial neural nets) has yet been obtained for real neural networks.

OLIVIER KOENIG

SELECTED BIBLIOGRAPHY

Arbib, M. (Ed.). (2003). *The handbook of brain theory and neural networks* (2nd. ed.). Cambridge, MA: MIT Press.
De Wilde, P. (1997). *Neural network models: Theory and projects* (2nd ed.). London; New York: Springer.
Frackowiak, R., Friston,, K., Dolan, R., Mazziotta, J., & Frith, C. (Eds.). (1997). *Human brain function.* San Diego, CA: Academic Press.
Haykin, S. (1994). *Neural networks: A comprehensive foundation.* New York: Macmillan.
Plaut, D., & Shallice, T. (1994). *Connectionist modelling in cognitive neuropsychology: A case study.* Hove, England; Hillsdale, NJ: Erlbaum.
Rumelhart, D., & McClelland, J. (Eds.) (1986). *Parallel distributed processing: Explorations in the microstructure of cognition.* Cambridge, MA: MIT Press.

NEUROPSYCHOLOGY

Neuroscience. — *Neuropsychology* is the study of higher mental functions and their relationships to the brain (→ FUNCTION, LOCALIZATION OF FUNCTION). Historically, this discipline has been both clinical and experimental. It began its rise in the second half of the nineteenth century with scientists such as Paul Broca, Hughlings Jackson, Jean-Martin Charcot, and many others.

Neuropsychology is first and foremost a clinical discipline. Its primary aim in this case is to understand the deficits of a patient as a whole. The patients examined are individuals with focal lesions of the brain caused by a vascular accident, an injury, a tumor, or similar anomalies. Also included are patients with more diffuse brain deterioration such as that found in degenerative disorders (e.g., Alzheimer's disease) (→ AGING). Diagnosing the disorder is very time-consuming, and every mental function can be altered: language in cases of *aphasia* (→ LANGUAGE); recognition in various types of *agnosia*, which depend on the modality (auditory agnosia and visual agnosia) or on the type of information processed (object agnosia, face agnosia, spatial agnosia) (→ PERCEPTION, SPACE); *memory* in cases of amnesia (→ MEMORY); elaborate gestures in *apraxia* (→ ACTION); and reasoning and executive functions in *frontal syndromes*, and so on (→ CONTROL, REASONING AND RATIONALITY). Diagnosis is fundamental for determining appropriate treatment and follow-up care for patients, since it cannot be reduced to disorder-specific functional rehabilitation. Other tasks are understanding how patients function in the activities of daily living and evaluating their spared functions in view of reintegration into the working world. Hence the importance of having a good team of clinical neuropsychologists with all the necessary specializations.

Neuropsychology is also an experimental discipline. The study of brain-damaged patients has always been the favored experimental approach. This type of study is reinforced by collaboration with clinicians. Unless they are clinical neuropsychologists themselves, experimentalists need the competence of practitioners, and reciprocally, the neuropsychology clinic obviously needs experimental discoveries. In fact, today's core knowledge of the links between the brain and higher mental functions has been acquired through the study of the performance of brain-damaged patients, at least in the human branch of neuropsychology.

This means that there must be a theory of the deficits themselves. As a general rule, it is assumed that the mental functions of a brain-damaged patient correspond to those of a normal subject with one parameter removed, the one corresponding to the mental operation subtended by the lesioned area. But things are usually not so simple, since compensatory strategies develop to reorganize mental functions. Experimental neuropsychology is currently delving into some very advanced methodological issues. To choose the most appropriate tasks, patients' deficits are described using the tools of cognitive psychology. Determining the link to the brain relies on the precise anatomical characterization of each lesion (with the help of brain scans and various morphological imaging techniques).

The most widespread neuropsychological method is *double dissociation*. It is based on the following principle: finding a patient who performs perfectly on task A and fails on task B, and another patient who performs in the opposite way, authorizes the conclusion that tasks A and B necessitate processing by independent functional modules ($\rightarrow$ COMPUTATIONAL ANALYSIS, MODULARITY). If the lesions are located in different regions, one can draw a map of the cerebral organization of the concerned modules. However, the success of the double dissociation method should not cause us to overlook another method, *symptom association*. Finding that a certain symptom is frequently associated with another functionally different one, although essentially of nosological and thus didactic interest, also has theoretical merit; it guides future research toward a better understanding of why two apparently different functions are so close anatomically. This may be purely coincidental, but it may also be a fundamental factor in the biological determinism of mental functions.

Experimental human neuropsychology is not based solely on lesion research, however. Studies on *hemispheric differentiation* make use of techniques in which information is presented to a single hemisphere of normal subjects (for example, dichotic listening, tachistoscopic presentation by hemifield). *Evoked potential studies*, which cover an entire field of neuroscientific research, provide a means of visualizing temporal differences between two cognitive tasks. Specific waves produced at different moments after the presentation of a given piece of information indicate the involvement of brain processes at different times, for example, between 100 ms and a second or more. Finally, studies using *functional brain imaging*, particularly positron emission tomography (PET) and functional magnetic resonance imaging (fMRI), are beginning to supply some very interesting indications on cerebral activity during cognition (→ FUNCTIONAL NEURO-IMAGING).

In addition to these various approaches using human subjects, animal studies are also making a useful contribution (→ ANIMAL COGNITION). They provide insight into certain aspects of human neuropsychology, whether in the field of perception, attention (→ ATTENTION), or memory. The methods are numerous and have different implications. Among the most informative are lesion studies and single-cell recording studies.

Neuropsychology is thus a multifaceted discipline with strong clinical roots and the immense task of being the key interface between the neurosciences and the cognitive sciences. This position affords certain advantages, but also incurs a number of disadvantages, particularly concerning the field's definition and its place in educational and health-related institutions. In the minds of neuropsychologists, however, the fundamental asset of the discipline lies in its dual basis as both clinical and experimental.

ÉRIC SIÉROFF

SELECTED BIBLIOGRAPHY

Farah, M., & Feinberg, T. (Eds.). (2000). *Patient-based approaches to cognitive neuroscience.* Cambridge, MA: MIT Press.

Kertesz, A. (Ed.) (1994). *Localization and neuroimaging in neuropsychology.* New York: Academic Press.

McCarthy, R., & Warrington, E. (1990). *Cognitive neuropsychology: A clinical introduction.* San Diego, CA: Academic Press.

Mesulam, M. (Ed.). (2000). *Principles of behavioral and cognitive neurology* (2nd. ed.). New York: Oxford University Press.

Plaut, D., & Shallice, T. (1994). *Connectionist modelling in cognitive neuropsychology: A case study.* Hove, England; Hillsdale, NJ: Erlbaum.

Shallice, T. (1988). *From neuropsychology to mental structure.* Cambridge, England; New York: Cambridge University Press.

NORMATIVITY

Philosophy. — *Normativity* is the property of activities or states of affairs that makes them subject to rules and capable of being evaluated. Prescriptions and assessments pertaining to what a person should do (moral norms) or what a person should think (epistemic norms; → EPISTEMIC) can be distinguished from those relating to the way a biological or social structure is expected to function (functional norms).

When content is being attributed to propositional attitudes (for example, when one is determining what Jean thinks or what Pierre desires) (→ PROPOSITIONAL ATTITUDE, THEORY OF MIND), normativity appears in the form of a principle of "charity" or a principle of rationality (→ REASONING AND RATIONALITY). By virtue of the first principle, the interpreter must assume that most of the interpreted person's beliefs are true ($\rightarrow$ BELIEF, INTERPRETATION, TRUTH). By virtue of the second, the interpreter must assume that the interpreted person is rational. Donald Davidson considers these two principles to be among the constituents of our capacity to interpret the beliefs of others.

JOËLLE PROUST

SELECTED BIBLIOGRAPHY

Davidson, D. (1984). *Inquiry into truth and interpretation*. Oxford, England: Clarendon Press.
Millikan, R. (1984). *Language, thought, and other biological categories*. Cambridge, MA: MIT Press.

NUMBER

Psychology. — Among the issues under debate in psychology, there is one particularly heated topic: How do numbers come to humans? Jean Piaget's answer was that number is constructed in children through the logicomathematical synthesis of classification and seriation operations ($\rightarrow$ COGNITIVE DEVELOPMENT, CONSTRUCTIVISM, LOGIC). In this view, number borrows its *inclusion* structure from classes (1 is included in 2, 2 in 3, etc.) ($\rightarrow$ CATEGORIZATION), but because it disregards qualities by transforming objects into units, it also brings into play *serial order*—the sole means of distinguishing one unit from the next: 1 then 1, then 1, etc. The serial ordering of units is combined with the inclusion of the sets that result from their union (1 is included in $1 + 1$, $1 + 1$ is included in $1 + 1 + 1$, etc.) to constitute number. The task Piaget used was conservation of number. When shown two rows of objects that contain an equal number of objects but differ in length (because the objects in one of the rows have been spread apart), young children think the longer one has more objects. Piaget's interpretation was that preschool children are still fundamentally intuitive, or, as he called them, *preoperational*, and hence limited to a perceptual way of processing information (here, based on length, or, in certain cases, on density). When they are about six or seven, children understand the equivalency of quantities, regardless of apparent transformations. At this point they are called *operational* or *conserving*—the criterion for mastery of number. Piaget also worked on determining whether the conservation of number develops simultaneously with inclusion (classification) and order relations (seriation). Given that the child's behaviors are observed in a variety of situations (different materials, different questions, different concepts assessed), this approach is resolutely structuralist.

Following this founding work on the genesis of number, research in this area proliferated, and criticisms of Piaget's theory were far from scarce. First, the synchronous development of classification, seriation, and conservation was not validated in experimental verifications. Second, it became increasingly clear that Piaget's view of the logicostructural aspect of number is overly polarized and overshadows other, more functional aspects of numerical development such as counting. However, there is one Piagetian author, Pierre Greco, who did show that counted quantities are conserved before uncounted ones.

A radical change in perspective began with Rochel Gelman, who not only turned the focus toward counting, but also postulated the early existence of five fundamental principles of counting: *stable order* (order of the number words), *strict one-to-one correspondence* (between the number words and the items counted), *cardinality* (the number word corresponding to the last item counted is equal to the total number of items), *abstraction* (any kind of item can be counted), and *order irrelevance* (items can be counted in any order). Gelman demonstrated the presence of these principles in young children by having them say whether they thought a doll was counting correctly or incorrectly. Knowledge or lack of knowledge of a given principle was deduced from whether the child detected the corresponding type of counting error (unstable order, violation of the one-to-one correspondence, cardinal number referred to by an ordinal word number, etc.). The results indicated that three year olds have already acquired the basic principles of counting. This led Gelman to distinguish three components in the ability to count: a *conceptual component* ("knowing why," or understanding the five principles), a *procedural component* ("knowing how," or understanding the structure and order of counting actions; → ACTION), and a *utilization component* ("knowing when," or understanding the relevance of using the first two components in a given context; → CONTEXT AND SITUATION). Defending the principles-before-skills hypothesis, Gelman suggested that the numerical difficulties of preschool children lie essentially in the procedural and utilization components. Another of Gelman's original contributions was her use of the "magic task" to demonstrate that three to four year olds are surprised by transformations that affect the cardinal number of a set (adding and subtracting members) but not by transformations that do not (spreading and grouping). She concluded that, despite their failure in Piaget's conservation of number task, children at this age are already capable of seeing through irrelevant transformations and treating the number of items as invariable.

Gelman's views are extreme and have therefore remained highly controversial. Many experimental findings cast doubt on young children's possession of principles as precisely defined as hers. But do the authors who refute the existence of these principles (and thus of the conceptual component) make a clear distinction, in their analysis of children's failures, between the three components of counting skills: conceptual, procedural, and utilization? Whatever the case may be, Gelman's contribution lies in the impetus her work gave to the study of early numerical activities, particularly counting.

Other functional approaches have focused on the acquisition of the counting word sequence. Karen Fuson, for instance, distinguishes four developmental stages between the ages of two and six years (her categories roughly correspond to the unit levels proposed by Leslie Steffe, shown in parentheses): the *string* (perceptual unit items; → PERCEPTION), the *unbreakable list* (figurative unit items), the *breakable chain* (the initial number sequence), and the *numerable chain*, a unitized seriated embedded bidirectional cardinalized sequence (the tacitly nested and later explicitly nested sequence). Even though Fuson's approach concentrates on how children learn the word-name sequence, it is much closer to Piaget's view than Gelman's is. In fact, the last step described (the numerable chain) has much in common with the Piagetian view, where number acquisition is a synthesis of classifications and seriations.

But what happens in infants, before verbal counting is possible and before the first steps are taken to construct the counting sequence described by Fuson and Steffe (→ INFANT COGNITION)? The most striking example—and one that has sparked heated debates—is found in Karen Wynn's work. Wynn recorded the looking time of four and five month olds in the "impossible-event" procedure (or violation-of-expectation procedure), and showed that infants were surprised by (looked longer at) impossible numerical events (e.g., $1 + 1 = 1$ and $1 + 1 = 3$, or $2 - 1 = 2$), but were not surprised at the corresponding possible events ($1 + 1 = 2$ and $2 - 1 = 1$) (the events were staged with Mickey Mouse figures). She concluded that infants are endowed with a mechanism that calculates the exact result of simple arithmetic operations. She even claimed that infants at this age are already able to encode ordinal information and possess genuine numerical concepts (→ CONCEPT) that cannot be reduced to holistic percepts derived from a pattern recognition process. Like Gelman's, Wynn's position is extreme and seems to run counter to what we know about the numerical difficulties of preschool children. It continues to be subject to disagreement, mostly regarding the cognitive status of the postulated numerical abilities: Are they protooperations (even protoconcepts), or are they the mere intake of perceptual and attentional information (→ ATTENTION, INFORMATION, PERCEPTION)?

The task of future research will be to devise a developmental model of numerical operations (conservation, counting, elementary arithmetic) that accounts for both early abilities (Gelman, Wynn, etc.) and late inabilities (Piaget, Fuson, Steffe, etc.), without denying the reality of the former but raising the question of the factors that explain the latter.

OLIVIER HOUDÉ

Neuroscience. — In cognitive neuroscience, the question of number is addressed through studies that attempt to determine the cerebral bases of elementary mathematics. With the methods developed in cognitive psychology, neuropsychology, and functional brain imaging, it is now possible to state which brain regions are active during arithmetic operations (→ FUNCTIONAL NEUROIMAGING, NEUROPSYCHOLOGY). Research deals in particular with the simplest, but also the most fundamental, of all mathematical objects: integers (Michael McCloskey and Jordan Grafman in the United States; Stanislas Dehaene, Laurent Cohen, and Xavier Seron in Europe).

Briefly, it has been shown by measuring the amount of time we take to compare two numbers that the brain examines number words and Arabic numerals (symbolic expressions) by referring to a mental representation of numerical quantities thought to resemble a line along which the numbers succeed each other in increasing order (→ REPRESENTATION, SYMBOL). This mental representation and the manipulation of numbers rely predominantly on the inferior parietal region of the cortex. A selective lesion in this area causes *primary acalculia*, a disorder whose victims no longer know how to perform calculations but can often still name and write numbers. Depending on whether the arithmetic operation is comparison, subtraction, or multiplication, the inferior parietal region is activated in one or the other hemisphere, and its activity is coordinated with other specialized areas throughout the brain, particularly those that control language production (→ LANGUAGE).

In reference to Dehaene and Cohen's *triple-code model*, the regions involved in number processing are as follows. Visual recognition activates the ventral occipitotemporal region of the left hemisphere for written counting words, and both sides of this structure for Arabic numerals (→ PERCEPTION). The recognition and production of spoken counting words activate the perisylvian region of the left hemisphere. Numerical quantities are represented in the inferior parietal region of both hemispheres, especially in the depths of the intraparietal sulcus. Finally, the prefrontal cortex is in charge of memorizing intermediate results, and for controlling the strategies implemented in the posterior regions (→ CONTROL, MEMORY). During a calculation, all of these regions exchange information (→ INFORMATION).

Recent brain imaging data have revealed the complexity of number processing in the brain. Here are a few illustrations. If we measure brain activity during various arithmetic tasks (reading, comparison, addition, subtraction, multiplication, etc.), it is the right parietal cortex that gets activated during number comparisons, whereas multiplication generates activity almost totally localized in the left hemisphere; subtraction triggers bilateral activation. We also know that another region, the left lenticular nucleus, is activated more when two numbers are being multiplied than when they are being compared, and neuropsychological data indicate that brain damage in this region can cause a loss of memory for the multiplication table. Convergent findings from patients and normal subjects help delineate the neural circuits associated with each operation.

Other interesting findings concern the steps involved in performing numerical operations, particularly the sequence of brain activations that takes place when we compare two numbers. When the brain's electrical activity is measured using electrodes spread over the surface of a person's scalp while he or she is comparing the number 5, for example, with one of the Arabic numerals 1, 4, 6, or 9 and one of the number words *one, four, six,* or *nine,* the following results are obtained: about 100 ms after the appearance of the number on the computer screen, a positive electric potential on the posterior electrodes indicates activation of the primary visual area. Then, at approximately 150 ms, a difference in the topography appears, depending on whether an Arabic numeral or a number word is presented, each being identified by anatomically different networks. As stated above, numerals are recognized by the ventral occipitotemporal regions of both hemispheres, whereas number words implicate only the left side. At this stage, however, no numerical distance effect is noticeable (an effect whereby the farther apart two numbers are, the faster they are compared): only the identity of the symbols has been recognized at this point, not their meaning. At about 190 ms, the distance effect shows up: subjects are consistently slower at comparing 4 and 6 than 1 and 9. In addition, the potential measured on electrodes across from the inferior parietal cortex varies with the difference between the test number and 5. Finally, the topography of this effect is similar for numbers presented in Arabic numerals and ones spelled out in words, which means that the inferior parietal region does not encode numbers as symbols in a particular numeration, but uses an abstract quantitative code that is independent of the input notation.

Another finding worth mentioning is the fact that when we multiply two small integers, say 2×3, parietal activation is highly lateralized on the left and is short-lived. If, on the contrary, the multiplication is less common, say 8×7, activation seems to begin in the left hemisphere before moving over into the right parietal region, where it lasts several hundred milliseconds. Thus, the size of the numbers manipulated and the type of operation carried out appear to determine which of the brain's pathways are involved in a given computation.

The existence of brain regions specialized in the processing of numbers raises the question of the origin of numerical specialization. Is the inferior parietal region already partly operational in infants, and does this already give them an approximate sense of quantity (→ COGNITIVE DEVELOPMENT)? Organisms as varied as the rat, the pigeon, the dolphin, the chimpanzee, and the human infant, all without speech, mentally represent the cardinal number of a set of visual objects or sounds, and can even make elementary arithmetic deductions (→ ANIMAL COGNITION, INFANT COGNITION). For instance, four- and five-month-old infants expect a set of two objects from which one was taken away to have only one object left: they mentally carry out an operation on concrete objects that is analogous to the abstract arithmetic operation $2 - 1 = 1$ (see *psychology* above). Brain circuits prespecified for representing numbers are thus thought to exist right from birth, independently of the child's mathematical education. Early learning how to recite the names of numbers (*one, two, three, . . .*) and how to recognize the visual form of the Arabic numerals (1, 2, 3, . . .) enables children to later associate symbolic enumeration systems with this "sense of quantity" (→ LEARNING). In other words, the child makes the connection between the word *four*, the numeral 4, and the corresponding quantity.

Whatever the validity of this view, a general principle of cerebral organization emerges here: the *modularity* of brain networks (→ MODULARITY). Without our awareness, dozens of specialized brain areas distributed across the two hemispheres are being activated when we engage in mental arithmetic (→ CONSCIOUSNESS). The information goes effortlessly from the visual representation areas specialized in numeral identity to the language areas, where numbers are encoded as word strings, and to the areas in charge of quantitative sense, where number quantities and relations of numerical proximity are found. We are beginning to uncover the principal nodes of this network, but two questions remain unanswered: What are the mechanisms that ensure the coherence of the numerical information distributed and give us the subjective impression of having performed a single operation? How do these elementary calculation mechanisms gradually give way, as mathematical knowledge is acquired, to mental representations of much more elaborate mathematical objects, to the point of reaching the extraordinary calculative fluidity and mathematical creativity of an Albert Einstein, a Henri Poincaré, or a Srinavasa Ramanujan Iyengar (→ CONSTRUCTIVISM, REALISM)?

STANISLAS DEHAENE

SELECTED BIBLIOGRAPHY

Carey, S. (2001). Bridging the gap between cognition and developmental neuroscience: The example of number representation. In C. Nelson & M. Luciana (Eds.), *Developmental cognitive neuroscience* (pp. 415–431). Cambridge, MA: MIT Press.

Dehaene, S. (1997). *The number sense: How the mind creates mathematics.* New York: Oxford University Press.

Dehaene, S., Spelke, E., Pinel, P., Stanescu, R., & Tsivkin, S. (1999). Sources of mathematical thinking: Behavioral and brain-imaging evidence. *Science, 284,* 970–974.

Gelman, R., & Meck, E. (1983). Preschooler's counting: Principles before skills. *Cognition, 13*, 343–359.

Houdé, O. (2000). Inhibition and cognitive development: Object, number, categorization, and reasoning. *Cognitive Development, 15*, 63–73.

Houdé, O., & Tzourio-Mazoyer, N. (2003). Neural foundations of logical and mathematical cognition. *Nature Reviews Neuroscience, 4*, 507–514.

Piaget, J. (1952). *The child's conception of number* (C. Gattegno & F. M. Hodgson, Trans.). New York: Humanities Press; London: Routledge and Kegan Paul. (Original work published 1941.)

Wynn, K. (1998). Psychological foundations of numbers: Numerical competence in human infants. *Trends in Cognitive Sciences, 2*, 296–303.

O

OBJECT

Psychology. — The concept of object has been approached in cognitive psychology primarily in work on perception and space (→ PERCEPTION, SPACE). Our presentation here will be confined to the question of *object permanence* as it is studied in developmental psychology (→ COGNITIVE DEVELOPMENT).

We are indebted to Jean Piaget for his clear statement of the problem of how objects act as the basic unit for constructing reality (→ CON-STRUCTIVISM): Does an object continue to exist for infants once it is out of sight? Does it have permanence outside of immediate experience (→ EXPERI-ENCE)? Six stages stand out from Piaget's observations. They mark off the laborious path toward object permanence taken by the infant, essentially during the first year of life.

According to Piaget, the systematic search for a disappeared object does not begin until Stage IV of sensorimotor development, at approximately eight or nine months. This stage still suffers from the "location error," which can be demonstrated using the following device: the experimenter puts the infant in front of two screens (A and B) that are equally easy to reach, and hides an object under A. The eight to nine month old has no trouble finding the object. After a few repetitions of this situation, the object is very conspicuously transferred from under A to under B (A → B). If there is a delay before the infant can respond, he or she continues to look for the object under A: this is the "A-not-B error." The Piagetian interpretation is that infants have not yet mastered true object permanence. It is not until the end of the first year that this concept is acquired, and hence the disappearance of the A-not-B error at about twelve months (with a few remaining refinements during the second year). This interpretation is contested today in the light of new data on the existence of object permanence by the early age of four or five months. The new data came with a change of methodology from the Piagetian study of the infant's actions (→ ACTION) to the cognitivist study of the infant's gazing behavior, that is, analysis of perceptual activity measured by visual fixation time (→ INFANT COGNITION).

With this new approach, Renée Baillargeon provided evidence of the early existence of object permanence using the "impossible event" paradigm (or violation-of-expectation paradigm). The experimental procedure is run in two phases. (1) The infant is facing a presentation device with a screen fastened to its base by a hinge in such a way that the screen can be rotated 180° along the horizontal axis. The infant is habituated to the alternating backward-forward rotation. (2) Next a box is placed behind the screen's rotation axis in such a way that the screen can now only be rotated 112° degrees, at which point it completely hides the box (the disappeared object). The infant is then shown a possible event, a 112° rotation of the screen, and an impossible event, a 180° rotation. In Phase 2, four and five month olds look longer at the impossible event than at the possible one, even though the impossible event is identical to the habituation situation (180° rotation) and the possible event is new (identical results have been found at three-and-a-half months, but not in all infants). Baillargeon concluded that four and five month olds realize that the event is impossible, which suggests that they can conceive of the violated property, namely, the permanence of the box hidden by the screen. By this young age (the beginning of Piaget's Stage III of sensorimotor development), object permanence may therefore already be in place, along with the cohesion principle (other experiments on this problem were conducted by Baillargeon and other investigators). Moreover, Karen Wynn showed that in protonumerical activities, a permanent object (one completely out of sight) can be integrated by four or five month olds as a physical entity connected to other discrete and quantifiable entities (→ NUMBER).

The divergence between the experimental data just presented and Piaget's theory, closely tied to the paradigms used, is highly problematic for infant psychologists. If by four or five months there is object permanence, how can one explain the A-not-B error classically found in eight to twelve month olds? For some authors, this question is not a critical one. For others, on the contrary, it is one of the fascinating puzzles of the psychology of cognitive development. A range of interpretations has been proposed, along with ingenious experimental situations: the role of memory capacity (→ MEMORY), spatial organization, motor programming constraints (motor perseveration and inhibition) (→ ACTIVATION/INHIBITION, CONTROL), and so forth. One of the most impressive interpretations was proposed by Adele Diamond in conclusion of a comparative study in neurocognitive animal psychology conducted on monkeys following prefrontal cortex ablation

($\rightarrow$ ANIMAL COGNITION, NEUROPSYCHOLOGY). Diamond suggests that the location error made by eight to twelve month olds is due to ineffective inhibition of a prepotent gesture (moving toward A) brought about by the insufficient development of the prefrontal cortex. Single-cell recordings in monkeys, as well as the neural models devised by Jean-Pierre Changeux and Stanislas Dehaene, corroborate Diamond's hypothesis that the frontal system plays a decisive role. Complementary studies by Marta Bell and Nathan Fox established a relationship between electroencephalographic recordings (EEGs) of the frontal system and the cognitive development of infants, in particular, their performance in the A $\rightarrow$ B situation. The recordings confirmed the existence, in infants, of the link between the A-not-B error and the frontal system established by Diamond for nonhuman primates. The authors concluded that success in the A $\rightarrow$ B situation is achieved through inhibition of the initial programmed gesture, in conjunction with a sufficient memory capacity and the ability to resist distraction during the delay.

Some experimental findings, however, argue against the hypothesized role of frontal inhibition (and thus of the perseveration of a to-be-inhibited gesture) as the sole explanatory factor. This inconclusive state of affairs exists for every other factor put forward to account for the A-not-B error, for example, memory capacity, whose role is supported by certain findings but seems to contradict others. Future research will be aimed at theoretically and experimentally delineating the simultaneous effects of several factors, including memory, spatial organization, and frontal inhibition, from the angle of their links to motor programming. An attempt in this direction was made by James Russell, who introduced the concept of *agency*, a broader concept than Piagetian action that also encompasses selective-attention mechanisms ($\rightarrow$ ATTENTION).

OLIVIER HOUDÉ

Artificial intelligence. — In computer science the notion of *object*, which permeates every branch of the field today, appeared in the 1970s under the impetus of two research trends: (1) a new approach developed in programming and software engineering, where programs were no longer conceived of as sequences of instructions but rather as interacting entities, and (2) the notion of semantic network, developed at the same time in artificial intelligence (AI) ($\rightarrow$ SEMANTIC NETWORK). Databases were added later to the first two innovations.

A computer object is an "individualized" object, in the sense that two objects created independently remain distinct for their entire lifetime. It is said to be "complete" in that it includes both a static part, which represents its state and the links that connect it to other objects, and a dynamic part, which describes its behavior, that is, the set of operations applicable to it. In spite of many variations, the notion of object can be defined in terms of three principal concepts: *class-instance structuring, activation by message sending*, and *hierarchical classification by inheritance*.

(1) Class-instance structuring is what groups together objects with a shared structure and shared behavior, in the form of a general model called a *class*. A class is a sort of mold from which the objects or instances of that class are generated ($\rightarrow$ CATEGORIZATION). The model contains the list of attributes the instances possess, along with the set of operations, called *methods*, that characterize their behavior. (2) Activation by message sending is the dynamic aspect of objects. When an object receives a message, it applies the appropriate method defined in its class. The advantage of this technique is its polymorphism: one and the same message sent to two objects belonging to different classes can trigger two different methods and thus cause the execution of two different behaviors. (3) Hierarchical classification by inheritance supplies a generalization-specialization hierarchy ($\rightarrow$ INHERITANCE). The most abstract classes are found at the top of the hierarchy, and the most concrete classes, the most practical ones, correspond to the leaves in this treelike structure.

The concept of object cannot be reduced to a mere computer technique. It is rooted in a general and much earlier understanding of knowledge in which the knowledge at a subject's disposal—which is also the knowledge that must be made available to any cognitive artifact—can be represented by entities that possess the above three characteristics.

Using objectlike representation techniques, investigators in the United States set out to compile all basic knowledge possessed by a six-year-old child ($\rightarrow$ REPRESENTATION). Despite the relative failure of this undertaking, it led to an upsurge of projects to develop large knowledge bases covering more limited domains, now improperly called "ontologies" ($\rightarrow$ DOMAIN SPECIFICITY, KNOWLEDGE BASE).

While the notion of object reigns today in all branches of computer science, artificial intelligence no longer claims that it holds the key to the ideal representation of knowledge. Several criticisms can rightfully be directed against it. Objects are based on a symbolic, cognitive representation of knowledge ($\rightarrow$ COGNITIVISM, SYMBOL), and, by that token, one can raise the objection that knowledge, albeit structured, is defined externally and is not the result of acquired experience ($\rightarrow$ EXPERIENCE). Second, the definition of inheritance in object-oriented languages is too elementary to be useful for classifying even slightly complex concepts ($\rightarrow$ CONCEPT, LANGUAGE). Finally, the compromise obtained in object-oriented languages between description by attributes and activation by methods is now often split into two models: the purely representational facet is more effectively described by techniques like semantic networks, whereas the activation facet has given rise to a new line of computer systems called *multiagent systems* (→ DISTRIBUTED INTELLIGENCE).

Nevertheless, by virtue of the capabilities they offer, both for programming and for describing well-structured, not too complex knowledge sets, objects have become an essential tool in knowledge programming and representation.

JACQUES FERBER

SELECTED BIBLIOGRAPHY

Baillargeon, R. (1995). Physical reasoning in infancy. In M. Gazzaniga (Ed.), *The cognitive neurosciences* (pp. 181–204). Cambridge, MA: MIT Press.

Baillargeon, R., & Wang, S. (2002). Event categorization in infancy. *Trends in Cognitive Sciences, 6*, 85–92.

Bell, M. A., & Fox, N. A. (1992). The relations between frontal brain electrical activity and cognitive development during infancy. *Child Development, 63*, 1142–1163.

Blum, A. (1992). *Neural networks in C++: An object-oriented framework for building connectionist systems*. New York: Wiley.

Dehaene, S., & Changeux, J.-P. (1989). A simple model of prefrontal cortex function in delayed-response tasks. *Journal of Cognitive Neuroscience, 1*, 244–261.

Diamond, A. (1991). Neuropsychological insights into the meaning of object concept development. In S. Carey & R. Gelman (Eds.), *The epigenesis of mind: Essays on biology and cognition*. Hillsdale, NJ: Erlbaum.

Diamond, A. (1998). Understanding the A-not-B error. *Developmental Science, 1*, 185–189.

Houdé, O. (2000). Inhibition and cognitive development: Object, number, categorization, and reasoning. *Cognitive Development, 15*, 63–73.

Johnson, M. (2001). Functional brain development in humans. *Nature Reviews Neuroscience, 2*, 75–483.

Piaget, J. (1954). *The construction of reality in the child* (M. Cook, Trans.). New York: Basic Books. (Original work published 1937.)

Russell, J. (1997). *Agency: Its role in mental development*. Hove, England: Erlbaum.

Spelke, E., Vishaton, P., & von Hofsten, C. (1995). Object perception, object-directed action, and physical knowledge in infancy. In M. Gazzaniga (Ed.), *The cognitive neurosciences* (pp. 165–179). Cambridge, MA: MIT Press.

Tello, E. (1989). *Object-oriented programming for artificial intelligence: A guide to tools and system design*. Reading, MA: Addison-Wesley.

Tracy, K., & Bouthoorn, P. (1997). *Object-oriented artificial intelligence using C++*. New York: Computer Science Press.

ORAL

Psychology. — The *oral* modality is one of the modalities of language, the other being writing (→ LANGUAGE, READING, WRITING). Strictly speaking, the oral modality ensures speech production by means of the articulatory system, and speech reception by means of the auditory system (→ PERCEPTION); the written modality involves the use of a graphemic representation system (→ REPRESENTATION). The oral mode is often associated with informal communication, and the written mode, with formal communication (→ COMMUNICATION). Although the opposition between speaking and writing is correlated with different levels or types of discourse (→ DISCOURSE), the correlation is not absolute (for example, a formal written discourse can be presented orally).

Depending on the theoretical approach adopted, one can envisage language from two angles by making the distinction, along with Ferdinand de Saussure, between *language* (*langue* in French), which corresponds to the abstract structure of the language, and *speech* (*parole* in French), which corresponds to how the language is actually used in a given situation (→ CONTEXT AND SITUATION). An analogous contrast is made between the different types of cognitive capabilities that characterize the knowledge speakers have of their native language. In Noam Chomsky's terms, a speaker's *competence* corresponds to his or her virtual knowledge of the grammatical structure of the language, whereas a speaker's *performance* refers to the current actualization of that competence at the behavioral level (→ COMPETENCE/PERFORMANCE).

Speech implies a linear organization of the flow of information over time (→ INFORMATION, TIME AND TENSE). This imposes processing constraints on the cognitive system that are specific to the oral modality and that bring into play various components of cognition—for example, working memory, long-term memory, and real-time semantic and pragmatic cue processing (→ MEMORY, PRAGMATICS, SEMANTICS)—whose relationship to grammatical knowledge is a subject of controversy (Brian MacWhinney and Elisabeth Bates, William Marslen-Wilson and Lorraine Tyler). The linear unfolding of speech determines not only its phrasal structure, but also the way utterances are strung together to form larger discourse units (narratives, conversations, etc.).

Speech is also closely tied to the context of utterance (Émile Benveniste, Roman Jakobson). It is accompanied by *contextual information* that is fundamental to oral communication because of the various functions it fulfills, that is, conveying the propositional content of utterances, assigning them interpersonal functions, indicating the speakers' intentions, incorporating certain sociolinguistic characteristics (e.g., group membership), and the like (→ PROPOSITIONAL FORMAT, SOCIAL COGNITION, THEORY OF MIND). Contextual information is of various kinds. It may be (1) *extralinguistic*, in which case it conveys information about the parameters that define the situation (identity of the interlocutors and of other referred-to entities, place and time of utterance) (→ SPACE) or about nonverbal messages (gestures, direction of gaze, facial expressions) (→ EMOTION); (2) *discursive* (discourse type and topic, relationships to past and future utterances produced by the speaker and listeners); or (3) *suprasegmental* (pronunciation, prosodic features such as stress or intonation). In all languages, the production and comprehension of certain linguistic devices, particularly deictics (pronouns, place and time markers), are intrinsically dependent upon shared knowledge of the situation, assumed or constructed by the interlocutors.

MAYA HICKMAN

SELECTED BIBLIOGRAPHY

Benveniste, É. (1971). *Problems in general linguistics* (M. E. Meek, Trans.). Coral Gables, FL: University of Miami Press. (Original work published 1966–1974.)

Chomsky, N. (1986). *Knowledge of language: Its nature, origin, and use*. New York: Praeger.

Hauser, M., Chomsky, N., & Fitch, W. (2002). The faculty of language: What is it, who has it, and how did it evolve? *Science, 298*, 1569–1579.

Jakobson, R. (1971). *Selected writings: Word and language* (Vol. 2). The Hague, The Netherlands: Mouton.

MacWhinney, B., & Bates, E. (1989). *The cross-linguistic study of sentence processing*. Cambridge, England: Cambridge University Press.

Marslen Wilson, W., & Tyler, L. (1980). The temporal structure of spoken language understanding. *Cognition, 8*, 1–71.

Pinker, S. (1994). *The language instinct: How the mind creates language*. New York: W. Morrow.

Saussure, F. de (1959). *Course in general linguistics* (C. Bally, A. Sechehaye, & A. Reidlinger, Eds.; W. Baskin, Trans.). New York: McGraw-Hill. (Original work published 1916.)

P

PATTERN RECOGNITION

Artificial intelligence. — The overall goal of work on *pattern recognition* is to build automatic perception systems that are capable of identifying patterns collected by sensors, which act as sensory organs (→ PERCEPTION). This approach is complementary to those aimed at endowing a machine with cognitive skills such as reasoning or decision-making (→ REASONING AND RATIONALITY). Pattern-recognition techniques are close to a number of other data-processing methods, in particular *data analysis* (factor analysis, discriminant analysis, principal component analysis, etc.), which attempts to transform and simplify pattern-representation and data-representation spaces (→ REPRESENTATION), and *automatic sorting*, which takes a set of patterns or forms in a given representation space and tries to define a *partition*, or set of classes (→ CATEGORIZATION). These methods are sometimes used in conjunction with pattern-recognition algorithms.

A standard pattern-recognition system has three major components. (1) First, there are *sensing subcomponents* (for example, microphones for speech; diode matrices for written character recognition; cameras for object recognition in scenes; pressure sensors, temperature gauges, and gas composition detectors to describe the state of an industrial installation, etc.) that capture the pattern, filter it, and preprocess it to make it usable by a program (→ LANGUAGE, READING). (2) Next, a *parameterization component* extracts a relevant set of representative features from the pattern (for example, formant frequencies for speech, a set of black and white dots for a printed character, lines representing the outline of an object in a picture, etc.). This stage reduces the amount of information carried by the pattern (→ INFORMATION). (3) Finally, a *decision-making component* identifies the pattern (assigns it to a class). This is done by comparing it to a set of prototype patterns incorporated into the system during prior learning phases (→ LEARNING), based on a metric or distance defined in advance by the properties of the patterns processed so far.

An important step in the development of a pattern-recognition system is finding an adequate definition of how to represent the prototype patterns in a way that can account for the variability and diversity of the patterns studied, and guarantee a certain amount of immunity to noise that is liable to taint them. Two major families of methods have been used: *structural* and *statistical*. Structural or syntactic methods look at the structure of the patterns and describe them in terms of assemblies of primitive patterns (→ SYNTAX). These methods are akin to formal language models and formal grammars (→ GRAMMAR). Statistical methods are based on statistical figures (means, standard deviations, etc.) that describe the patterns studied. Methods of the latter type are currently exhibiting the highest performance in various domains of application. *Hidden Markov models* (HMM) are a good example and are now widely used in speech recognition and written character recognition. An HMM can be described as an automaton that represents a pattern to be recognized (a word, a phoneme, etc.) and whose changes in state are governed by probabilities. The states of the automaton contain statistical information about a small portion of the represented pattern. In the case of speech, for example, recognition amounts to searching for the HMM that has the greatest probability of having produced the acoustic pattern of the input.

A variety of decision-making methods are employed, including *Bayesian decisions*, where an unknown pattern is classified in the category that incurs the lowest risk of error based on the probability distributions of the pattern classes (often approximated by Gaussian functions); sorting based on surfaces in the parameter space (or rather on hypersurfaces, which are analogous to mathematical surfaces for spaces of any dimension), where each region of the space delineated by the surfaces corresponds to a class; *nearest-neighbor decisions*, which assign an unknown pattern to the category of its nearest neighbor(s) whose class is known, with nearness being defined by the distance between the two patterns in the parameter space; and finally, classification by a *connectionist* or *neural network* (→ CONNECTIONISM, NEURAL NETWORK), where the necessary decision-making functions are learned by a network made up of interconnections between a large number of formal neurons, designed to simulate the functioning of the brain (following the work by Warren McCulloch and Walter Pitts). The last method is becoming increasingly popular today, especially with multilayer perceptrons, Hopfield networks, and Kohonen's cards.

A major obstacle in making pattern-recognition decisions is the existence of nonlinear distortions within a given pattern category (for example, variations in rhythm and duration affecting the same word pronounced at different instants or by different speakers, differences in the size of written characters, etc.). They make comparing two patterns a delicate process. The use of dynamic programming offers an optimal solution to this problem.

A crucial task that strongly determines the performance of a pattern-recognition system is *learning*, the initial phase during which the system memorizes the discriminating features of families of to-be-recognized patterns (→ MEMORY). Statistical methods propose learning algorithms that converge mathematically, provided the system is given a sufficiently large number of representative patterns. This is true in particular of hidden Markov models and neural networks, a fact that certainly accounts for their success. But their use in some domains may be precluded due to the massive amounts of data needed for learning (for example, several hours of recorded speech for a robust system capable of recognizing the ten numerals pronounced by several speakers).

Many practical applications of pattern recognition have been developed and are now in routine operation in various branches of the economy. For the most part, they fall into two main categories: (1) recognition of signals of various types, including speech signals (speech recognition, speaker identity verification), radar signals, sonar signals, biomedical signals (electroencephalography, electrocardiography, etc.), and seismic or industrial signals; and (2) recognition of two- or three-dimensional images, such as optical reading of printed characters, robotic vision (→ ROBOTICS), object detection on satellite images, quality control on assembly lines, and biomedical imaging (anatomical cross sections, X-rays, etc.) (→ FUNCTIONAL BRAIN IMAGING).

Very often, the recognition of a pattern is accompanied by a cognitive process of interpretation and understanding (→ INTERPRETATION). This is the case for spoken sentence recognition and understanding, and for the interpretation of radiographic images, sonar signals, computer vision, and so on. The interpretation process requires a body of specific knowledge that is difficult to account for using tools derived from "blind" mathematical models. Developing a pattern-recognition system may also call upon additional techniques used in explicit knowledge-based systems (→ KNOWLEDGE BASE). This poses the classic problems of knowledge representation, reasoning, strategies, and so on, encountered in artificial intelligence. Designing architectures that support optimal coordination of different kinds of knowledge is an important problem, analogous to that posed, for example, in natural language understanding. The blackboard model, and more generally *multiagent system architectures* (→ DISTRIBUTED INTELLIGENCE) in which different knowledge sources communicate and cooperate by means of various mechanisms (message sending, information sharing), have interesting properties for solving such problems.

JEAN-PAUL HATON

SELECTED BIBLIOGRAPHY

Bechtel, W., & Abrahamsen, A. (2002). *Connectionism and the mind: Parallel processing dynamics and evolution* (2nd ed.). Oxford, England: Blackwell.

Bishop, C. (1995). *Neural networks for pattern recognition*. Oxford, England: Clarendon Press; New York: Oxford University Press.

Horn, B. (1986). *Robot vision*. Cambridge, MA: MIT Press.

Lew, M. (Ed.). (2001). *Principles of visual information retrieval*. Berlin, Germany: Springer-Verlag.

Paulus, D., & Hornegger, J. (1998). *Applied pattern recognition: A practical introduction to image and speech processing in C++* (2nd ed.). Wiesbaden, Germany: Verlag Vieweg.

Tarr, M., & Bulthoff, H. (1998). *Object recognition in man, monkey, and machine*. Cambridge, MA: MIT Press.

PERCEPTION

Psychology. — *Perception* is a process by means of which the organism becomes aware of its environment on the basis of information taken in by its senses (→ COGNITIVISM, CONNECTIONISM, EXPERIENCE, INFORMATION, PSYCHOPHYSICS). From the cognitive standpoint, one of the functions of perception is to interpret sensory data, and hence to process information (→ FUNCTION, INTERPRETATION). This function is assumed to involve two types of processing: data-driven (*bottom-up processing*) and concept- or representation-driven (*top-down processing*) (→ CONCEPT, REPRESENTATION). The part played by each type depends on whether the processing bears primarily on sensory information drawn directly from stimuli, or on the subject's knowledge, expectations, motivations, and so on. The cognitive approach requires identifying different processing *levels*, starting from the analysis of sensory stimulation and ending with its identification (perceptual semantics; → SEMANTICS).

Information taken in by the sensory systems provokes a sensation. Each system detects only information that is specific to it, and for this reason, it remains incomplete and fragmented. At this level, processing is automatic, prewired, essentially inaccessible to consciousness, and thus *modular* (→ AUTOMATISM, CONSCIOUSNESS, MODULARITY). Before the stimulus is identified, various grouping together and breaking down processes are performed on the sensory flow according to the perceiver's knowledge. This knowledge is what drives the perceptual structuring process and enables object identification (→ OBJECT, PATTERN RECOGNITION). Attentional processes also play a major role by determining what information gets selected (→ ACTIVATION/INHIBITION, ATTENTION). The identification of an object generates a series of multimodal representations (visual, auditory, somesthetic, and possibly gustatory and olfactory), as well as motor, lexical, and semantic representations (→ ACTION, LEXICON).

Analyzing the relationships between these processing levels and their impact on object identification is not always a straightforward endeavor. Similarly, while modularity is an undeniable characteristic of sensory processing, its applicability to higher perceptual processing levels cannot be ruled out (now a topic of some fairly lively theoretical discussions). Generally speaking, the perceptual processes implemented to identify objects or scenes (→ SPACE) vary with the degree of familiarity and the circumstances in which the objects or scenes are perceived. In familiar situations, most perceptual processes require little attentional effort, but as soon as any incongruities, difficulties, or novelties appear, additional attentional resources are allocated and reasoning processes are triggered (→ CONTROL, REASONING AND RATIONALITY).

As far as perception theories are concerned, the views of the *gestaltists* (Max Wertheimer, Kurt Koffka, and Wolfgang Köhler) radically oppose the elementarist views of the *associationists* (John Locke, William James, George Berkeley, David Hume, and Donald Hebb), for whom perceptions are learned and are the result (sums and associations of elementary sensations) of an organism's multiple encounters with its environment. By focusing on the geometric and structural aspects of stimuli (→ MORPHOLOGY), gestaltists refuse the sensation/perception distinction stipulated by the associationists. They see an isomorphism between the structure of the stimulus and the corresponding percept, and from there, deduce an isomorphism with the underlying physiological mechanisms. Their position is necessarily globalistic and emphasizes the idea that subjects organize and structure (shape) the environment (contrary to the associationist idea of an environment that acts upon the subject). The observation that separate elements appear all at once as belonging to the same entity or structured whole, a gestalt or configuration, leads them to define a series of principles (veritable structure generators), the most important being the laws of proximity, similarity, continuation, closure, and the minimum principle or best possible form (*Prägnanz*). These laws determine how the forces within a perceptual field interact and, according to the isomorphism postulate, they take effect at three levels, physical, cerebral, and perceptual.

In line with the gestaltists, James Gibson also rejects the sensation/perception distinction, along with any approach where the subject contributes by performing associational, mediational, or processing operations. This "direct perception" view is based on the argument that the physical environment composed of surfaces and textures provides a wealth of organized information, and that the perceptual flow coming from the stimuli is structured in a correlated fashion with the environment. Accordingly, even a very young perceiver has the capacity to detect the structure of information flowing in from the environment, and can therefore immediately perceive objects (→ INFANT COGNITION). And if perception is isomorphic to reality, it is not because of some hypothetical harmony between the subject's structures and those of reality, as suggested by the gestaltists, but because reality determines the percept by means of a causal relationship of specification. In the description of perceptual development proposed by Eleanor Gibson, young children discover increasingly greater amounts of information and select the part that best fits their actions and everyday frames of reference (→ COGNITIVE DEVELOPMENT). This progression leads to finer and finer perceptual differentiation as new encounters with the environment take place. The organism begins to respond in a differentiated manner to sets of stimuli that initially triggered a generic response. Going beyond the problem of perception per se, James Gibson added an ecological dimension to his theory by introducing the concept of *affordance*. An affordance is an objective property of a stimulus whose meaning for a given organism depends on the organism's needs and ability to detect that property (→ MEANING). In this way, a subject's actions are constrained by his or her ecological niche and by the affordances the environment offers to that particular individual.

The cognitive theory of perception is clearly illustrated by David Marr's *computational approach* (→ COMPUTATIONAL ANALYSIS). Inspired by research in artificial intelligence, the aim of this approach is to develop a model of visual perception that can be implemented (in the sense that it can be used to run simulations). More than others, this approach deals directly with the problem of three-dimensional object recognition, and clearly distinguishes early vision and visual recognition. Marr defines three levels of representation, or *sketches*. (1) The *primal sketch* is a breakdown of the properties of surfaces that contains symbols or place tokens indicating the presence of edges, angles, lines, points of different sizes, and so on (→ SYMBOL). Many of these elements remain invariable under changes in brightness or contrast. (2) The *2½-D sketch* is the core of the theory, since this level acts as the interface between perception and cognition. It is a representation of the surfaces of the object that are visible when the observer is looking in a particular direction from a strategic viewpoint. No top-down processing enters into this sketch. Perceptually, it is the most elaborate level; it is the level that takes the information supplied by the preceding level and determines the contour, distance, and orientation of the surfaces with respect to the observer, and depth cues. Finally, (3) the *3-D sketch* is based on a coordinate system with the object at the origin (not the observer) and a stationary view of the object. This level is a structural description of the shape of the object and the arrangement of its parts. It includes the object's volumetric characteristics and permits access to its meaning.

ARLETTE STRERI

Neuroscience. — Among the many cognitive processes, the perceptual processes have no doubt been studied the most in cognitive neuroscience. This is due, of course, to the importance of perception in our daily lives, especially visual and auditory perception, and to the dramatic consequences of impaired vision. But it is also because perception is "the doorway to cognition."

Remarkable progress has been made toward understanding the mechanisms of perception, not only through animal research (→ ANIMAL COGNITION), but also because of human neuropsychology research (→ NEURO-PSYCHOLOGY) and brain imaging studies, which will receive particular attention here (→ FUNCTIONAL BRAIN IMAGING). It is perhaps in the area of visual perception that our knowledge is the deepest. This domain has benefited considerably from studies on monkeys, whose visual system is very close to ours, and brain imaging research of this type is flourishing. To illustrate how perceptual activities are analyzed in cognitive neuroscience, the emphasis will be placed here on visual information intake.

Research in neuroscience has shown that visual perception, like other cognitive processes, is not performed by a unitary, undifferentiated system. The visual perception system is composed of many specialized subsystems, each in charge of specific information-processing stages (→ INFORMATION). It is precisely for visual perception that Marr demonstrated the importance of the computational approach (→ COMPUTATIONAL ANALYSIS), which is aimed at specifying the processing stages necessary to any system accomplishing a given task (see *psychology* above).

Brain imaging studies have confirmed the retinotopical structure of the primary visual cortex, and the functional specialization of the extrastriate cortex for analyzing movement and color. *Retinotopy* refers to the precise topographical mapping between a cell of the retina and a corresponding cell in the primary visual cortex. A consequence of this mapping is that the structure of the image perceived is maintained in the primary visual area. This principle has been demonstrated in positron emission tomography experiments where subjects have to stare at the center of different-sized rings displayed on a computer screen. The results have shown that the more the rings activate the periphery of the retina, the farther the brain activity is from the posterior part of the striate cortex. In addition, when only the upper quadrants of the visual field contain a stimulus, activation appears below the calcarine sulcus; when something is in the lower quadrants, activation appears above it. Similarly, stimuli in the quadrants of the left visual field trigger activation of the right hemisphere, whereas stimuli in the quadrants of the right visual field activate the left hemisphere. Other investigators have used the same technique to locate color processing in the brain (→ LOCALIZATION OF FUNCTION). When subjects stare at a figure composed of a mixture of colored rectangles (or the equivalent figure in shades of gray), activation specific to color processing is found in the inferior occipital cortex. This zone is thought to correspond in monkeys to area V4, whose cells respond to color. Still other studies (again, using positron emission tomography) have pointed out what brain regions are involved in the perception of movement. In one study where the brain activity of subjects was recorded as they looked at a series of stationary or moving dots displayed on a screen, movement-specific activation was found in the posterior parietal lobe, at its junction with the occipital lobe.

These few results of imaging studies clearly show that different parts of the brain are implicated in different aspects of visual perception. But functional specialization goes far beyond the examples presented here. For instance, Mortimer Mishkin and his collaborators showed, again in monkeys, that the shape of objects (the "what?") is treated separately from their spatial location (the "where?") (→ SPACE). Shape processing takes place in the temporal cortex (in the so-called ventral system), whereas location processing occurs in the parietal cortex (in the so-called dorsal system). Many neurophysiological studies have confirmed these findings by showing that the neurons of these two systems respond selectively to information about shape or location.

Functional specializations specific to different types of perceived stimuli—or to the processing they trigger—have also been demonstrated. Once again, brain imaging research has proven highly useful in identifying the cognitive operations involved. Studies that use words as stimuli seem to show that our visual system carries out two distinct sets of operations when we perceive words (→ LANGUAGE, READING). The first set analyzes the visual characteristics of the stimuli while disregarding the fact that they represent words composed of letters (real words give rise to the same results as comparable stimuli made up of pseudoletters). Processing at this level seems to take place in various extrastriate areas of both hemispheres. A second set of operations analyzes the visual shape of words. These operations are initiated only by stimuli that conform to the orthographic and phonological rules of the language. They generate specific activation in the internal part of the left hemisphere.

Similar findings have been obtained for face processing: brain regions situated in the ventromedial part of the right hemisphere (lingual gyrus and posterior part of the fusiform gyrus) seem to be specialized in the processing of face configurations and invariant features that determine a person's physiognomy. Other regions, such as the parahippocampal gyrus of the right hemisphere and the anterior part of the temporal lobes of both hemispheres, seem to be in charge of face-identity processing. Combined with the data obtained from brain-damaged patients, these findings suggest that the parahippocampal gyrus is implicated in the retrieval of memories associated with the representation of a face, while the anterior temporal region contains the biographical information needed to identify a face.

This brings up an important point: any perceptual activity that leads to recognition, identification, and naming necessarily requires the activation of representations stored in memory (→ MEMORY, REPRESENTATION). Recent brain imaging studies seem to confirm the existence of separate networks for storing perceptual and semantic representations (→ SEMANTICS). In the case of visual perception, perceptual representations of objects are thought to be stored specifically in the (inferior temporal) ventral system, whereas semantic representations are thought to have several storage areas, including the angular gyrus and the superior temporal cortex of the left hemisphere, the middle temporal cortex, and the inferior prefrontal cortex. Unlike the perceptual representations involved solely in visual perception, semantic representations may be activated regardless of the information intake modality and independently of the perceptual medium (words or pictures). Although our example here is visual perception, it should be noted that certain "high level" perceptual mechanisms are not specific to the visual modality alone.

Representations are thought to be activated on the basis of similarities between the activity patterns triggered by the perceptual stimulus and the formats in which the representations are stored (→ ACTIVATION/INHIBITION). This process is made possible by a mechanism called *constraint satisfaction* (→ CONSTRAINT), which activates the representation that best fits the specific properties of the perceptual input.

OLIVIER KOENIG

Philosophy. — In the ordinary sense, perception is an experience through which a subject becomes aware or cognizant of objects and properties that exist at a given time in his or her environment (→ CONSCIOUSNESS, EXPERIENCE, OBJECT). Perceptual experience is often seen as having two facets. On the one hand, it has *phenomenal properties* or *qualia* that are immediately available to the conscious subject and define what Thomas Nagel expressed as "what it is like" to have that experience (→ QUALIA). On the other hand, perceptual experience has *intentional content*: it presents perceiving subjects with entities localized in space and (often) separate from themselves (→ INTENTIONALITY, SPACE). It is the task of any philosophical analysis of perception to describe these two facets and explain their relationship.

One might contend that perception does not really have phenomenal properties. It would therefore be transparent, in the sense that it would give the subject access only to whatever is part of the perceived scene. In this case, its phenomenal properties would in reality be the properties (apparently) present in the experience but entirely determined by intentional content. *Direct realism, phenomenalism,* and *indirect realism* are three theories that acknowledge the transparency of perception (→ PHENOMENALISM, REALISM). They differ solely in the ontological nature of what is perceived. For the direct realist, we perceive real entities that do not depend on our experience (colored tables, persons, etc.). The phenomenalist contends that we perceive a body of phenomenal sensory data that exists only through the experience we have of it. The indirect realist introduces a distinction between the immediate objects of perception and other objects. In the classical version of indirect realism, immediate objects are phenomenal sensory data, and other objects are perceived in an indirect manner, being mediated by our perception of immediate objects: we perceive our environment indirectly, behind the veil of appearance, by directly perceiving phenomenal entities.

Adverbial theory proposes another conception of the relationship between the two facets of perception. According to this theory, the phenomenal properties of experience at least partly determine its apparent intentional content. For example, seeing a red sphere means first seeing in a certain way, "spherically and redly." These adverbs are supposed to characterize the phenomenal properties of experience. The apparent reference to intentional objects gives way to a direct characterization of what it is like to have that experience.

Another debate concerns the nature of intentional content. According to one point of view, perception has *conceptual content* (→ CONCEPT). One cannot perceive an object without possessing or even using some sort of concept of that object. This theory runs up against several obstacles. It makes no provisions for the perceptual capacities of animals and prelinguistic children (→ ANIMAL COGNITION, INFANT COGNITION). In addition, even adult humans seem to be capable of perceiving complex scenes without bringing to bear an interrelated set of concepts corresponding to all perceived aspects of the scene. Finally, it is not clear that there is such a thing as "what it is like" to grasp conceptual content (either that is the case, or the effect is the same for all contents of this kind).

If the intentional content of perception were entirely conceptual, phenomenal properties would at best play a minor role in the perceptual relationship between the subject and the environment. According to an opposing theory, the intentional content of perception is nonconceptual: it is possible to perceive a complex scene without possessing (and a fortiori without using) a concept for each aspect perceived. With the notion of nonconceptual content, one can account for the "phenomenal density"of a scene in intentional terms. There is a potential application of this notion in developmental psychology (→ COGNITIVE DEVELOPMENT), where some authors hypothesize that a system of concepts can "emerge" from intentional contents that are not strictly conceptual (→ EMERGENCE). Such an explanation is possible only if the nonconceptual content present in perception exhibits some degree of autonomy with respect to the conceptual content of other intentional states.

JÉRÔME DOKIC

SELECTED BIBLIOGRAPHY

Bechtel, W., & Abrahamsen, A. (2002). *Connectionism and the mind: Parallel processing dynamics and evolution* (2nd ed.). Oxford, England: Blackwell.

Farah, M. (2000). *The cognitive neuroscience of vision.* Malden, MA: Blackwell.

Gazzaniga, M. (Ed.). (2000). *The new cognitive neurosciences* (Section III, *Sensory systems*) (2nd ed.). Cambridge, MA: MIT Press.

Gibson, J. (1987). *The ecological approach to visual perception* (3rd ed.). Hillsdale, NJ: Erlbaum.

Kosslyn, S., & Koenig, O. (1992/1995). *Wet mind: The new cognitive neuroscience.* New York: Free press.

Marr, D. (1982). *Vision.* San Francisco: Freeman.

McAdams, S., & Bigand, E. (Eds.). (1993). *Thinking in sound: The cognitive psychology of human audition.* Oxford: Clarendon Press; New York: Oxford University Press.

Mesulam, M. (Ed.). (2000). *Principles of behavioral and cognitive neurology* (2nd ed.). New York: Oxford University Press.

Nagel, T. (1979). *Mortal questions.* New York: Cambridge University Press.

Searle, J. (1983). *Intentionality: An essay in the philosophy of mind.* New York: Cambridge University Press.

Zeki, S. (1999). *Inner vision: An exploration of art and the brain.* Oxford, England; New York: Oxford University Press.

PHENOMENALISM

Philosophy. — *Phenomenalism* is a form of antirealism (→ REALISM). It contends that the only knowable objects are experiences and the logical constructions that follow from them (→ EXPERIENCE, LOGIC, OBJECT). In the phenomenalist view, then, there is nothing to perceive beyond experience (→ PERCEPTION). By considering real things to be on "the other side of the veil of perception," to use John Locke's terms, phenomenalists argue that nothing can give us access to what is on the other side of that veil. Like the advocates of the theory of direct perception, phenomenalists see the objects of experience as being perceived directly, but they do not see perceived objects as being physical.

Like *idealism*, phenomenalism does not necessarily conclude that reality can be reduced to that which is perceived by the mind (→ MIND); unlike idealism, it has to come up with a definition of the physical world in phenomenal terms. Twentieth century phenomenalism, largely inspired by the work of the Vienna Circle, was rejected because its project to reduce all knowledge to the logical construction of elementary experiences imposed unacceptable limitations on the sciences. Empiricist philosophers like Willard Quine abandoned the idea that sensations are the primitive materials of conceptual elaboration (→ CONCEPT). Roderick Chisholm showed that the alleged "reductions" of phenomenalism depend on the physical circumstances in which perception takes place, which lie outside the realm of such reductions.

JOËLLE PROUST

SELECTED BIBLIOGRAPHY

Chisholm, R. (1948). The problem of empiricism. *Journal of Philosophy, 45*, 512–517.
Quine, W. (1960). *Word and object*. Cambridge, MA: MIT Press.

PHYSICALISM

Philosophy. — *Physicalism* is an ontological doctrine according to which the constituents of reality are physical entities or are determined solely by physical entities. One can interpret physicalism as a response to the challenging fact that mental entities seem indeed to exist and to interact causally with the physical world: the mind is causally affected by sensations and becomes effective through actions (→ ACTION, CAUSALITY AND MENTAL CAUSATION, MIND).

Defending an ontological thesis, physicalists do not necessarily claim that scientific explanations can, or could some day, settle for describing phenomena using physical terminology supplemented by the laws of physics. Physics, assumed to be perfectly complete, nevertheless plays a key role as an arbitrator that makes the final decisions about the existence of entities of a given type. Physicalism does not imply *reductionism*, a stronger approach (→ REDUCTIONISM): the latter not only requires all elements of reality to belong to the domain of physical entities, but also necessitates a theory that encompasses physics and all other sciences; any reduction is fundamentally tied to the theory that accomplishes it.

Eliminativism, a radical form of physicalism, argues that the existence of the mental states will prove illusory, and that alleged explanations in mental terms will be replaced by explanations in physical terms (→ DUALISM/ MONISM). The *psychophysical identity thesis* contends that every mental property is identical to a brain property (in the "type physicalism" version; → TYPE/TOKEN). Weaker versions of physicalism posit only the identity of a mental property and a particular brain event (token physicalism). They share the idea that mental properties *supervene* on physical properties: there can be no mental difference without a physical difference (→ SUPERVENIENCE).

Functionalism, anomalous monism, and *epiphenomenalism* are forms of physicalism: they bring all causality down to the physical level (→ EPIPHE-NOMENALISM, FUNCTIONALISM). Functionalism identifies mental events on the basis of their interactions and their relationships with perceptual input and behavioral output (→ PERCEPTION); their identity is not determined by their physical realization, although the latter does determine their causal interactions. Anomalous monism insists upon the identity between any (given) mental event and a physical event, and stipulates that causal laws exist only at the physical level. Epiphenomenalism denies all causal efficacy to whatever is mental, for the mental is but an inefficacious effect of the physical.

MAX KISTLER

SELECTED BIBLIOGRAPHY

Gillett, C., & Loewer, B. (2001). *Physicalism and its discontents*. New York: Cambridge University Press.

PRAGMATICS

Psychology. — *Pragmatics* is the cognitive, social, and cultural study of language and communication. It strives to answer the question: How can language use be defined and studied (→ COMMUNICATION, LANGUAGE)?

Charles Morris formulated the founding definition of pragmatics: the study of the relationship between signs and interpreters (→ INTERPRETATION, SIGN). An interpreter is a user of the language who, in a particular context, determines the link between a linguistic sign and an object (→ CONTEXT AND SITUATION). Morris's definition situates pragmatics relative to *syntax* (the study of how the signs are related to each other) and *semantics* (the study of how the signs are related to the objects) (→ SEMANTICS, SYNTAX). This view was directly inspired by Charles Peirce's theory of signs (*semiotics*), in particular the tripartite subdivision of signs into symbols, icons, and indices (→ SEMIOTICS, SYMBOL).

In psychology, pragmatic research has been based on theoretical proposals that enable the investigator to set forth hypotheses about the subject's underlying mental processes and test them experimentally. Some examples are the *cooperative principle*, postulated by Paul Grice, and *speech-act theory*, proposed by John Austin and then by John Searle, where speech acts are defined as social acts. Very generally, nonliteral uses of language (indirect speech acts, metaphors, idioms, irony, etc.) provide excellent material for studies in pragmatics. Cognitive psychology and developmental psychology are two examples of subdisciplines that have incorporated pragmatics into their fields.

In cognitive psychology, the first important question that pragmatics could help answer was: How do human beings construe the meaning of an utterance in a particular context? The meaning a subject ascribes to a statement (for example, *This man is a lion* or *Can you pass me the salt?*) often goes beyond its purely linguistic meaning (→ MEANING). The solution to this type of problem requires studying the inferences subjects make on the basis of the context and their own general knowledge (→ REASONING AND RATIONALITY). Andrew Ortony's work on understanding metaphors is a good illustration of this approach. A second question relating more directly to the communication process itself was addressed next: What representations and processes are involved in the use of language (→ REPRESENTATION)? For Herbert Clark, the essential prerequisite for communication is a representation of the knowledge and beliefs shared by speaker and listener and known to be so by both parties (→ BELIEF). In this light, the meaning of an utterance is the outcome of a collaborative process, and as such, communication is more a matter of creating meaning than of "selecting" it. In present-day cognitive psychology, three lines of pragmatic research are essential. (1) The first concerns *when* contextual factors are brought to bear. Is it after a purely linguistic phase, or at the very onset of utterance interpretation? A modular approach leans in the direction of the former (→ MODULARITY), whereas recent findings in developmental psychology tend toward the latter (see below). (2) The second line of inquiry is aimed at developing models of cognitive representations in which each of the communicating partners is taken into account, in addition to their individual representations of the representations of others (as in *theory-of-mind* models) (→ SOCIAL COGNITION, THEORY OF MIND). (3) The third deals with the nature of representations of meaning: if meaning is highly flexible and context-dependent, then one can wonder whether a core meaning that is linguistically defined still exists.

Pragmatic developmental psychology was founded by Susan Ervin-Tripp and Claudia Mitchell-Kernan. The principal question raised concerns how children become aware of the correspondence between utterance forms and communication contexts. Studies that attempt to answer this question look at natural conversations, larger analysis units than the word or sentence (for example, the speaking turn or the speech act), the extralinguistic context, variability across individuals or social groups (→ DIFFERENTIATION), and the diverse functions of language, a domain where Michael Halliday's pioneering work has been highly influential (→ FUNCTION). In this approach, language is not a mere grammar (→ GRAMMAR); it is also a set of strategies used by children to structure their social actions and to monitor and carry out their communicative activities. Pragmatic developmental psychology, defined as such and issued from the philosophy of language, has much in common with Lev Vygotsky's theory (from which Jerome Bruner drew a number of elements), especially Vygotsky's ideas on the social nature of linguistic signs. Studies in language production and in language comprehension have demonstrated the critical role played by the context of communication, at least until the age of six or seven years. After that, linguistic markers, when needed, are gradually taken into account. More recent research has also shown that by the age of two, children produce nonverbal messages whose form varies with the communicative context in a way comparable to the verbal messages produced later. Today, new research paths are emerging: the study of the sources of structural or pragmatic development, research into certain brain disorders and other types of pathology (→ NEUROPSYCHOLOGY), the study of children growing up in bilingual and/or bicultural settings, and comparisons of children and primates (→ ANIMAL COGNITION).

Pragmatics is a domain where inderdisciplinarity is the rule (psychology, linguistics, philosophy, artificial intelligence, anthropology, cognitive neuroscience, etc.), and where the role of psychologists is to provide evidence of the mental processes underlying the use of language, by both adults and children.

JOSIE BERNICOT

Linguistics. — Although the term *pragmatic* has been in use in everyday language for quite some time (in expressions like *a pragmatic man, a pragmatic attitude*, etc.), pragmatics is a new discipline. Developed first in the philosophy of language in the framework of speech-act theory, and then in the theory of *implicatures*, it became a field of interest for linguists following the introduction of the *performative hypothesis* by generative semanticists. It finally made its way into the cognitive sciences, in particular through relevance theory ($\rightarrow$ RELEVANCE, SEMANTICS).

The first definition of the term, which dates back to 1938, was given by Morris. He described pragmatics as one of the three dimensions of semiotics ($\rightarrow$ SEMIOTICS). The pragmatic dimension is the relationship between the signs and the interpreters, and the study of this dimension is pragmatics ($\rightarrow$ INTERPRETATION) (see *psychology* above).

In linguistics, this definition did not trigger any significant developments. There are three main reasons for this. First of all, it became clear that pragmatic information cannot take effect only during the last stage of utterance processing (after syntax and semantics), but interacts instead with syntactic information ($\rightarrow$ INFORMATION, LANGUAGE, SYNTAX). Some examples that support this observation are linguistic phenomena such as chaining via pragmatic connectives like *because* and *since* (for example, *What are you doing tonight? Because I've got a nice chicken in the refrigerator;* or, *I'm leaving, since we promised we'd tell each other everything*) and the so-called performative uses of *if* (for example, *If you're thirsty, there are some drinks in the refrigerator*), where the link is made at the speech-act level, not in the proposition expressed by the sentence. *Integrated pragmatics*, a linguistic theory developed by Oswald Ducrot, is an approach in pragmatics where the linguistic description of an utterance includes its pragmatic features.

Second, Morris's definition assumes that the truth conditions of sentences determine the pragmatic sense of the utterance ($\rightarrow$ TRUTH). Yet the Oxonian tradition, represented by Austin and pursued by Searle, hypothesizes that utterances do not represent states of affairs, and that the very fact of uttering a sentence accomplishes an *illocutionary act*, comprised of an *illocutionary force marker* (the performative preface) and a propositional content. An utterance like *I promise to come home early* is said to be an explicit performative in that its sense (a promise) is stated and is self-referential. In contrast, an utterance like *I'll come home early*, understood to be a promise, is an implicit performative (or indirect speech act) because its sense (a promise) is not signaled linguistically but communicated indirectly or non-literally. In generative semantics, it is hypothesized that the deep structure of a sentence contains a performative preface. Speech-act theory thus runs counter to the view that the pragmatic stage is the last one in utterance processing: on the contrary, illocutionary force indicators are conventional indicators that form the basis of the semantic rules governing speech acts (preparatory rules, propositional-content rule, sincerity rule, essential rule) and underlie the syntactic structure of sentences.

The third reason for refusing Morris's definition can be found in Grice's work in philosophy. Grice's thesis is that in attempting to understand the mechanisms by means of which speakers communicate and understand each other's communicative intent, it is false to assume that communication is based on the application of logical principles (the deductive rules of propositional calculus) (→ LOGIC) or on the code model proposed by communications engineers (→ COMMUNICATION). On the contrary, communication can be explained only if one assumes that the interlocutors obey the cooperative principle, which stipulates that speakers' contributions must be in keeping with the purpose and direction of the exchange in which they are engaged. A contribution is cooperative if it abides by, or deliberately violates, the *maxims of conversation*, that is, the two *submaxims of quantity* (give as much information as required and do not give more information than required); the *maxim of quality* (make your contribution true), which can be divided into two submaxims (do not say what you believe to be false and do not say things for which you lack adequate evidence); the *maxim of relation* (be relevant); and the *maxim of manner* (be clear), which has four submaxims (avoid obscurity, avoid ambiguity, be brief, and be orderly).

Information that is not communicated literally but recovered via a conversation maxim is called a *conversational implicature*. Depending on whether the implicature is triggered by the sense of the words alone, or by both their sense and their form, it will be called *particularized* or *generalized*. Finally, an implicature attached to a particular word not triggered by a maxim is called *conventional*. Conventional implicatures are not calculated, nor can they be canceled, whereas conversational implicatures are calculated and cancelable. For example, the implicatures triggered by the word *even* in *Even Paul came* are conventional (*other persons came* and *Paul was the least likely person to come*), the implicature triggered by *and* in *Lucky Luke mounted his horse and disappeared in the sunset* is conversational and generalized (the word *and* means *and then*), and finally asking for the salt by saying *The soup needs salt* is conversational and particularized.

The Gricean trend is conventionally called *radical pragmatics*, wherein sense is preferentially explained at the pragmatic level and semantics is reduced to truth conditions. In addition, the Gricean approach is *monoguist* (it does not strive to multiply the senses of expressions, abiding by Grice's modified version of the Occam's razor principle) and opposes ambiguist semantic theories.

In the late 1980s, Grice's theory of implicatures gave rise to a new theory in pragmatics, founded on a single principle: the principle of *relevance* (Dan Sperber and Deirdre Wilson). This principle stipulates that speakers produce the most relevant utterance, and that listeners can rightfully assume its optimal relevance. An utterance's relevance is a comparative notion measured by its productivity: the greater the contextual effects an utterance produces (addition of a proposition by contextual implication, modification of the strength of belief in a proposition, deletion of a proposition; → BELIEF, CONTEXT AND SITUATION), the more relevant it is; the greater the processing effort an utterance requires (utterance length to be processed, long-term memory retrieval, number of inferential rules at stake; → MEMORY), the less relevant it is. Relevance (or *relevant*) theory predicts that the first interpretation that comes to the listener's mind and balances the cognitive load is the one that is consistent with the relevance principle and corresponds to the speaker's communicative intent, if the communication was successful.

One can see, then, that in the tradition of speech-act theory, and in implicature or relevance theory as well, pragmatics has a very different status from that granted to it by Morris's semiotic theory. In all cases, the emphasis is on nonliteral communication and the inferential principles that permit access to the speaker's communicative intentions (→ REASONING AND RATIONALITY). Only the explanatory principles change: generalizations of semantic rules for indirect speech acts, conversation maxims for conversational implicatures, and the relevance principle for determining the full interpretation of an utterance. In addition to the priority it gives to nonliteral communication, pragmatics has been assigned a special task, at least in relevance theory: that of accounting for disambiguation, referent assignment, and the processes that determine the implicatures and illocutionary force of an utterance.

JACQUES MOESCHLER

SELECTED BIBLIOGRAPHY

Austin, J. (1962). *How to do things with words*. Cambridge, MA: Harvard University Press.

Cruse, D. A. (2000). *Meaning in language: An introduction to semantics and pragmatics*. Oxford, England; New York: Oxford University Press.

Ducrot, O. (1984). *Le dire et le dit* [Saying and what is said]. Paris: Minuit, 1984.

Ervin-Tripp, S. M., & Mitchell-Kernan, C. (Eds.). (1977). *Child discourse*. New York: Academic Press.

Grice, H. P. (1989). *Studies in the way of words*. Cambridge, MA: Harvard University Press.

Searle, J. (1969). *Speech acts: An essay in the philosophy of language*. London: Cambridge University Press.

Sperber, D., & Wilson, D. (1986). *Relevance: Communication and cognition*. Oxford, England: Blackwell; Cambridge, MA: Harvard University Press.

Yule, G. (1996). *Pragmatics*. Oxford, England: Oxford University Press.

PROBLEM SOLVING

Artificial intelligence. — Problem solving is studied in several disciplines of the cognitive sciences, particularly in psychology, where it is addressed in conjunction with cognitive functions such as attention, control, learning, reasoning, and so on (→ ATTENTION, COGNITIVE DEVELOPMENT, CONTROL, LEARNING, REASONING AND RATIONALITY) using a symbolic and/or connectionist approach (→ COGNITIVISM, CONNECTIONISM, SYMBOL).

After having somewhat naively developed only very general problem-solving systems, artificial intelligence research in problem solving began to make a number of important conceptual and algorithmic contributions. The processes involved in describing and solving a large class of problems were formalized, and a precise algorithmic meaning was given to the notion of *heuristic*. Solving procedures comprising several paradigms were also devised, and the scope and limitations of each were specified.

The class of problems discussed here falls between problems for which solution algorithms are known, and problems that have not yet been formalized. These problems are well defined in the sense that for each one, there is a *test procedure* capable of recognizing any solution to the problem and an *enumerative procedure* capable of generating potential solutions to submit to the test. This is not accomplished randomly or without taking the results of former tests into account: the testing and enumeration procedures are incorporated into a *constructive procedure* that proceeds by eliminating alternatives and reducing the set of potential solutions.

Several paradigms are available for designing a constructive procedure. In one paradigm, partial solutions are completed and tested one by one, and then those partial solutions that seem likely to lead to a complete solution are chosen. The choice is based on a local measure of each partial solution using what is called a *heuristic*. In case of failure, the choice may be questioned. For example, suppose we want to find a chessboard layout where there are eight queens all located on safe squares (no queen is on *take*). Applying this paradigm, we would proceed at each stage by placing a kth queen on a safe square of a chessboard that has $k-1$ queens. One heuristic would be to choose the partial solution that leaves the greatest possible number of safe squares on the board. A more precise heuristic would be to start from the fact that each remaining piece must necessarily be placed in an empty column (otherwise it could be taken). In this case, one would choose a solution where the minimal number of empty squares in the $8 - k$ columns remaining to be filled is the greatest. This popular heuristic is called the *minimax* heuristic.

Another paradigm involves breaking down the initial problem into simpler subproblems, and then repeating this until one ends up with only immediately solvable problems. The respective solutions to these problems are then recombined to obtain the answer to the initial problem. Choosing a heuristic amounts to choosing among the alternative ways of breaking down the problem. By way of illustration, consider a counterfeit coin problem where one wants to determine, using the smallest possible number of weighings, which one of n coins is counterfeit, and whether it is lighter or heavier than the others. Each weighing breaks down the problem into subproblems. For example, weighing three coins against three others reduces the $2n$ initial possibilities (the ith coin is heavier, lighter, etc.) to 6, $2n - 12$, or 6 possibilities, respectively, depending on whether the scale tilts to the left, is balanced, or tilts to the right. One continues with each of these three subproblems until all branches are reduced to a single possibility. When working on a given subproblem, the weighing chosen is the one that provides the greatest amount of information ($\rightarrow$ INFORMATION). This heuristic is often used in devising testing plans (for $n = 8$, the above three-against-three weighing would be chosen because it supplies the most information). Note that the minimax heuristic is also applicable here: one would choose the weighing that minimizes the maximum number of suspects for its three branches. In general, this heuristic is more efficient than one based on the amount of information. Other paradigms exist, such as reducing the domain of possible values taken on by the variables describing the problem ($\rightarrow$ CONSTRAINT).

In sum, two ingredients are necessary for implementing a problem-solving procedure: (1) a number of different ways of transforming an initial situation or any other situation (subproblem, partial solution, set of potential solutions) into one or more other situations, (2) a means of testing the resulting situations relative to the goal, and (3) a heuristic for choosing the most appropriate means of transforming the current situation.

If the operators and the initial state are given, the *set of possible problem states* is implicitly defined. This set has a particular structure that depends on what operators are used. It can be a graph (as in the first paradigm described above): a node is a partial solution, an arc is the application of an operator to that solution, and the successor node is the extension obtained. Solving the problem entails finding a path on this graph between the initial state and a solution state. Depending on the type of representation used, this graph may have important properties for efficiently solving the problem, such as finiteness, connectivity, absence of circuits, a tree structure, small size, and so forth. The properties of the heuristic are also essential in determining the performance and behavior of the solving procedure. One strives to implement a procedure (1) that is complete (it finds a solution if there is one), (2) that finishes (is complete and necessarily stops if there is no solution), and (3) is admissible (finishes and puts out an optimal solution relative to a given criterion). Unfortunately, these techniques are usually not very efficient for reasons of intrinsic complexity.

MALIK GHALLAB

SELECTED BIBLIOGRAPHY

Bechtel, W., & Abrahamsen, A. (2002). *Connectionism and the mind: Parallel processing dynamics and evolution* (2nd ed.). Oxford, England: Blackwell.

Brookshear, J. (2003). *Computer science: An overview* (7th ed.). Boston: Addison-Wesley.

Dale, N., Weems, C., & Headington, M. (2002). *Programming and problem solving with C++* (3rd ed.). Boston: Jones and Bartlett.

Kosslyn, S., & Rosenberg, R. (2001). *Psychology: The brain, the person, the world*. Boston: Allyn & Bacon.

Luger, G. (2002). *Artificial intelligence: Structures and strategies for complex problem-solving* (4th ed.). Harlow, England; New York: Pearson Education.

Newell, A., & Simon, H. (1972). *Human problem solving*. Englewood Cliffs, NJ: Prentice Hall.

Solso, R. (2001). *Cognitive psychology* (6th ed.). Boston: Allyn & Bacon.

PROPOSITIONAL ATTITUDE

Philosophy. — The term *propositional attitude* is a generic term that encompasses all beliefs (→ BELIEF), desires (→ DESIRE), intentions, fears, hopes, wishes, and so on that share the property of being identified by their propositional content: the belief that Aristotle is a philosopher is identified by the proposition that Aristotle is a philosopher (→ PROPOSITIONAL FORMAT).

In ordinary situations, these notions play a critical role in explaining, justifying, and predicting behavior (→ ACTION, CAUSALITY AND MENTAL CAUSATION, THEORY OF MIND). But are they acceptable in naturalistic scientific psychology (→ NATURALIZATION)? The current debate pits philosophers such as Paul Churchland, Willard Quine, Dan Dennett, and Stephen Stich, who refuse to grant a scientific status to propositional attitudes—even though some of these philosophers nevertheless acknowledge the practical utility of attitude attributions in interpreting behavior—against realist philosophers such as Jerry Fodor, Fred Dretske, and Ruth Millikan, who argue that propositional attitudes are real mental states that, by virtue of their content, play a causal role in explaining behavior (→ INTERPRETATION, REALISM). From a naturalistic perspective, realist philosophers need to explain how the physical states that realize these mental states can have representational properties (→ REPRESENTATION) and can have a causal efficacy that is a function of their content.

ÉLISABETH PACHERIE

SELECTED BIBLIOGRAPHY

Dennett, D. (1987). *The intentional stance*. Cambridge, MA: MIT Press.
Fodor, J. (1987). *Psychosemantics: The problem of meaning in the philosophy of mind*. Cambridge, MA: MIT Press.

PROPOSITIONAL FORMAT

Psychology. — *Propositional format* in cognitive psychology is an abstract way of representing knowledge (→ REPRESENTATION) that can be formalized according to a *predicate logic* (→ INFORMATION, LOGIC, SYMBOL). It is qualified as "abstract" for two reasons. (1) The mental representation of a propositional *function*, that is, a psychological predicate associated with one or more arguments—for example, *ON* (*x, y*)—is a way of conceptualizing objects and their relations in terms of classes—in our example, the set of all (*x, y*) pairs that make the function *ON* (*x, y*) true—and hence, without reference to particular instances (→ CATEGORIZATION, CONCEPT, FUNCTION). (2) Even when the predicate function is instantiated in a given context—say, *ON* (*vase, table*)—the resulting proposition is not in verbal or image format (→ LANGUAGE, MENTAL IMAGERY). In our example, we are not talking about the image of a vase on a table, nor about the image of the proposition describing a vase on a table. Moreover, even though propositions are linear strings of symbols in a mental language whose lexicon strictly but not totally corresponds to that of natural language, they are still not sentences; the syntax differs (→ LANGUAGE OF THOUGHT, LEXICON, SYNTAX).

Being neither pictorial nor verbal, propositional format in fact acts as the infrastructure (or part of the infrastructure) that supports pictorial and verbal symbolization in long-term memory (→ MEMORY). According to Stephen Kosslyn's original model, generating the mental image of a nonvisible object requires not only a representation of the "skeletal image" of the object, but also propositional representations of the object's parts and their locations and of the object's relationships with superordinate object categories. As in the study of text processing (see *linguistics* below), some authors argue that the semantic and pragmatic dimensions of linguistic representations are based on a pretextual or preverbal propositional structure (→ PRAGMATICS, SEMANTICS, TEXT). Radical propositionalists such as Zenon Pylyshyn defend the view that the sheer fact of acknowledging that a representation format (for example, the analogical format of mental imagery) has an abstract substrate reduces it to an epiphenomenon.

OLIVIER HOUDÉ

Linguistics. — In cognitive linguistics, as in psychology, some models rely on symbolic propositional expressions to describe the structure of the mental states behind the comprehension or production of linguistic utterances (→ LANGUAGE, LANGUAGE OF THOUGHT, LOGIC, SYMBOL). These models make use of all or part of the following principles. (1) Propositions belong to a system endowed with rules that govern the formation and derivation of other propositions, and this system is different from the language. This postulate is accepted implicitly by Ray Jackendoff, Walter Kintsch, and Steven Pinker. For Jackendoff and Kintsch, propositions serve primarily to disambiguate and interpret linguistic statements by assigning them a propositional structure (→ INTERPRETATION). The latter can carry nonverbal contextual information (→ CONTEXT AND SITUATION, INFORMATION). For Pinker, symbolic representations are used to describe the semantic constraints that determine how speakers learn verb classes, defined by certain syntactic variations (→ LEARNING, SEMANTICS, SYNTAX). (2) The sense of a propositional expression is identical to its corresponding mental representation. For Jackendoff, it is brain states, whose structure is homologous to the structure of the descriptive symbols used, that are meaningful. For Kintsch, the links between mental symbols and perception are the basis of their meaning (→ MEANING, PERCEPTION). (3) In the case of expressions about the world, the sense of an expression contains the conditions that make it *true* to say that it applies to the world (→ SENSE, TRUTH). This truth-conditional foundation is evident in George Miller's and Philip Johnson-Laird's work. One of its consequences is that categorizing an object amounts to correctly applying "objective" criteria to it (with respect to an unspecified reference discourse) in order to decide whether it belongs to a given category (→ CATEGORIZATION). (4) Semantic variations in lexemes are part of the propositional-conceptual representation of these expressions (→ CONCEPT). This principle seems to be accepted by the leading advocates of cognitive linguistics (Jackendoff, George Lakoff, Ronald Langacker) and is opposed to a conception of meaning that accommodates assimilating and dissimilating effects of context.

JEAN-MICHEL FORTIS

SELECTED BIBLIOGRAPHY

Jackendoff, R. (1983). *Semantics and cognition*. Cambridge, MA: MIT Press.
Jackendoff, R. (1990). *Semantic structures*. Cambridge, MA: MIT Press.
Kintsch, W. (1974). *The representation of meaning in memory*. Hillsdale, NJ: Erlbaum.
Miller, G., & Johnson-Laird, P. (1976). *Language and perception*. Cambridge, MA: Harvard University Press.
Pinker, S. (1989). *Learnability and cognition: The acquisition of argument structure*. Cambridge, MA: MIT Press.
Pylyshyn, Z. W. (1973). What the mind's eye tells the mind's brain: A critique of mental imagery. *Psychological Bulletin, 80*, 1–24.
Pylyshyn, Z. W. (1986). *Computation and cognition*. Cambridge, MA: MIT Press.

PSYCHOPHYSICS

Psychology. — *Psychophysics* is the discipline that studies quantitative relationships between physical stimuli and the sensations they generate, and more generally, between physical stimuli and the observable and measurable performance of subjects.

Already in the eighteenth century, advances in physics had given scientists the idea that it might be possible to understand human functions, particularly human perception, by developing methods derived directly from physics (→ PERCEPTION). As suggested by its name, coined in 1860 by Gustav Fechner in his *Elemente der Psychophysik*, psychophysics attempts to develop measurement methods for psychology modeled after physics. The measures are defined statistically from the subjects' response distributions.

Since Fechner, three types of performance measures have been used in psychophysics, and more generally in experimental psychology. They can be distinguished essentially on the basis of the tasks involved: *detection, scaling*, and *measurement of reaction time*. (1) Detection occurs when the intensity of the stimulus is such that it can be perceived at a given probability level; *discrimination* occurs when the difference between the intensities of two stimuli can be detected at a given probability level. In both cases, the subject chooses a response. (2) In scaling, scales that relate the intensity of stimuli to an operationalization of the corresponding sensations is constructed by the juxtaposition of different *levels* (Fechner's scales), *ratings* ([Lionel] Thurstone's scales), or *ratio judgments* ([Stanley] Stevens's scales). *Fechner's law* states that there is a logarithmic relation between stimulus intensity and subjective sensation, whereas Stevens proposed a *power law* to describe this relation. These methods are also applicable to cases where the "physical" scale of the stimuli is unknown (for example, crime-severity scales, attitude or preference scales). (3) Reaction time is a measure of the time lapse between the beginning of the stimulation and the moment when the subject responds. (Henri) *Pieron's law* describes a hyperbolic type of relation between stimulus intensity and reaction time.

There are a range of views as to what the observed psychophysical measures (performance) actually reflect. In the *behaviorist* view, only performance counts. No conclusions are drawn about the processes implemented. Psychophysics in this case serves to describe stimulus-response relationships and to study their stability. This conception is mainly founded on operationalism.

For other authors (such as Stevens) whose perspective is *introspectionistic* (→ INTROSPECTION) or *subjectivistic*, observed responses are a reflection of sensations. The experimenter measures stimuli, but the subject measures sensations. In other words, the subject acts as an instrument that gives a measure mediated by his or her sensations, which form the measurement scale. If this is true, then there should be only one psychophysical law to describe how sensations vary as stimulus intensity increases. For Fechner, this law is logarithmic; for Stevens, it is a power law.

Psychophysics grew out of a physicalist endeavor to measure mental activities (Fechner). The project was pursued by authors like Thurstone and Stevens. The aim was—and often still is today—to obtain perceptual (or subjective) scales with known formal properties. This approach underlies practically every applied study that calls upon psychophysics methods, particularly for the sensory analysis of products (aromas and flavors). From this perspective, it follows that variability in the results is regarded as undesirable "noise" that must be reduced using suitable methods. From a fundamental standpoint, several authors have attempted to show that there is only one law in psychophysics. Kenneth Norwich, for example, demonstrated that all psychophysical laws are formally unifiable under one and the same *law of conservation*, which is a law of informational entropy. Stephen Link contends that all of these laws assess the same sensory capacity, discrimination.

By contrast, a cognitive approach to the behavior of subjects performing psychophysical tasks leads to the view that performance can be broken down into component parts (→ COMPUTATIONAL ANALYSIS). It is determined both by the mechanisms of sensory *information processing* (→ INFORMATION) and by the effects of the *decision-making processes* involved in producing the response. The factors that influence the former and the latter are different. In this approach, the type of psychophysical law (logarithmic or power) may be contingent upon the operations that take place between the stimulation and the response. This approach allows one to go beyond a simple behaviorist description, and to avoid erroneously considering responses to be a direct reflection of the to-be-measured sensations. The concept of information processing and the idea of elucidating the processes required by a given task captured little if any interest in psychophysics until recently, despite the pioneering proposals of authors like Frans Donders. The view of perception as an information-processing system spurred a real paradigm revolution, taking psychophysics from the search for descriptive laws to the search for processes.

Signal Detection Theory (SDT; David Green and John Swets) opened up an entirely new research area by establishing the idea that all performance obtained in a psychophysics task should be broken down into the two main functional components mentioned above. Models are needed that enable the observed performance measures to be used to estimate the parameters of the sensory component, both those that depend on the characteristics of the stimulus, and of course, those that depend on the characteristics of the processing system under study. The other component of the response is subject-dependent, since it is decisional and more generally cognitive in nature ($\rightarrow$ CONTROL). This component may not involve intentional strategies, but includes everything that falls under the heading of context effects ($\rightarrow$ CONTEXT AND SITUATION). Saying that subjects have control over this component does not mean they can change its effects at will, let alone avoid them. Coming up with an operational distinction between these two components is not always a straightforward task, despite available models for grounding its rationality.

The idea, then, is to take the observed responses and their variations and single out what results from the effects of "purely" sensory processing systems and what results from the effects of factors that modify the subject's response system (stimulus frequency effects, sequence effects, etc.). Any experimental approach to perception that does not take this distinction into account is potentially fallacious. In short, it is posited here that in principle, a subject's response can never be taken to directly reflect the processes or mechanisms one is claiming to study. Phenomenal judgments can at best reflect only our most elaborate representations, and they have very little chance of permitting access to preattentional processing levels, which, by definition, are unconscious ($\rightarrow$ ATTENTION, AUTOMATISM, CONSCIOUSNESS, REPRESENTATION). The fact that these judgments might be quantitative (e.g., judgments of magnitude) in no way changes their status.

Seen from this angle, psychophysics is an integral part of cognitive psychology, for one of its aims is to develop models and methods for gaining insight into the different levels of processing under study.

CLAUDE BONNET

SELECTED BIBLIOGRAPHY

Algom, D. (Ed.). (1992). *Psychophysical approaches to cognition*. Amsterdam; New York: Elsevier.

Donders, F. C. (1969). On the speed of mental processes. Trans. and reprinted in W. G. Koster (Ed.). Attention & Performance II, *Acta Psychologica, 30,* 412–431.

Fechner, G. (1966). *Elements of psychophysics* (D. Howes & E. Boring, Eds.; H. Adler, Trans.). Austin, TX: Holt Rinehart & Winston. (Original work published 1860.)

Gescheider, G. (1988). Psychophysical scaling. *Annual Review of Psychology, 39,* 169–200.

Gescheider, G. (1997). *Psychophysics: The fundamentals*. Mahwah, NJ: Erlbaum.

Green, D. M., & Swets, J. A. (1966). *Signal detection and psychophysics*. New York: Wiley.

Link, S. W. (1992). *The wave theory of difference and similarity*. Hillsdale, NJ: Erlbaum.

Norton, T., Corliss, D., & Bailey, J. (2002).*The psychophysical measurement of vision*. Burlington, VT: Elsevier/Butterworth-Heinemann.

Norwich, K. H. (1987). On the theory of Weber fraction. *Perception & Psychophysics, 42,* 286–298.

Stevens, S. S. (1975). *Psychophysics: Introduction to its perceptual, neural and social aspects*. New York: Wiley.

Thurstone, L. L. (1959). *The measurement of values*. Chicago: University of Chicago Press.

Wickens, T. (2002). *Elementary signal detection theory*. Oxford, England; New York: Oxford University Press.

Q

QUALIA

Philosophy. — The technical term *quale* (*qualia* in the plural form) is conventionally used to refer to some or all of the qualitative elements of conscious experience (→ CONSCIOUSNESS, EXPERIENCE). This characterization is vague and the definitions proposed in the literature are not universally accepted. Sometimes the word *qualia* is used to refer to events like the manifestations of a particular pain, and sometimes it is used to refer to the properties of those events like the intensity or type of pain. Difficulty treating qualia in the framework of a mechanistic theory of nature is at the roots of the Galilean distinction between objective or primary qualities (form, dimension) and subjective or secondary qualities (colors, sounds). But this distinction can be generalized, because a qualitative aspect can be discerned even in impressions of form and dimension. Another generalization extends the concept of qualia to all conscious phenomena.

Explaining the nature of qualia is the psychologist's task, but difficulty doing so has made qualia into a critical testing ground for different philosophical conceptions of the nature of mental properties and events.

1. The simplest qualia are classified into spaces on the basis of similarity (color qualia, sound qualia, etc.), such that each space has its own topology and metrics (for example, the quale *orange* is located between *yellow* and *red*, and is closer to *green* than *blue*). Based on this classification, attempts are made to identify the physiological structures that account for the properties of the various spaces (for example, the antagonistic processes at play in color perception) (→ PERCEPTION). This theoretical reduction concerns only the structural properties of

qualia (explaining, for example, why the quale *orange* falls between the qualia *yellow* and *red*). But it does not provide a complete explanation of qualia, unless we agree that qualia themselves are fully defined by their structural properties. In particular, for our example here, this kind of theoretical reduction would not be capable of explaining (a) why there are qualia at all, (b) why it is that the qualia *red, yellow*, and *orange* are located in that structure instead of other color qualia that have the same relationships between them as do red, yellow, and orange, and (c) why the qualia in question are not noncolor qualia related to each other in the said way. Clearly, one might argue that these three questions are illegitimate by saying that the standard they impose on psychological explanation is too strict—in the same way as it would be asking too much of physics to require an explanation for the fundamental properties of the ultimate components of matter. This nevertheless amounts to assigning qualia the role of primitives in psychological explanation, that is, to accepting a form of dualism ($\rightarrow$ DUALISM/MONISM).

2. An extreme position, motivated by these difficulties, denies the existence of qualia altogether. It seems, though, that this would require too radical a revision of the role of elementary phenomenology.

3. The possibility of an inverse color space (where all colors are replaced by their complements, but the topological and metric properties of the space remain the same) would alleviate the need for a functional definition of qualia, thereby supplying a counterargument against functionalism ($\rightarrow$ FUNCTIONALISM). Take the far-fetched case of imaginary subject A who is completely deprived of qualia but is nevertheless capable of the same behavioral responses as qualia-endowed subject B under the same stimulation conditions. If the only noticeable difference between A and B is the fact that A possesses qualia, then not only are qualia useless in a psychological explanation, they cease to be definable from the functional standpoint.

4. Another interesting case of the imaginary complement is subject C who possesses all relevant physical and psychophysical information about color perception ($\rightarrow$ INFORMATION, PSYCHOPHYSICS), but who, having grown up in an achromatic room, is not confronted with a red object until adulthood. If we agree that C acquires the quale *red* only after seeing the red object, then we must also admit that psychophysical descriptions cannot fully characterize qualia, which, as such, become epiphenomenal ($\rightarrow$ EPIPHENOMENALISM).

5. According to the *representational* theory of conscious mental phenomena, qualia are representations of properties, some external to the body (like colors), some internal (like pain) ($\rightarrow$ REPRESENTATION). In this view, the nature and identity of qualia are completely determined by the fact that they are representations, and by the type of object they

represent. However, the existence of "common sensibles"—that is, physical properties represented by different qualia (such as geometric shape, which can be seen and touched)—rules out a potential correspondence between representations and represented properties, and thereby constitutes an objection for the representational viewpoint.

ROBERT CASATI

SELECTED BIBLIOGRAPHY

Clark, A. (1993). *Sensory qualities.* Oxford, England: Clarendon Press; New York: Oxford University Press.
Jackson, F. (1986). What Mary didn't know. *Journal of Philosophy, 83,* 291–295.
Levine, J. (2000). *Purple haze: The puzzle of consciousness.* Oxford, England; New York: Oxford University Press.
Shoemaker, S. (1982). The inverted spectrum. *Journal of Philosophy, 79,* 357–381.

QUALITATIVE PHYSICS

Artificial intelligence. — The idea of a qualitative representation of the world is not new, nor are attempts to reason qualitatively about the world (→ REASONING AND RATIONALITY, REPRESENTATION). Well before its appearance in artificial intelligence (AI), the word *qualitative* was already being employed in various scientific communities (in economics in the 1960s with sign-based qualitative analysis, in ecology in the 1970s with the use of signs for effects between variables, and in dynamic system theory and automatic control [→ DYNAMIC SYSTEM]). These approaches were motivated by the lack of quantitative data that would have enabled the use of conventional numerical models, by the desire to distinguish between what depends on the particular numerical configurations of a given model and what is related to the overall structural features of the system, or, sometimes, simply by the desire to find explanations that are understandable to human beings (→ EXPLANATION).

A radical change came about in the 1970s when the AI community in the United States began working on what was called *qualitative physics* in view of developing computer systems capable of reasoning about physical systems in ways that more or less resemble human reasoning. Patrick Hayes's work on naive physics marked the starting point of the discipline. Hayes posed the problem of the axiomatization of our commonsense knowledge of the physical world. In his famous *Naive Physics Manifesto*, published in 1979 and revised in 1983, he raised the issue of "intelligent" machines endowed with a model of the surrounding world and capable of foreseeing what may or may not happen. His axiomatization of naive physics was based on first-order logic (→ LOGIC). Hayes introduced the key concept of *qualitative quantity space*, that is, a space that is discretized by a few ordered symbols with a physical meaning (→ SYMBOL). In his *Ontology for Liquids*, he illustrated his ideas about the logical axiomatization of the intuitive behavior of liquids. The project was ambitious, especially in light of the quantity of knowledge to be grasped. The challenge was to develop a system capable of stating whether a situation is "reasonable" and of predicting the qualitative characteristics of possible evolutions of the world. Despite the attractiveness of such a project and the considerable impact of Hayes's seminal work, naive physics and commonsense reasoning remained largely unexplored and were practically dropped altogether after 1985.

In essence, the AI community began to follow a different path. Interest was now directed at the possibility of having engineers use qualitative techniques to solve their problems (→ PROBLEM SOLVING). The goals were now more in line with those of the "artificial engineer project" launched in 1977 at the Massachusetts Institute of Technology than with Hayes's call for research programs. By the end of the 1970s, Johan de Kleer had developed a system for qualitatively solving simple mechanics problems. He introduced the concept of *envisioning* (prediction of behavior over time; → TIME AND TENSE), represented by a state transition graph that captures all physically possible sequences of qualitative behaviors. He also devised programs that used qualitative knowledge to set forth causal hypotheses for reasoning about electric circuits, for example, for troubleshooting (model-based diagnosis) or explaining how a circuit performs its function (→ CAUSALITY AND MENTAL CAUSATION, FUNCTION, MODEL).

Under the name *qualitative physics* and then *qualitative reasoning*, the discipline began to focus in particular on solving problems that would assist engineers in their daily tasks. In this respect, the year 1984 marked the birth of the qualitative reasoning community, with the publication of three key contributions presenting the basic concepts still valid today: ENVISION systems (de Kleer and John Brown), which use only the sign of variations, and the QSIM (Benjamin Kuipers) and QPT (Kenneth Forbus) systems, which utilize finer-grained quantity spaces with greater expressive and predictive power (→ EXPRESSIVENESS). The same year, a first special issue of the journal *Artificial Intelligence* was published (followed by a second in 1991, both of which also appeared in book format).

From the modeling standpoint, ENVISION is *component-based*: the physical system is described by components (instances of generic models) and their specific connections, governed by the principle of "no functions in the structure" (the laws describing the behavior of a part must not be based on any assumptions about the functioning of the whole). QPT is *process-based* and is thus more general, insofar as the processes that act upon the components are explicitly modeled. QSIM is *constraint-based* and is relatively independent of the choice of model (→ CONSTRAINT). The notion of envisioning is central in all three approaches: the temporal evolution of the system is specified by ordering the qualitative solutions, each of which constitutes a possible state (time is thus only implicitly represented). But one of the main difficulties is the existence of solutions that do not correspond to any real behavior: qualitative simulations are complete but incorrect. Finding ways to eliminate at least some of these incorrect solutions has been the aim of many studies.

Opposed to (or sometimes combined with) these approaches, where causality is not explicit (although some studies attempt to automatically derive causal influences from noncausal equation models), are the *causal approaches*, where the model is an oriented graph of effects whose arcs can carry various qualifiers of causality. A causal model is more suited to the explanation process, the abductive search for the primary causes of abnormalities ($\rightarrow$ ABDUCTION), and it supplies a natural framework for expressing empirical knowledge about poorly formalized physical systems (e.g., ecological systems).

Qualitative reasoning in the service of the engineering sciences continued to grow after that, with applications in diagnosis, supervision, and design. In doing so, it came closer to quantitative reasoning (use of numerical intervals), but moved even farther away from the original naive physics, while offering new perspectives to other communities that had not contemplated using models at a higher level of abstraction than the numerical level. This way of designing and implementing models is justified for high-level tasks requiring conceptual schemas similar to those of human operators ($\rightarrow$ CONCEPT). Such an interface with human beings leads us to foresee a partial "return to the source," with the cognitive dimension being considered once again. Research in functional and teleological modeling, causality, and explanation all attest to this. Computer-aided model acquisition, in critical demand today, will surely require incorporating this dimension.

PHILIPPE DAGUE

SELECTED BIBLIOGRAPHY

Aubin, J.-P. (1996). *Neural networks and qualitative physics: A viability approach*. Cambridge, England; New York: Cambridge University Press.

Bobrow, D. (Ed.). (1985). *Qualitative reasoning about physical systems*. Cambridge, MA: MIT Press.

De Kleer, J., & Williams, B. (Eds.). (1991). *Qualitative reasoning about physical systems, II*. Amsterdam, Elsevier.

Kuipers, B. J. (1994). *Qualitative reasoning: Modeling and simulation with incomplete knowledge*. Cambridge, MA: MIT Press.

Weld, D., & De Kleer, J. (Eds.). (1990). *Readings in qualitative reasoning about physical systems*, San Mateo, CA: Morgan Kaufmann.

R

READING

Psychology. — Research in the cognitive psychology of reading has mainly been devoted to building models of the cognitive functioning of skilled readers during the reading process. The models describe the various processing steps that take place between perception of the written form and word recognition (→ LANGUAGE, PERCEPTION).

A heated debate in the 1970s opposed strictly *bottom-up* views of reading to essentially *top-down* ones (→ INFORMATION). In the bottom-up approach, defended in particular by Kenneth Forster, processing is sequential in nature, going from the perception of the written form to the identification of words in memory (→ MEMORY). In the top-down approach, whose best-known spokesmen are Kenneth Goodman and Frank Smith, even the very first step that generates the perceptual image is dependent upon knowledge possessed by the reader: all steps thus involve strategies for retrieving the meaning of what is being read (→ SEMANTICS). This debate is outdated today, and most authors now agree upon a more interactive conception in which bottom-up processing, necessary at the outset if not elsewhere, is influenced by the subject's prior knowledge.

In line with Max Coltheart's model, the overall architecture of the cognitive system in charge of written word processing is usually described as consisting of two coexisting routes for accessing the *mental lexicon* (the set of all words in the reader's vocabulary) (→ LEXICON). The so-called indirect route relies on phonological mediation, whereas the direct route permits recognition without converting the written word into its oral counterpart (→ ORAL). Adopting a very different perspective, *connectionist* models (→ CONNECTIONISM) describe the parallel operation of networks in which propagation systems cause some configurations to be activated and others to be inhibited (→ ACTIVATION/INHIBITION). In Mark Seidenberg and James McClelland's model, the networks involve interacting units of orthographic, phonological, and semantic knowledge, along with transformation processes that spread the activation and inhibition across the different knowledge units. The system is not only at work when individuals are reading, but also when they are hearing or thinking about a word. From this angle, recognizing a word is not finding an entry in a mental dictionary, but activating the particular pattern of knowledge (orthographic, phonological, and semantic) that corresponds to that word.

The processes at play in written-word identification can be severely impaired by brain lesions (see *neuroscience* below). In such cases, called *acquired dyslexia*, the deficit may affect the very first steps of visual percept processing (*peripheral dyslexia*), or it may alter the formation of the mental representation in its orthographic, phonological, and/or semantic aspects (*central dyslexia*) (→ REPRESENTATION).

Studies in the cognitive psychology of reading also look at access to meaning (→ MEANING AND SIGNIFICATION). There are two complementary lines of research in this area. The first focuses on the syntactic computation of sentence meaning (→ SYNTAX) and sees access to meaning as an additional step in the reading process, beyond lexical processing. The second strives to explain how, starting from the text and knowledge acquired beforehand, readers elaborate a structured body of information corresponding to what they understand (→ TEXT).

Research on how children learn to read began to expand considerably in the 1980s (→ LEARNING). Uta Frith identified three major steps in the reading acquisition process. During the initial step, the *logographic phase*, children use cues to guess words: the cues are present in the environment (as in an advertising logo), but they are also taken from the word itself (usually certain letters). In this "reading-guessing" process, linguistic information is treated as a picture. During the second step, or *alphabetic phase*, the learner's efforts are mostly devoted to applying grapheme-phoneme conversion rules. During the third and last step, the *orthographic phase*, words are broken down into orthographic units, without mandatory recourse to phonological conversion. Morphology is thought to play an important role in this final step (→ MORPHOLOGY). Moreover, as Usha Goswami showed, it seems that before the alphabetic phase per se, children engage in a kind of reading-by-analogy in which they read new words based on their knowledge of how other words are pronounced. For example, a child who can read the words *hat* and *cat* will use this knowledge to read the word *sat*.

An important aspect of learning to read is *automatization* (→ AUTOMATISM), both automatization of word-recognition processes, which frees up cognitive resources for understanding, and automatization of some of the processes that compute and build meaning, which enhances the reader's text-handling skills.

In the area of learning disabilities, substantial progress has been made toward understanding developmental dyslexia, a disorder strictly limited to reading (and spelling) and independent of a child's intelligence and social and/or affective life. Since Frank Vellutino's book in 1979, the hypothesis of a biologically rooted dysfunction in certain information-processing mechanisms (particularly phonological ones) has gained more and more support. Such cases represent approximately 25 percent of poor readers. For the remaining 75 percent (which Jean-Émile Gombert calls "dissynopsics"), failure in reading is most likely caused by environmental factors.

JEAN-ÉMILE GOMBERT

Neuroscience. — The study of reading disabilities caused by acquired brain damage in adults has always captured the attention of neuropsychologists (→ NEUROPSYCHOLOGY). One reason for this interest is that in understanding the biological laws of evolution, it is very informative to discover brain regions whose only (or nearly only) role—despite the recency of written language in the history of humankind—is to accomplish fundamental reading operations (→ LANGUAGE, LOCALIZATION OF FUNCTION). The hypothesized existence of such regions seems to be supported by the fact that certain brain lesions result in a virtually isolated reading disorder. A second reason is that acquired lesion-linked reading deficits are very common and come in a variety of forms. Studies on reading performance in brain-damaged patients, which have been crucial in developing models of the reading process in normal subjects, are at the origin of the cognitive approach in neuropsychology.

The description of acquired reading disorders dates back to the nineteenth century and owes much to authors like Jean-Martin Charcot and Jules Dejerine. The two major syndromes at the time were *alexia* without *agraphia* and alexia with agraphia (→ WRITING): some patients are no longer able to read but can still write, while others have lost all use of written language. Reading disorders may also arise in association with other deficits, whether related to language or spatial information processing (→ SPACE). In the case of alexia without agraphia, the purest syndrome, the responsible lesions are always situated in the left temporal-occipital lobe. Brain metabolism studies have confirmed the presence of activation in this area of normal subjects' brain as they read (→ FUNCTIONAL NEUROIMAGING). It seems to be a critical region for decoding letters, or for assembling letters in order to identify whole words.

Around 1970, John Marshall and Freda Newcombe inaugurated what can today be called the "cognitive revolution in neuropsychology." They set out to describe precisely the deficits of brain-damaged patients suffering from certain reading disabilities, and to analyze and differentiate the types of errors they make. These patients are quite different from patients with classical alexia in that their speech is often impaired (→ ORAL) and above all, reading is not impossible for them. They can read, but they make mistakes. The authors found at least two types of patients: those who made pronunciation errors on phonologically similar words (for example, a patient reads *insist* when shown the word *insect*) and those who made mistakes involving words from the same semantic category (for example, the word *crocodile* is read aloud as *turtle*). This double observation led to the idea that there are two parallel reading pathways: one that goes directly from the orthographic code to the semantic code (this is the damaged pathway in the first case) (→ SEMANTICS) and a pathway that converts the orthographic code into a phonological code (damaged in the second case). Since then, the situation has become much more complex, but reading disorders are still approached within this same basic framework.

At the current time, in cases of acquired brain lesions in adults, two main types of alexia or dyslexia (the two terms are used in a nearly synonymous way) are distinguished. (1) Peripheral dyslexia is a reading disability affecting the initial steps in the visual processing of verbal information (→ INFORMATION). Two major syndromes are described here. Letter-by-letter alexia resembles alexia without agraphia (less frequent), although in a less severe form. It is caused by a left temporal-occipital lesion. These patients read painstakingly, one letter at a time. *Neglect dyslexia* is a reading disorder that arises within a more spatial kind of deficit. The lesions are parietal and more often on the right than on the left. (2) Central dyslexia is a reading disability that shows up "later" in the reading process. Dyslexics categorized as *profound* make semantic errors when reading words, whereas *surface* or *lexical dyslexics* have trouble reading irregular words. The lesions are in the left hemisphere. *Semantic dyslexia* can be added to the above. These patients (often with degenerative lesions) can read words aloud, even irregular ones, but cannot understand them.

A final important discovery in neuroscience concerns *developmental dyslexia*. In the 1980s, Norman Geschwind and Albert Galaburda showed that developmental dyslexia is often linked to neuronal dysfunction. Several patients who had had problems learning to read were found to exhibit neuron migration abnormalities (migration occurring before birth) in the left temporal lobe regions specifically involved in phonological encoding, notably the temporal plane.

As a whole, these findings and others (from evoked-potential and neuroimaging studies, for example) give us a glimpse of the complex but differentiated way in which the processes responsible for written-word comprehension are organized in the brain.

ÉRIC SIÉROFF

SELECTED BIBLIOGRAPHY

Farah, M., & Feinberg, T. (Eds.). (2000). *Patient-based approaches to cognitive neuroscience.* Cambridge, MA: MIT Press.

Frackowiak, R., Friston,, K., Dolan, R., Mazziotta, J., & Frith, C. (Eds.) (1997). *Human brain function.* San Diego, CA: Academic Press.

Goswami, U., & Bryant, P. (1990). *Phonological skills and learning to read.* Hillsdale, NJ: Erlbaum.

Goswami, U., McGurk, H., & Butterworth, G. (1992). *Analogical reasoning in children.* Hove, England: Erlbaum.

Jackson, N., & Coltheart, M. (2001). *Routes to reading success and failure: Toward an integrated cognitive psychology of atypical reading.* New York: Psychology Press.

Kintsch, W. (1998). *Comprehension: A paradigm for cognition.* Cambridge, England; New York: Cambridge University Press.

McCandliss, B. D., Cohen, L., & Dehaene, S. (2003). The visual word form area: Expertise for reading in the fusiform gyrus. *Trends in Cognitive Sciences, 7,* 293–299.

Paulesu, E., McCrory, E., Fazio, F., Menoncello, L., Brunswick, N., Cappa, S., Cotelli, M., Cossu, G., Corte, F., Lorusso, M., Pesenti, S., Gallagher, A., Perani, D., Price, C., Frith, C., & Frith, U. (2000). A cultural effect on brain function. *Nature Neuroscience, 2,* 91–96.

Petersen, S., Fox, P., Posner, M., Mintun, M., & Raichle, M. (1988). Positron emission tomographic studies of the cortical anatomy of single-word processing. *Nature, 331,* 585–589.

Plaut, D., McClelland, J., Seidenberg, M., & Patterson, K. (1996). Understanding normal and impaired word reading: Computational principles in quasi-regular domains. *Psychological Review, 103,* 56–115.

Posner, M., & Raichle, M. (1994/1997). *Images of mind.* New York: Freeman.

Seidenberg, M., & McClelland, J. (1989). A distributed, developmental model of word recognition and naming. *Psychological Review, 96,* 523–568.

Vellutino, F. (1979). *Dyslexia: Theory and research,* Cambridge, MA: MIT Press.

REALISM

Philosophy. — The *realist* position consists in contending, relative to a given discourse domain, that the entities associated with that domain are real. Accordingly, commonsense realism maintains that tables and chairs are real, and scientific realism, that electrons or genes are real. Psychological realism argues that the entities upon which psychological discourse bears, such as pain and beliefs, are real (→ BELIEF). In particular, this implies that their existence and their properties are objective, that is, they are independent of the epistemic attitudes and affirmations one forms about them (→ EPISTEMIC). To the extent that a thing is real, knowledge of it must be the product of a discovery rather than an invention. In particular, this implies that it is possible to be unaware of something even though it is real, and that one can be mistaken about it: the knowledge acquisition process may encounter obstacles.

Epistemological realism posits that independently of perception, there exists a world of physical objects whose nature can be known to humans (→ EPISTEMOLOGY, PERCEPTION). It comes in a range of versions. According to *direct realism*, the properties of objects are identical to the properties we attribute to them on the basis of perception, whereas *critical realism* contends that objects do not possess all of the properties they appear to have. Realism is opposed to idealism and phenomenalism (→ PHENOMENALISM).

In *folk psychology*, the entities used in causal explanations are beliefs and desires, or *propositional attitudes* (→ CAUSALITY AND MENTAL CAUSATION, DESIRE, PROPOSITIONAL ATTITUDE). I answer the phone because I believe it is ringing and I want to talk to the person who is calling me. We call *intentional realism* the view that ascribes a causal role to propositional attitudes by virtue of their content. Intentional realism thus defends the following theses: (1) there exist mental states that, owing to their presence and their mutual interactions, can be counted among the causes of behavior (→ FUNCTIONALISM); (2) these states have *content:* they can be evaluated semantically (synonymous expressions) (→ SEMANTICS); and (3) their causal effectiveness is determined by their content; hence their causal role is approximately the one that generalizations of folk psychology attribute to beliefs and desires.

MAX KISTLER

Psychology. — In addition to the question of beliefs and desires in folk psychology (see *philosophy* above), the issue of realism in its oppositional relationship to *constructivism* (→ CONSTRUCTIVISM) is raised in cognitive psychology mainly with regard to logicomathematical objects (→ CATEGORIZATION, NUMBER, REASONING AND RATIONALITY, SPACE). The question is an ontological one: What is the nature of the objects studied? This is not a new question; it dates back to Plato's Ideas and to medieval philosophy, where the quarrel about universals pitted Thomas of Aquinas's realism against William of Occam's *nominalism*. In the former, universals are part of the real world and are accessible to human reasoning. In the latter, the real is made up only of particular objects that we experience through our senses (→ EXPERIENCE): classes, kinds, and universals are nothing more than a series of names that have no direct counterpart in reality. In a contemporary version of this debate, waged by the mathematician Alain Connes and his neurobiologist opponent Jean-Pierre Changeux, Connes argued that a raw and immutable reality exists outside of humans, and that we perceive it only by way of our brain, through a "rare mixture," as the poet Paul Valéry said, of concentration and desire. The proof that this reality exists would be the fact that we have trouble delineating it. This is true of numbers, for instance: to any person who claims to have found the largest prime number, it is easy to explain that there is a way to find a larger one (Euclid's proof). Mathematical objects "are there"—prime numbers, the infinity of prime numbers, and so forth—and the only thing the mind does is unveil a reality that initially escaped it (→ MIND). This kind of realism is opposed to the constructivism of other mathematicians, called *formalists*, who see logicomathematical objects as subtle inventions "secreted" by the brain, not as discoveries of preexisting material.

The constructivist position, by definition, looks at what genetic mechanisms ("genetic" in the sense of genesis, development) underlie logicomathematical constructions, a problem rooted both in the history of science and in cognitive psychology. As the logician Jean-Blaise Grize stressed, a representation of a piece of knowledge in a logicomathematical language is the result of a thought process from which the subject has withdrawn; the building is there but the architect and the workers have left (→ LANGUAGE, LOGIC, REPRESENTATION). Stated in a different way, this time as a question: Doesn't removing all content—which is where logicomathematical objects seem to operate—amount to increasing the level of abstraction, as Jean Piaget thought, via an activity whose roots are far more concrete? Think of the relationship established by historians between trade and the origins of number, or between land surveying and the origins of geometry.

The same question can be asked about individual history, and this is where cognitive psychology enters the picture, that is, developmental psychology (→ COGNITIVE DEVELOPMENT). Relating psychogenesis to the logicomathematical systems already in place is in fact the very foundation of the Piagetian approach. In this way, Piaget drew a line that connects the most abstract kind of thinking—for example, thoughts that can be described by propositional calculus—to the sensorimotor development of infants (→ INFANT COGNITION), after passing through a preparatory stage where concrete operations set in. Right through to his last posthumous book, published in 1990, Piaget never stopped denouncing the realist conception of logicomathematical truth, which he deemed fit for preexisting beings (be they, as he said, Platonic Ideas or something else). No matter what criticisms might be made of Piaget's theory today, his postulate of a link between normativity (→ NORMATIVITY) and psychogenesis (in the sense defined above) remains valid in current psychology and cognitive science. This is true for new trends in developmental psychology (neostructuralism and developmental cognitivism); it is also true in the neural constructivism of logicomathematical objects, defended by Changeux against contemporary realism (→ NEURAL DARWINISM).

OLIVIER HOUDÉ

SELECTED BIBLIOGRAPHY

Alston, W. (Ed.). (2002). *Realism and antirealism*. Ithaca, NY: Cornell University Press.

Bosley, R., & Tweedale, M. (Eds.). (1997). *Basic issues in medieval philosophy: Selected readings presenting interactive discourses among the major figures*. Peterborough, Ontario; Orchard Park, NY: Broadview Press.

Changeux, J.-P., & Connes, A. (1998). *Conversations on mind, matter, and mathematics* (M. B. DeBevoise, Ed. and Trans.). Princeton, NJ: Princeton University Press. (Original work published 1989.)

Dennett, D. (1987). *The intentional stance*. Cambridge, MA: MIT Press.

Fischer, K., & Kaplan, U. (2003). Piaget, Jean. In L. Nadel (Ed.), *The encyclopedia of cognitive science* (Vol. 1, pp. 679–682). London: Nature Publishing Group, Macmillan.

Fodor, J. (1985). Fodor's guide to mental representation. *Mind, 94*, 76–100.

Fodor, J. (1987). *Psychosemantics: The problem of meaning in the philosophy of mind*. Cambridge, MA: MIT Press.

Grize, J.-B. (1993). Pensée logico-mathématique et sémiologie du langage [Logico-mathematical thought and semiology of language]. In O . Houdé & D. Miéville (Eds.), *Pensée logico-mathématique* [Logico-mathematical thought]. Paris: Presses Universitaires de France.

Katz, J. (1998). *Realistic rationalism*. Cambridge, MA: MIT Press.

Papineau, D. (Ed.). (1996). *The philosophy of science*. Oxford, England; New York: Oxford University Press.

Piaget, J., Henriques, G., & Ascher, E. (1992). *Morphisms and categories: Comparing and transforming* (T. Brown, Trans. and Ed.). Hillsdale, NJ: Erlbaum. (Original work published 1990)

Piaget, J., & Inhelder, B. (1969). *The psychology of the child* (H. Weaver, Trans.). New York: Basic Books. (Original work published 1966.)

Putnam, H. (1988). *Representation and reality*. Cambridge, MA: MIT Press.

Rey, G. (1996). *Contemporary philosophy of mind: A contentiously classical approach*. Oxford, England: Blackwell.

REASONING AND RATIONALITY

Psychology. — Right from the beginning of cognitivism, the brain was treated as a deductive machine whose constituents (neurons) embody logical principles (→ COGNITIVISM, LOGIC). This view led to the idea of the "logical mind" (→ MIND), and the brain was metaphorically likened to the inference system of a computer. In the psychology of reasoning, *inference-making processes*, the foundation of deduction, have been widely studied within this framework. But have the studies demonstrated the deductive competence of the logical mind? Apparently not. While certain inference schemas are well mastered by all subjects, others have been shown to trigger frequent errors. This finding has raised the question of the rationality of human subjects: Is there a *mental logic*, and if so, how can we explain reasoning errors? This, essentially, is the core of the cognitivist debate, with one side arguing for the theory of mental logic and the other for approaches revolving around mental models, pragmatic schemas, and reasoning biases.

According to Martin Braine, human subjects possess a universal mental logic or natural logic, defined as a set of very simple, often automatized *inference rules* (→ AUTOMATISM) that is fully mastered by adults and, for the most part, understood early by children (→ COGNITIVE DEVELOPMENT). Accompanied by an executive program, natural logic would enable information to be processed by a "direct reasoning routine." Although Braine's view is a logical-mind view, he does not attribute absolute deductive competence to the ordinary subject. He makes the distinction between two skill levels in propositional calculus: *primary skills* and *secondary skills*. Primary skills correspond to the logical inferences required to understand discourse and reason about everyday practical things (→ DISCOURSE, LAN-

GUAGE); they are universal (overarching all languages) and independent of the individual's education in logic and mathematics. By contrast, secondary skills follow directly from logical and mathematical instruction: they are almost totally academic and necessitate elaborate analytical reasoning that is not universal. It is generally at this level that subjects make errors and that psychologists experimentally test their competence (→ COMPETENCE/PERFORMANCE). The originality of Braine's contribution is that he places natural logic among the primary skills and contends that reasoning errors in tasks requiring those skills are the only errors apt to cast doubt on the hypothesis of a universal mental logic.

The question that arises regarding this theory is whether the existence of a logic system is a prerequisite to successful deductive reasoning. Philip Johnson-Laird's answer is an unhesitating *no:* a mental model-building process suffices to account for the deduction capabilities of human subjects. He illustrates this position using categorical syllogisms. For Johnson-Laird, syllogistic reasoning is the result of a three-step process: (1) build a mental model representing a semantic interpretation of the premises, (2) draw a conclusion from that model, and (3) search for other models that meet the requirements of the premises but produce counterexamples of the tentative conclusion (→ INTERPRETATION, REPRESENTATION, SEMANTICS). On the last step, if the subject finds alternative incompatible models, the inference is declared invalid; otherwise, the conclusion is said to be true and the inference valid. This reasoning process is a form of "thought experiment."

What makes Johnson-Laird's theory fundamentally different from the mental-logic approach is that it does not involve syntactic inference rules (→ SYNTAX), but rather a semantic construction process that builds mental models of the premises and the conclusion. In this framework, reasoning errors are ascribed to two factors: the limited capacity of working memory (problems that require the greatest number of mental models in memory are the ones with the greatest risk of error) (→ MEMORY) and the *belief-bias effect* (→ BELIEF) according to which subjects lack the motivation to look for counterexamples whenever a model that appears appropriate is compatible with the premises; in this case, they decide to believe the model without conducting an exhaustive search for alternatives. Johnson-Laird attempted to apply his theory to domains other than categorical syllogisms, namely propositional calculus and inductive reasoning.

In an approach akin to the preceding one, this time proposed by Patricia Cheng and Keith Holyoak, subjects are thought to reason not with formal rules, but by using general pragmatic schemas like the ones that structure daily-life experiences: permission schema, obligation schema, causality schema, etc. (→ PRAGMATICS). Still another approach is the one put forward by Jonathan Evans, who concentrates solely on logic errors and their underlying reasoning biases and sees bias as a systematic tendency to take irrelevant factors into account while ignoring relevant factors. For Evans, reasoning biases are rooted in heuristics (a form of everyday reasoning) whereas deductive competence stems from analytic processes; two forms of rationality are thus defined.

In looking at the different cognitivist approaches to reasoning (mental logic, mental models, pragmatic schemas, and reasoning biases), a question that arises concerns their compatibility and hence their respective domains of relevance. The two broadest points of view are those of Braine and Evans. Braine specifically places mental logic at the primary-skill level, although without denying the psychological reality of another level of functioning where, in the face of more complex problems, subjects often commit errors and must rely on different strategies. He thus acknowledges the importance of approaches based on mental models and pragmatic schemas in accounting for the various components of the ability to reason. In a complementary perspective, Evans centers his analysis on errors and reasoning biases, while emphasizing the need to study the mechanisms of rational behavior, whether optimal, logical, or otherwise. By contrast, Johnson-Laird's position is more clear cut. He firmly rejects the idea of formal rules that define a mental logic, stating that mental models suffice to account for the diversity of reasoning behavior. This position is currently contested for its monistic character.

Although deduction has been the main topic in the psychology of reasoning, the study of *induction* and *abduction* has also gained a firm footing (→ ABDUCTION). Other forms of reasoning such as reasoning-by-analogy are under investigation as well. Another approach is *connectionism*, where reasoning is described as a propagation mechanism operating in a subsymbolic network (and not in reference to symbolic units like the formal rules of mental logic or mental models) (→ CONNECTIONISM). The task of current research is to account for the polymorphism of human reasoning and the cognitive architecture within which it takes place in the brain.

OLIVIER HOUDÉ AND SYLVAIN MOUTIER

Neuroscience. — Simplifying, one can say that to reason is to set a goal and imagine one or more means of reaching it. This process is extremely complex and necessitates the participation of many subsystems, including those involved in analyzing the situation perceptually, retrieving information from memory, and making decisions, not to speak of planning, controlling, and executing the response (→ CONTROL, INFORMATION, MEMORY, PERCEPTION).

Reasoning is often mediated by plans or solving procedures stored in memory. Such plans define a set of operations carried out by various processing subsystems, and the mechanism that selects a plan is a critical part of the reasoning process. Results of positron emission tomography research (→ FUNCTIONAL NEUROIMAGING) indicate that the dorsolateral frontal cortex is implicated in this mechanism. But selecting a suitable plan often requires inhibiting competing plans (→ ACTIVATION/INHIBITION), which the frontal cortex appears to handle too. Studies on monkeys have shown that frontal-lesioned animals are deficient at inhibiting recently awarded dominant responses (→ ANIMAL COGNITION, NEUROPSYCHOLOGY). This behavior can be compared to the perseveration behaviors observed in patients with frontal brain damage, who have difficulty switching to a new sort criterion (in the Wisconsin card-sorting task, for example).

Given the large number of subsystems involved at various levels of reasoning (in the broad sense), it is not surprising that reasoning disorders sometimes appear subsequent to a multitude of cognitive dysfunctions linked to different lesion sites. Some of the major neuropsychology research areas concerned with reasoning are working memory, calculation, and pragmatics (→ NUMBER, PRAGMATICS).

OLIVIER KOENIG

Artificial intelligence. — The classical tradition would have us base the principles used to justify reasoning on the idea of *validity*. In other words, if in a reasoning process the premises are posited as true, then the conclusion must also be true. This is obviously a requirement of mathematical reasoning, but it is unwise to make this deductive form of reasoning the archetype of all forms of reasoning. In artificial intelligence (AI), "valid" reasoning is too slow to be compatible with any decision-making process (→ COMPLEXITY, EXPRESSIVENESS). It is impossible, then, to grant the status of "norm of rationality" to a form of reasoning that responds so poorly to the intuitive criteria of rationality. Adaptations have been made (for example, limited rationality for Herbert Simon or Christopher Cherniak), but it is far from evident that they might suffice to resolve this inherent incompatibility. Moreover, there are other, invalid forms of reasoning, such as generalizing induction or abduction (Charles Peirce) (→ ABDUCTION), that are indispensable in accounting for the diversity of human reasoning. Research on learning, which is almost as old as computer science, attempts to simulate inductive reasoning using symbolic or connectionist means (→ CONNECTIONISM, LEARNING, SYMBOL). More recently, automatic diagnosis techniques have provided interesting results in the area of abductive reasoning. Case-based reasoning, which involves finding analogies between a to-be-solved problem and a set of already-solved problems, has also been widely studied.

However, in simply making the distinction between various forms of reasoning, we are sidestepping some important issues. For one thing, different forms of reasoning need to be combined and controlled by strategies, which are reasoning processes that bear on the progression of the problem-solving process rather than on the problem itself (→ CONTROL, METACOGNITION, PROBLEM SOLVING). *Heuristic search* is a possible strategy that was studied extensively in the 1970s. In its standard version, heuristic search amounts to assigning, to each intermediate state of a problem solution, a numerical estimate assessing the distance between that particular state and the final goal. However, apart from a few rare cases, this strategy does not seem to shorten the solving time enough to be considered effective. Other ideas currently being explored include dividing the solving process among various software agents each specialized in a different domain of expertise (→ DISTRIBUTED INTELLIGENCE, DOMAIN SPECIFICITY). It has been clear for quite some time that attempts to create universal problem solvers such as the General Problem Solver (or GPS, proposed by Allen Newell and Herbert Simon in 1960) will never be successful, and that a given reasoning system can be productive only if it uses knowledge specific to the domain of application. Domain-specific knowledge must be in a format that permits its rapid utilization, and forms of reasoning well suited to certain types of representation have now been developed (→ REPRESENTATION). Propagation in semantic networks, for instance, which corresponds more or less to the notion of spreading activation proposed in cognitive psychology, is a very incomplete but highly efficient reasoning method (→ SEMANTIC NETWORK).

An issue of increasingly obvious importance in AI—even though we are still not really able to solve it—concerns the fit between the problem posed and the (artificial) language used to represent the knowledge (→ LANGUAGE). In other words, this is an ontological endeavor, one that strives both to conduct the step-by-step proof process that takes the reasoner from the premises to the conclusion (→ LOGIC) and, at the same time, to check the adequacy of the mapping of the elements whose existence is presumed by the question posed, to the elements used to express the knowledge assumed to be relevant to answering it.

Finally, if a reasoning process is characterized by the existence of a justification, available upon request, of its end product (and not by the mere inferences that are performed during it), it is necessary to give *explanatory* capabilities to any system alleged to model reasoning (→ EXPLANATION). The expert systems developed in the 1980s generally possess such capabilities in an embryonic state. To go further, it is necessary to incorporate a finer-grained view of the cognitive faculties of the users to whom the explanations are geared, and to make use of techniques (in particular, the principles of argumentation pragmatics;

→ PRAGMATICS) for stating explanations in an effective and understandable manner.

DANIEL KAYSER

Philosophy. — Human beings are rational animals, and one of the things that makes them so is their ability to reason. Since Aristotle, logicians have been codifying the rules and norms of correct deductive reasoning (→ LOGIC, NORMATIVITY), and since Blaise Pascal and Daniel Bernoulli, mathematicians have been doing the same for probabilistic reasoning. But reasoning in a natural setting is usually ridden with errors and paralogisms. (Logic is something that has to be taught.) Psychologists have shown that human agents make systematic errors (see *psychology* above), both in simple deductive reasoning (like that required to resolve the kind of *If p then q* conditional statements found in Philip Wason's card-selection task) and in probabilistic reasoning, also simple (when in situations like Daniel Kahneman and Amos Tversky's, for example, we tend to consider a conjunction of events to be more probable than one of the events alone, thereby falling prey to the conjunction fallacy). Should these facts (reviewed for example by David Over and Keith Mantkelow) be taken as experimental proof that human agents consistently deviate from the norms of rationality defined by logic or probability theory, and hence that they are irrational?

The answer to this question depends first on the meaning one wishes to give to the polysemous term *rationality*, which has at least two major meanings: (1) agents are rational in their thinking if they are capable of abiding by the norms of correct reasoning, and (2) agents are rational in the instrumental sense if they maximize their utility through their actions (→ ACTION). In the first meaning, one can contend that the systematic reasoning errors noted by psychologists simply reveal that an agent's performance is altered, not his or her competence, to borrow Noam Chomsky's famous distinction (→ COMPETENCE/PERFORMANCE). But how can that competence be characterized?

Philosophers have proposed two types of arguments to show that one must, a priori, attribute rationality to all human agents. The first argument relies on the idea, advanced in particular by Willard Quine, Donald Davidson, and Daniel Dennett, that any interpretation of the behavior of human agents, be it their inferences or their actions, presupposes being able to attribute to the agent a set of true beliefs that conforms to minimal norms of rationality and logical coherence by relying on a principle of "charity" (→ BELIEF, INTERPRETATION). Such a presumption of rationality can also be applied to the second of the two meanings above, by bringing to bear the notion of *optimization by natural selection*: a species capable of surviving and maximizing its fitness must have a majority of true beliefs and correct reasoning schemas. Another argument in support of this presumption is based on the concept of *reflective equilibrium* (used in moral theory by John Rawls): norms of rationality must pass the test of our individual intuitions about specific ways of reasoning, which in turn can be assessed only on the basis of the norms in question, in such a way that any test of rationality or irrationality must be circular and presuppose the validity of rationality norms.

But these arguments in favor of an a priori rationality are questionable. First of all, does the principle of charity conform to our everyday practices of interpretation? Basing their thinking on developmental studies of children's theories of mind (→ THEORY OF MIND), some philosophers express their doubts about such a claim, pointing out that our interpretations rest instead on a psychological simulation of others that does not presuppose the truth or rationality of the simulated beliefs. Second, the evolutionary-optimization argument applies, strictly speaking, only to human reasoning capacities. These capacities must have been selected rather than particular forms of reasoning. A final point is that we are far from reaching a consensus regarding norms of logical and probabilistic rationality. Traditional psychological research on reasoning assumes the validity of classical norms of logic and of Bayesian canons of probabilistic reasoning, but there is no evidence that these norms and canons are actually used by agents. There are several competing theories in the psychology of natural reasoning. They seem to show that logical reasoning tasks presented to agents in the form of verbal tests are subject to all sorts of determinants, including biases and heuristics (→ LANGUAGE). Probability norms are also under debate, and can be interpreted in particular in a subjectivistic way or in a frequentist way. Neither norms nor the intuitions of agents have a clear status, making the general hypothesis of the rationality or irrationality of human inferential behavior difficult to test empirically. Today's challenge is to assess the hypothesis of an a priori rationality, and also the opposing "pragmatist" hypothesis (Stephen Stich) according to which there are many competing norms of rationality.

PASCAL ENGEL

SELECTED BIBLIOGRAPHY

Braine, M., & O'Brien, D. (Eds.). (1998). *Mental logic*. Mahwah, NJ: Erlbaum.

Dennett, D. (1987). *The intentional stance*. Cambridge, MA: MIT Press.

Engel, P. (1991). *The norm of truth: An introduction to the philosophy of logic* (M. Kochan & P. Engel, Trans.). Toronto, Ontario; Buffalo, NY: University of Toronto Press. (Original work published 1989.)

Evans, J. (1989). *Biases in human reasoning*. Hillsdale, NJ: Erlbaum.

Goel, V., Gold, B., Kapur, S., & Houle, S. (1997). The seats of reason? An imaging study of deductive and inductive reasoning. *NeuroReport, 8*, 1305–1310.

Holyoak, K., & Cheng, P. (1995). Pragmatic reasoning about human voluntary action. In S. Newstead & J. Evans (Eds.), *Perspectives on thinking and reasoning* (pp. 67–89). Hillsdale, NJ: Erlbaum.

Houdé, O., & Tzourio-Mazoyer, N. (2003). Neural foundations of logical and mathematical cognition. *Nature Reviews Neuroscience, 4*, 507–514.

Houdé, O., Zago, L., Mellet, E., Moutier, S., Pineau, A., Mazoyer, B., & Tzourio-Mazoyer, N. (2000). Shifting from the perceptual brain to the logical brain. *Journal of Cognitive Neuroscience, 12*, 721–728.

Johnson-Laird, P. (1995). Mental models, deductive reasoning, and the brain. In M. Gazzaniga (Ed.), *The cognitive neurosciences* (pp. 999–1008). Cambridge, MA: MIT Press.

Kahneman, D., Slovic, P., & Tversky, A. (Eds.). (1982). *Judgment under uncertainty: Heuristics and biases.* Cambridge, England: Cambridge University Press.

Kahneman, D., & Tversky, A. (Eds.). (2000). *Choices, values, and frames.* New York: Russell Sage Foundation; Cambridge, England: Cambridge University Press.

Kolodner, J. (1993). *Case-based reasoning.* San Diego, CA: Morgan Kaufmann.

Luger, G. (2002). *Artificial intelligence: Structures and strategies for complex problem-solving* (4th ed.). Harlow, England; New York: Pearson Education.

Mantkelow, K., & Over, D. (Eds.). (1993). *Rationality: Psychological and philosophical perspectives.* London: Routledge.

Newstead, S., Evans, J., & Byrne, R. (1993). *Human reasoning: The psychology of deduction.* Hove, England; Hillsdale, NJ: Erlbaum.

Russell, S. (1997). Rationality and intelligence. *Artificial Intelligence, 94*, 57–77.

Stich, S. (1990). *The fragmentation of reason.* Cambridge, MA: MIT Press.

Wharthon, C., & Grafman, J. (1998). Deductive reasoning and the brain. *Trends in Neurosciences, 2*, 54–59.

REDUCTIONISM

Philosophy. — *Reducing* a property or a proposition is giving an explanation of it that shows its equivalence to another or several other more fundamental properties or propositions.

A number of attempts have been made to reduce mental properties. The ontological status of mental properties is considered problematic, partly because they are not directly accessible to intersubjective observation—a feature they have in common with "theoretical" properties and the entities postulated in other sciences (e.g., physics)—and partly because, at present, there is no mature theory of mental properties.

Logical behaviorism is an important variant of mental-state reductionism. It is generally abandoned today in favor of *functionalism* (→ FUNCTIONALISM). According to behaviorism, mental states are dispositions to behave in a given way. But postulating that there is a conceptual link with behavior amounts to eliminating mental states from scientific research.

A more recent form of mental-state reductionism is the theory of an identity relationship between mental properties and the brain's underlying physical properties (→ PHYSICALISM). It is derived more directly from successful reductions achieved in other sciences, particularly physics. This theory assumes that there are bridge laws that subsume the regularities of psychology under those of neurophysiology, and those of the latter under chemistry and/or physics. Functionalism is compatible with reductionism (David Lewis, David Armstrong), but it has also been interpreted in an antireductionist manner (Hilary Putnam): in a functionalist analysis of mental states, it is conceivable that one and the same type of mental state can be realized in several manners at the physiological or physical level. The externalistic thesis on the identity of mental contents poses another major problem for the project of reducing the mental to the physiological (→ EXTERNALISM/INTERNALISM).

Contrary to what is sometimes suggested, the reduction of a property, mental or otherwise, does not lead to its elimination, but supplies scientific backing for its reality. On the other hand, properties that resist reduction are eliminated. Accordingly, since the revolution of chemistry in the eighteenth century, it is no longer believed that the alchemist predicate "phlogiston" (a putative fire element) denotes any real substance or property, precisely because it has proven impossible to reduce it to more basic predicates.

MAX KISTLER

SELECTED BIBLIOGRAPHY

Chalmers, D. (2002). *Philosophy of mind: Classical and contemporary readings.* New York: Oxford University Press.

Changeux, J.-P., & Connes, A. (1998). *Conversations on mind, matter, and mathematics* (M. B. DeBevoise, Ed. and Trans.). Princeton, NJ: Princeton University Press. (Original work published 1989.)

Charles, D., & Lennon, K. (Eds.). (1992). *Reduction, explanation, and realism.* Oxford, England: Clarendon Press; New York: Oxford University Press.

Clark, A., & Clark, W. (1990). *Psychological models and neural mechanisms: An examination of reductionism in psychology.* New York: Oxford University Press.

Faye, J. (2001). *The problem of the unity of science.* River Edge, NJ: World Scientific.

Hardcastle, V. (1996). *How to build a theory in cognitive science.* Albany, NY: State University of New York Press.

Putnam, H. (1988). *Representation and reality.* Cambridge, MA: MIT Press.

RELEVANCE

Linguistics. — The term *relevance* is used in logic in a technical sense (→ LOGIC). It is also at the heart of pragmatic views of language and communication (→ COMMUNICATION, LANGUAGE, PRAGMATICS).

Relevance logic (also called *relevant logic*) appeared in the 1950s in direct connection with the desire to propose a new and stronger definition of *material implication*. In a material implication relation, a proposition *if p, then q* is true both when *p* is false, and when *p* is true and *q* is also true. When *p* is true and *q* is false, the proposition is false. One possible criticism of this classical definition of implication is that *p* and *q* do not have to be related semantically or otherwise because it is based solely on the truth or falsity of *p* and *q* (→ SEMANTICS, TRUTH). To overcome this difficulty (extremely troublesome if one hopes to use logic to account for linguistic behavior, particularly natural-language conditionals), logicians like Alan

Anderson and Nuel Belnap developed relevance logic. Basically, there are two foundations of relevance logic: first, p and q must share variables, that is, there must be a semantic link between their propositional contents; second, there must be a dependency between p and q, in the sense that p must actually be used to obtain q in a relation of *entailment*. Note that while relevance logic now ranks among the newer widely accepted logics, it has still not achieved its ambition of replacing classical logic in the formalization of natural language.

In cognitive science, we owe another sense of the term *relevance* to the philosopher Paul Grice. In a certain way, Grice's preoccupations have much in common with those of relevance logicians, in that they go beyond traditional logic to account for language. However, rather than replacing classical logic by a new logic, Grice prefers to see speakers as complying with a general principle, the *principle of cooperation*, whereby a speaker is obligated to supply his or her interlocutors with whatever it takes to understand the statements being made. This principle can be broken down into several maxims: the *maxim of quantity* (give as much information as necessary, but no more; → INFORMATION), the *maxim of quality* (do not state what you think is false and things for which you lack proof), the *maxim of relation* (be relevant), and the *maxim of manner* (be clear: that is, avoid obscurity and ambiguity; be brief and orderly). Although the notion of relevance is central to relevance logic, it has a bearing on only one of the maxims (the maxim of relation) and is not given any particular technical definition (Grice settles for employing it in its ordinary sense). In addition, it is difficult to discriminate between the relevance maxim and the quantity maxim, insofar as a relevant utterance could be one that supplies the right amount of information.

Working within a post-Gricean, cognitivist framework, Dan Sperber and Deirdre Wilson developed a pragmatic theory called *relevance theory*. In line with Jerry Fodor, Sperber and Wilson consider pragmatics to be a central, nonspecialized process that takes effect after the strictly linguistic (syntactic and semantic) analysis of the utterance (→ MODULARITY, SYNTAX). The driving force of this process is a principle of relevance according to which each utterance carries with it the presumption of its *optimal relevance*. Optimal relevance is a function of the effort required to interpret the utterance and the effect it produces in that particular interpretation context (→ CONTEXT AND SITUATION, INTERPRETATION), namely: any contextual implications produced jointly by the utterance and the context, changes in the confidence level at which propositions in that context are entertained, and deletion of propositions that are contradictory to the one implied by the utterance. Each new utterance is thus interpreted relative to a context that is not given, but is constructed utterance by utterance. The context is selected via the principle of relevance; in other words, it is the one most consistent with that principle. The context is formed by propositions that follow from the interpretation of the immediately preceding utterances, encyclopedic knowledge available to the individual about the world, and knowledge directly accessed via the perception of the environment in which the communication process is taking place (→ PERCEPTION). Finally, the interpretation of an utterance cannot be reduced to a paraphrase of it, but includes the propositions (contextual implications) that one can draw from it. The principle of relevance thus governs which propositions will enter into the context, and when to stop the interpretative process: it ends when an interpretation that obeys the principle of relevance is obtained.

Sperber and Wilson's relevance theory has several original features relative to relevance logic and Grice's theory. Compared to relevance logic, its particularity is that it does not propose an alternative logic, but retains classical logic (except for the introduction rules) and Noam Chomsky's analysis, to which it adds an inferential analysis dictated by the principle of relevance. Compared to Grice's theory, relevance theory replaces the various maxims and the principle of cooperation with a single principle, that of relevance, which interlocutors may or may not choose to obey but which necessarily applies. In this way, Sperber and Wilson give an original definition of the concept of relevance that corresponds to the two foundations of relevance logic (shared content and dependency) and offers a solution to the problem of when to terminate the interpretation process.

JACQUES MOESCHLER AND ANNE REBOUL

Psychology. — In addition to its use in the psychology of language and communication (→ COMMUNICATION, LANGUAGE, PRAGMATICS), the notion of relevance in the sense employed in relevance logic (see *linguistics* above) is also applied to the study of cognitive development (→ COGNITIVE DEVELOPMENT).

Referring to the work by Anderson and Belnap, Jean Piaget and Rolando Garcia defined a *logic of meaning* that they presented as an intensional adjustment of classical operatory logic (Piaget and Jean-Blaise Grize), the latter being too close to traditional models of extensional truth-value logic (→ LOGIC, MEANING). The key operation in this logic of meaning, designed to formalize the cognitive activities of children, is *meaningful implication*, a form of relevance relation: p implies q (denoted $p \rightarrow q$) if a meaning s of q is among the meanings of p and if this common meaning s is transitive. In this case, inclusions of meanings in intension, which Piaget and Garcia called *inherent relations* (intimate and necessary links), correspond to nestings in extension (→ CATEGORIZATION). The logic of meaning is applicable to propositions or utterances (generated by the semiotic function during cognitive development), but according to the authors, it already exists in human infants at the sensorimotor stage, when implications between the meanings of actions set in (→ ACTION). Even in the most elementary, yet preprogrammed scheme, the sucking reflex, there would be implications (between movements and successes or failures): when the infant puts its mouth in the wrong place, it must move it to reach the nipple (→ INFANT COGNITION). This is not only an intensional revision of operatory logic (meaningful implications), but also an affirmation of the existence of a protologic right from the beginning of life (in line with Jonas Langer's observations on infant pragmatic logic).

From a psychological point of view, then, Anderson and Belnap's relevance logic—translated here into the terms of the logic of meaning—would be the substrate of Piaget's classical operatory logic; hence the utility of jointly studying these two kinds of logic.

OLIVIER HOUDÉ

SELECTED BIBLIOGRAPHY

Anderson, A. R., & Belnap, N. D. (1975). *Entailment: The logic of relevance and necessity*. Princeton, NJ: Princeton University Press.
Brady, R. (2003). *Relevant logics and their rivals*. Burlington, VT: Ashgate.
Grice, H. P. (1989). *Studies in the way of words*. Cambridge, MA: Harvard University Press.
Langer, J. (1980–1986). *The origins of logic*. New York: Academic Press.
Piaget, J., & Garcia, R. (1991). *Toward a logic of meanings* (P. Davidson & J. Easley, Eds. and Trans.). Hillsdale, NJ: Erlbaum. (Original work published 1987.)
Piaget, J., & Grize, J.-B. (1972). *Essai de logique opératoire* [Essay on operatory logic]. Paris: Dunod.
Priest, G. (2001). *An introduction to non-classical logic*. Cambridge, England; New York: Cambridge University Press.
Read, S. (1988). *Relevant logic: A philosophical examination of inference*. Oxford, England: Blackwell.
Sperber, D., & Wilson, D. (1986). *Relevance: Communication and cognition*. Oxford, England: Blackwell; Cambridge, MA: Harvard University Press.

REPRESENTATION

Psychology. — The idea that the human cognitive system functions by manipulating *representations* is no doubt an old one, at least in its implicit form. But more than anything else, the notion of mental representation rose to its status as an inner entity, the individual cognitive counterpart of external realities experienced by a subject (→ EXPERIENCE, MIND), with the development of cognitive psychology over the past few decades. Representation as a concept became a necessity in psychology as soon as the discipline started to question approaches based solely on behavior. Social psychology had been emphasizing both the variety and the individual particularities of representations. This approach is still relevant today and has been extended to the analysis of cross-individual invariants in mental representations and the mechanisms responsible for their construction ($\rightarrow$ COGNITIVE DEVELOPMENT).

It is no doubt regarding the concept of representation that psychology has had its most fruitful conceptual exchanges with other cognitive sciences. In doing so, though, it has obviously not disregarded the fundamental differences that exist between natural representations like the ones organisms equipped with a nervous system build of their environment, and artificial representations like those constructed in a rational way by engineers for use in information-processing systems (see *neuroscience* and *artificial intelligence* below). Exchanges across disciplines have also clearly brought out the distinction between representations as information-conveying structures ($\rightarrow$ INFORMATION), and mediums that do not themselves carry any information but serve as the bases upon which representations are inscribed. The idea introduced here is that there are different mediums for different types of information, and that each medium imposes specific constraints on the information-processing operations it supports. In this respect, the biological base of cognitive representations is characterized both by its processing capacities and also by certain limitations in those capacities.

As brief as it is, the history of psychology has shown that representations have not always been deemed necessary to account for cognitive performance (when, more radically, the concept hasn't been rejected altogether). Models of cognitive representation began to emerge with the increasingly widespread idea that through their experiences, individuals build internalized models of their environment, the objects they come across, and the interactions they have with those objects ($\rightarrow$ OBJECT). The study of representations then started to develop around the postulate that representations—cognitive entities that are not directly observable—could nevertheless be accessed by scientists if they could devise experimental procedures that brought behavioral observables to bear. This epistemological approach made it possible to discern the general properties of representations (seen as structures that store information, albeit in a reduced and more abstract format) and to include the study of representations in that of cognitive functioning, notably by determining the functions that representations fulfill: retaining information that is no longer directly available, guiding and controlling behavior, and planning action ($\rightarrow$ ACTION, CONTROL, MEMORY).

In this approach, it is indispensable to distinguish two states of cognitive representations: a state of *availability*, which means that there is information stored in long-term memory, and a state of *activation*, which occurs when stored information is actually being used ($\rightarrow$ ACTIVATION/INHIBITION). This is much like the distinction between representations as permanent cognitive entities and representations as temporary activations likely to be undergoing more or less durable manipulations. Psychological events occurring during such activations may give rise to a conscious cognitive experience the subject manifests by an explicit response (→ CONSCIOUS-NESS, METACOGNITION), but the temporary activation of a representation can also take place without any conscious experience on the subject's part. The latter situation provides the rationale for developing experimental procedures to indirectly detect the actual utilization of mental representations.

Finally, a crucial question here concerns the format in which mental representations are stored in long-term memory and temporarily activated by a processing mechanism. The hypothesis of a *language of thought* supports the idea that in the end, all information is coded in a highly abstract format (→ LANGUAGE OF THOUGHT). Other hypotheses emphasize the multimodal nature of cognitive representation. The human mind has the capacity to process information presented in extremely diverse forms and organized in a multitude of ways. Accordingly, it can construct and manipulate various types of representations, not only analogical ones like *mental images*, which preserve the structure of the objects represented (→ MENTAL IMAGERY), but also more abstract ones like *propositional representations*, which have a language-like structure (→ LANGUAGE, LOGIC, PROPOSITIONAL FORMAT). The capacity of human cognition to adapt to both the semantics of resemblance and a semantics based on arbitrary symbols (→ SEMANTICS, SYMBOL) offers the subject the capability of translating one representation format into another, each format being suited to the specific demands of the task at hand.

MICHEL DENIS

Neuroscience. — All perceptual activity involving recognition, identification, or naming requires the activation of representations stored in memory (→ ACTIVATION/INHIBITION, MEMORY, PERCEPTION). Stored representations also guide the execution of motor activities and mental-image generation (in any modality) (→ ACTION, MENTAL IMAGERY). The question of the format and nature of these representations is a fundamental but complex one that has been addressed in several disciplines, including cognitive neuroscience. It is hypothesized that representations contained in cortical neural networks are expressed in the form of patterns of weights assigned to connections between different units in the network (→ NEURAL NETWORK). These patterns (or *traces*) stored in memory are thought to approximately correspond to neural activity patterns triggered by stimuli during perception. Recognition is possible when the activity pattern created by a perceived stimulus is able to activate a stored pattern via a matching mechanism. A new representation or memory trace is formed whenever a new stimulus is perceived, and the repeated perception of this stimulus contributes to consolidating the corresponding activation pattern in memory. Such representations, whose format is thought to match the activity pattern generated by the stimulus being perceived, are called *perceptual representations*. They seem to be stored in the same regions as those where the perceptual encoding of the stimulus occurred, and for this reason, they are called *modality-specific*. The place where representations are stored is called a *perceptual representation subsystem* (Endel Tulving and Dan Schacter) or a *pattern activation subsystem* (Stephen Kosslyn and Olivier Koenig), depending on the author.

Perceptual representations are to be distinguished from other representations, called *semantic representations*, which are activated irrespective of the information-intake modality (→ INFORMATION, SEMANTICS). According to the above authors, semantic amodal representations are stored in an associative memory subsystem. Links between representations are a fundamental feature of this subsystem and account for the organization of the *semantic network* (→ SEMANTIC NETWORK). A topic of growing interest today is how representations are organized within such networks. The study of category-specific deficits in brain-damaged patients is likely to provide valuable information on this topic and to contribute to a finer understanding of the structure and organization of semantic representations (→ CATEGORIZATION, NEUROPSYCHOLOGY). Results obtained in functional neuroimaging studies strongly support a localized, dissociated view of mental representations rather than a distributed and thus nonlocalized one (→ FUNCTIONAL NEUROIMAGING, LOCALIZATION OF FUNCTION).

OLIVIER KOENIG

Artificial intelligence. — *This postcard represents the Chambord Chateau* is a readily verifiable statement for someone who knows that particular castle. The statement *This sketch represents the way to get there* can only be verified if the person to whom it is directed knows a few conventions, for in order to be useful, a sketch must be more than a simple photographic image. *This sequence in the machine represents the system's inference rules* is a statement whose verification necessitates a great deal of knowledge.

The three examples given above illustrate the idea that the relationship between a represented entity E and its representation R generally depends on elements that are not part of R or E. For a representation to be "accurate," in the sense that all properties of E are figured in R, R must be equal to E, which contradicts the very idea of representation. Indeed, representing E is useful only if E itself is unavailable or not suitable for the desired task. Thus, R must not possess all of E's characteristics; the ones that are legitimately omitted are contingent upon what need R is supposed to satisfy. Depending on the case, a finer- or coarser-grained representation that relies on analogical, symbolic, or hybrid techniques may be judged suitable (→ SYMBOL).

Computer science has at its disposal a wide range of techniques for representing entities of all kinds: images are coded as matrices of pixels and the information thus obtained can be reduced using data compression techniques (→ INFORMATION); sounds, like any other virtually periodic signal, can be sampled at appropriate intervals without loss of information, and each measure taken is coded by a number with a chosen level of precision; text is represented as coded sequences, some parts corresponding to the characters in the text and others capturing paging and formatting (→ TEXT). Several graphic representation techniques are also available.

But these often huge data sets are not true representations unless procedures exist for utilizing them. Here again, the range of available techniques is broad: text, sound, and image processors, extraction of terms in view of documentary searches, translation into logical format for inference making, and so on (→ LOGIC). This last technique, one of the most sophisticated services computer science can provide, requires highly specialized representations due to the intrinsic complexity of inference-making mechanisms (→ COMPLEXITY). Semantic networks, inspired by models in cognitive psychology, were widely studied in the 1970s (→ SEMANTIC NETWORK) but have been replaced today by logics of description.

Given that a representation is worthless without the processes that utilize it, one can contemplate coding the utilization of represented knowledge rather than the knowledge itself. This type of representation is called *procedural*. A heated debate in the early 1970s opposed it to *declarative representation*, but the latter came out ahead: one of the drawbacks of procedures is that they mix the general level (the inference-making process) with the specifics of the represented knowledge, causing low readability and major problems in developing and modifying the systems. What is more, a representation depends on the algorithmic notation chosen, itself linked to the state of the art in computer technology.

The expert systems of the 1980s claimed to have achieved a declarative expression of knowledge, that is, one totally independent of how knowledge is used. This claim was not fully true, however: it turns out that a representation that is only useful as input into one or more processes cannot be designed without taking those processes into account to a greater or lesser degree. Efforts to come up with representations that are as declarative as possible are beneficial nonetheless—from the theoretical standpoint, they can provide insight into the potentials of the representation language used (→ LANGUAGE); from the practical standpoint, they can help improve the effectiveness of generic inference methods.

The idea of a language of representation presupposes the existence of a sort of alphabet of representations and suggests that it is possible to represent knowledge as structured combinations of semantic primitives (→ SEMANTICS). A seemingly opposing approach consists in not assigning interpretations to primitive elements, qualified as *subsymbolic*. The representation function is ensured by techniques that make use of element connectivity (→ CONNECTIONISM). In this case, one speaks of a *distributed representation*. This idea is (rightly) compared to the hologram technique used in coherent optics: the parts of a hologram do not represent the parts of the image, but each one can be used (with a lesser degree of precision) to restore the whole image, and this guarantees greater robustness. Distributed representations have similar advantages but also have some drawbacks: they are not directly readable, they take up a considerable amount of space in memory (→ MEM-ORY), and the algorithms that use them necessitate powerful computing capabilities.

Insofar as no representation is perfect, the nature of the task is what de-termines whether it is preferable to choose a symbolic representation, a distributed representation, or a compromise located somewhere between these two extremes.

DANIEL KAYSER

Linguistics. — Representation is a core issue in a *mentalist* view of cognitive linguistics. Looking only at recent research trends, three types of considera-tions seem to have contributed in a critical way to the emergence of represen-tation as a concept in this discipline: the discovery that complex behavior sequences cannot be explained by chains of associations (Karl Lashley, Noam Chomsky), the idea that current stimulations or tasks underdetermine the range of possible behaviors, as in latent learning or pattern recognition in a noisy environment (→ LEARNING, PATTERN RECOGNITION), and finally, the need to devise algorithms designed to serve as formally explicit models for generating intelligent behaviors. These considerations have all concurred in defining representations as both the input and the output of computational transformations that produce the extra information needed to explain all pos-sible task-compatible behaviors (→ COMPUTATIONAL ANALYSIS, INFORMATION). One can argue accordingly that the ability to break down the nouns *writer* and *rider* and to associate them with the corresponding verbs provides sup-porting evidence of the existence of a phonological representation level that is different from the phonological surface form, and of rules for going from one level to the other. Ray Jackendoff illustrates this for American English with the *t/d* opposition, which is valid at the first level but neutralized at the surface level, and the short/long opposition, valid at the surface level only.

Insofar as perceptual representations are inferences that can be true or false, depending on the world they represent, one must explain how the content of a representation can be specified by its relationship to the world, not just by inferences that make up for the paucity of the initial informa-tion: it is agreed in this case that representations, even perceptual ones, are themselves sign-like in nature (→ PERCEPTION, SIGN). But then, reality would be the sum of all information that can be (nomologically) inferred from representations with external causes, that is, a *semiotic construction* (Jacques Bouveresse) (→ SEMIOTICS).

Some approaches set limits on the definition of representations as semiotic constructions, and define alternatives that challenge the notion of representation as a semiotic reference to an object. For one thing, the idea that semiotic relations constitute the sole way of assigning content to a representation can be questioned. The processes shared by the percept and the image would thus serve to specify the content of the latter as a function of the former (→ MENTAL IMAGERY). However, some authors do not agree that phenomenal forms of representations, such as mental images, can constrain both the processes applicable to them and the information they render accessible. According to these authors, representations activated during semantic tasks are organized into a propositional system (a language of thought) (→ LANGUAGE OF THOUGHT, PROPOSITIONAL FORMAT, SEMANTICS) and their conscious format is an epiphenomenon.

It is possible to conceive of the environment as a structured medium, and brain events as correlates of invariants present in the outside world. In this view, representations are not semiotic constructions, because they are neither organized into inferential processes nor interpreted.

Opposing the above points of view, certain theories clearly liken representations to signs. In this case, the entire content of a representation is included in the operations used to interpret it (→ INTERPRETATION). The approach to semantics called *procedural* thus consists in assigning to procedures, properties that can be defined by functions, particularly recursive ones (Philip Johnson-Laird) (→ FUNCTION). A procedure builds a unique model (in spatial format, for example) from the problem data and then tries to generalize the model by performing a series of successive verifications (→ REASONING AND RATIONALITY). Certain authors have attempted to extend this approach beyond reasoning tasks. Ronald Langacker tried to conceive of mental representations in terms of processes in his efforts to describe human cognition a priori and to identify the mental representations that exist when a linguistic meaning is being grasped. While still relying on schematic images to symbolize representations of sense (usually morphemes combined to make words), he stressed that such images are made up of infinitesimal processes, whereas image spatialization is the result of a summary scanning process (→ SENSE). These operations naturalize interpretative processes by anchoring them in the basic mechanisms of human perception (→ NATURALIZATION).

Most authors in cognitive linguistics conceive of the content of a representation as a structure that carries meaning—that is, a sign. Accordingly, models of language production or comprehension (→ LANGUAGE) often include a step involving message formulation, activation of semantic representations, or access to concepts ($\rightarrow$ CONCEPT). An alternative to this view is to consider, along with Ludwig Wittgenstein, that the experience of thought differs little from the experience of discourse ($\rightarrow$ DISCOURSE, EXPERIENCE), or rather, that it would simply be that experience, with a few additional concomitant processes.

JEAN-MICHEL FORTIS

Philosophy. — A representation can be defined as the function an object, event, or property has of standing for another object, event, or property ($\rightarrow$ FUNCTION). The function of representing can be granted by convention or be acquired naturally. In the first case, *intentionality*—that is, the capacity to convey representational content—is derived; in the second, it is intrinsic ($\rightarrow$ INTENTIONALITY). A sentence is a representation of the first type; a mental state is a representation of the second type ($\rightarrow$ LANGUAGE, MIND).

Charles Peirce was one of the first theorists to analyze the link between a representation and the entity it represents. He distinguished *icons*, which resemble what they represent (like a portrait), *indexes*, which are connected causally to their object (for example, smoke indicating fire) ($\rightarrow$ CAUSALITY AND MENTAL CAUSATION), and *symbols*, which are associated by convention to what they represent (like mathematical symbols) ($\rightarrow$ SYMBOL). In spite of the problems posed by the strict opposition between "resembling" representations and conventional representations, this opposition nevertheless evokes the important distinction between *analogical* and *digital* representations. Fred Dretske proposed an understanding of this distinction based on the characteristics of the information transmitted by the signal (by *information*, we mean the information conveyed by a particular signal, not a probabilistic conception of communication between a source and a receiver, as in Claude Shannon's theory) ($\rightarrow$ COMMUNICATION, INFORMATION). The coding of a property furnishes an analogical representation when it defines a mapping between two continuous properties; it furnishes a digital representation when it maps a discontinuous signal to a property that can be either discrete or continuous. Dretske extends this distinction to the representation of facts: every signal carries information that is both analogical and digital. The most precise information it transmits is the digital representation, and the categorization of the signal brought about by this type of coding necessarily implies a loss of information ($\rightarrow$ CATEGORIZATION).

The primary property of any representation is that it is supposed to convey information about a state of affairs. In this sense, it presupposes the existence of regular covariation relations among states of affairs or properties. However, representation does not necessarily imply informativeness: a false representation is a representation nonetheless. This possibility of misrepresenting prohibits conceiving of the relationship between a representation and what it represents as a causal covariation. On the other hand, a representation can be evaluated semantically (→ SEMANTICS), which means that the content of a particular *token* of a representation (for example, the content of the sentence *It is raining*, uttered in a given place at a given time) may fail to apply to the situation represented by that token, which determines its truth value: the token of the representation is false. This normative aspect of representations is the focus of teleological analyses of representation (→ NORMATIVITY). It is because a representation has a function by virtue of its *type* (that function being to represent an object as having such and such a property) that it can occasionally malfunction in certain tokens of application without losing the function it typically has.

JOËLLE PROUST

SELECTED BIBLIOGRAPHY

Abbott, L., & Sejnowski, T. (Eds.). (1999). *Neural codes and distributed representations: Foundations of neural computation*. Cambridge, MA: MIT Press.

Antoniou, N. (1998). *Learning and reasoning with complex representations*. Berlin, Germany: Springer-Verlag.

Bechtel, W., & Abrahamsen, A. (2002). *Connectionism and the mind: Parallel processing dynamics and evolution* (2nd ed.). Oxford, England: Blackwell.

Bouveresse, J. (1995). *Langage, perception et réalité* [Language, perception, and reality]. Nîmes, France: Chambon.

Chalmers, D. (2002). *Philosophy of mind: Classical and contemporary readings*. New York: Oxford University Press.

Dretske, F. (1981). *Knowledge and the flow of information*. Cambridge, MA: MIT Press.

Dretske, F. (1988). *Explaining behavior: Reasons in a world of causes*. Cambridge, MA: MIT Press.

Dretske, F. (2000). *Perception, knowledge and belief: Selected essays*. Cambridge, England; New York: Cambridge University Press.

Johnson-Laird, P. (1995). Mental models, deductive reasoning, and the brain. In M. Gazzaniga (Ed.), *The cognitive neurosciences* (pp. 999–1008). Cambridge, MA: MIT Press.

Kosslyn, S. (1994). *Image and brain: The resolution of the image debate*. Cambridge, MA: MIT Press.

Kosslyn, S., & Koenig, O. (1992/1995). *Wet mind: The new cognitive neuroscience*. New York: Free Press.

Kosslyn, S., & Rosenberg, R. (2001). *Psychology: The brain, the person, the world*. Boston: Allyn & Bacon.

Langacker, R. (1987–1991). *Foundations of cognitive grammar* (Vols. 1–2). Stanford, CA: Stanford University Press.

Luger, G. (2002). *Artificial intelligence: Structures and strategies for complex problem-solving* (4th ed.). Harlow, England; New York: Pearson Education.

Millikan, R. (1984). *Language, thought, and other biological categories*. Cambridge, MA: MIT Press.

Peirce, C. (1991). *Peirce on signs: Writings on semiotics*. Chapel Hill, NC: University of North Carolina Press.

Putnam, H. (1988). *Representation and reality*. Cambridge, MA: MIT Press.

Pylyshyn, Z. (1984). *Computation and cognition: Toward a foundation for cognitive science*. Cambridge, MA: MIT Press.

Thagard, P. (1996). *Mind: Introduction to cognitive science*. Cambridge, MA: MIT Press.

Tulving, E., & Schacter, D. L. (1990). Priming and human memory systems. *Science, 247*, 301–306.

ROBOTICS

Artificial intelligence. — The term *robotics* is usually used to refer to *manufacturing robotics*, where the goal is to automate tasks in a way that is flexible, robust, and not too costly in terms of programming (⟩ AUTO-MATISM). Manufacturing robotics draws from work done in environmental engineering and in task-specific instrumentation of articulated mechanical systems (for example, robot arms that execute repetitive tasks on assembly lines with preprogrammed arm positioning, or wire-guided elevating platforms that operate via the detection of special landmarks; → MEMORY). Robotics is also concerned with remote-controlled systems, where sensors on machines supply a distant operator with the information needed to control task execution (→ INFORMATION). Manual control of actuators is possible only if the time it takes to transmit and interpret information is very short relative to the task dynamic (→ CONTROL, INTERPRETATION).

Another form of robotics, *autonomous robotics*, has more in common with the cognitive sciences. The idea is to design intelligent machines equipped with the ability to perceive, act, and reason in view of performing a wide variety of tasks in a variable environment (→ ACTION, PERCEPTION, REASONING AND RATIONALITY). The scientific challenge is to be able to define the concept of "rational behavior" in a physical machine. Rationality is assessed here with respect to both the machine's performance on the set of tasks it can autonomously undertake and the variability of the environment in which it can accomplish those tasks in a robust way. This kind of rationality is necessarily limited (in the sense defined by Herbert Simon), not only by the complexity of time-constrained processing, but also by the inherent uncertainty of all sensory information and the incompleteness of the models and programs that describe it.

The most ambitious projects in this branch of robotics integrate movement and manipulation. These include elevating platforms equipped with manipulating arms and instrumented with various sensors (cameras, range sonars, laser range finders, radar, odometers, inertial or satellite positioning, etc.) and communication devices (→ COMMUNICATION). *Intervention robotics* is distinguished from *service robotics*. In intervention robotics (used, for example, in the exploration of hostile sites: planets, the ocean floor, the Antarctic), the environment is unstructured, poorly understood, and coarsely modeled. The emphasis is on issues such as moving, navigating, and perceiving, as well as on the autonomous modeling of the environment and communication. The tasks undertaken include drawing coherent maps and implementing task-specific instruments. In service robotics (handling, maintenance, and monitoring), the environment is well structured (workshops, hospitals, ports) and abundant knowledge is available. The variability, richness, and dynamics of the situation, along with the diversity of the tasks performed, are essential facets of this field. Some of the interesting problems are human-machine interaction and multirobot cooperation.

Active multisensory perception is an essential function in autonomous robotics. It poses the problem of how to merge information from various sensors, whether at the signal level or at the level of primitives and interpretation hypotheses. It is called active because it is not confined to finding the best interpretation of available data, but attempts instead to make use of perceptual cues to set forth relevant hypotheses and then select the appropriate sensors, the most advantageous viewpoints, and the best acquisition and processing modes to validate or refute the hypotheses. In attempts to model natural environments, some of the problems encountered are the choice of meaningful perceptual landmarks and the overall coherence of maps acquired locally and represented at various levels of granularity. In scene interpretation, the problems concern recognizing objects, but also maintaining a coherent interpretation of an evolving environment (→ PATTERN RECOGNITION).

The control of manipulators and mobile robots is based on control theory. Because of the integration of *exteroceptive sensory feedback* (as in a camera, as opposed to an odometer, which is a *proprioceptive* sensor that provides feedback on a machine's internal state), this field has been extended to reactive perception processes such as tracking a moving object. Motion planning in Euclidean space or in a space of configurations, performed in a cluttered environment by a kinematically constrained robot (called a *nonholonomic robot*), requires solving complex algorithmic geometry problems (→ SPACE). Uncertainty regarding the location of the robot and difficulty planning its trajectory in accordance with its sensory capabilities add to the problem. The planning and control of task execution, deliberate action, and reacting to the unexpected cannot be achieved using the classical plan-synthesis paradigm (instantaneous action based on state changes, static environments, and reliable and complete information). Uncertain and incomplete information requires perceptual action, which, by nature, is nondeterministic. The combinatorial impossibility of synthesizing conditional plans has led to approaches based on decision theory. Time is an essential factor and must be explicitly represented (→ TIME AND TENSE). Predicted or observed events contingent upon the robot's actions must also be taken into account. Some of the difficult learning problems include developing models of the environment and of the means available to the robot, and translating them into effective procedures, strategies, and heuristics for solving or reacting to the problems encountered (→ KNOWLEDGE ACQUISITION, LEARNING, PROBLEM SOLVING). The possibility of having robots that can plan and experiment has opened up an important line of research. Finally, human-robot interaction poses almost exactly the same problems as human-machine communication, in addition to the more particular problems of cooperatively defining and executing tasks in a coautonomous setting ($\rightarrow$ DISTRIBUTED INTELLIGENCE).

MALIK GHALLAB

SELECTED BIBLIOGRAPHY

Arkin, R. (1998). *Behavior-based robotics*. Cambridge, MA: MIT Press.

Ford, K., & Pylyshyn, Z. (1996). *The robot's dilemma revisited: The frame problem in artificial intelligence*. Norwood, NJ: Ablex.

Kitamura, T. (Ed.). (2001). *What should be computed to understand and model brain function? From robotics, soft computing, biology and neuroscience to cognitive philosophy*. Singapore; River Edge, NJ: World Scientific.

Kortenkamp, D., Bonasso, R., & Murphy, R. (Eds.). (1998). *Artificial intelligence and mobile robots: Case studies of successful robot systems*. Menlo Park, CA: AAAI Press; Cambridge, MA: MIT Press.

Murphy, R. (2000). *An introduction to AI robotics*. Cambridge, MA: MIT Press.

Wise, E. (1999). *Applied robotics*. New York: Delmar Learning.

Wise, E. (2002). *Applied robotics II*. New York: Delmar Learning.

S

SCHIZOPHRENIA

Psychology. — The term *dementia praecox* (early dementia), proposed by Emil Kraepelin to stress the overall state of deficiency to which this morbid process leads, was replaced with the term *schizophrenia* by Eugen Bleuler, who wanted to bring out the splitting (*Spaltung*) nature of the disorder, which affects not only the behavior but also the judgments and feelings of schizophrenics. For a long time, however, Bleuler's explanation ranked only as a mere pathogenic theory. It was not until the principles and methods of psychology and neurocognitive psychology were applied that Bleuler's view proved valid (→ COGNITIVE PSYCHIATRY, FUNCTIONAL NEURO-IMAGING, NEUROPSYCHOLOGY).

For more than thirty years now, the cognitive alterations of schizophrenia have been studied using experimental setups where schizophrenics are compared to controls or to patients with other illnesses. Three aims are pursued: to develop models of the cognitive dysfunctions specific to the disorder, to explain all or part of their symptomatology, and to relate these data to findings from studies on the brain.

The first step was to refute the hypothesis of a motivational disorder or general deficit. This was achieved primarily through the use of experimental devices that provided evidence of better performance in schizophrenics than in controls. The second step involved searching for cognitive alterations resulting from impairment of basic cognitive functions (→ COMPUTATIONAL ANALYSIS, FUNCTION). This research revealed attention deficits (hyperreactivity to stimuli, difficulty selecting relevant information) (→ ACTIVATION/ INHIBITION, ATTENTION), language disorders (lexical, syntactic, semantic, and pragmatic) ($\rightarrow$ LANGUAGE, LEXICON, PRAGMATICS, SEMANTICS, SYNTAX), and memory deficits (encoding, use of strategies) ($\rightarrow$ MEMORY).

Facing the diversity of these dysfunctions, investigators began to look for central dysregulations caused by an overall abnormality affecting systems such as the executive attention system (Michael Posner), contextual information processing, integration of past information (David Hemsley and Jeffrey Gray), and control and representation of action (Christopher Frith) ($\rightarrow$ ACTION, CONTEXT AND SITUATION, CONTROL, INFORMATION). Although the various executive models are largely cross-validating, a key question is whether schizophrenia can be regarded as a chain of abnormalities, each one triggering the next.

This integrative view needs to be articulated with neurobiological disorders affecting the prefrontal and diencephalic-nucleus loop. However, this type of study does not offer a currently convincing explanation of the illness, for it fails to address the question of environmental and affective factors. Furthermore, researchers have been unable to observe any consistent abnormalities within clinically identical populations, which also leaves unanswered the question of the specificity of the dysfunctions or of the illness itself.

DANIEL WIDLÖCHER

SELECTED BIBLIOGRAPHY

Bleuler, E. (1950). *Dementia praecox or the group of schizophrenias* (J. Zinkin, Trans.). New York: International Universities Press. (Original work published 1911.)

David, A., & Cutting, J. (Eds.). (1994). *The neuropsychology of schizophrenia*. Hove, England; New York: Psychology Press.

Frith, C. (1992). *The cognitive neuropsychology of schizophrenia*. Hove, England; Hillsdale, NJ: Erlbaum.

Green, M. (1998). *Schizophrenia from a neurocognitive perspective: Probing the impenetrable darkness*. Boston: Allyn & Bacon.

Halligan, P., & David, A. (2001). Cognitive neuropsychiatry: Towards a scientific psychopathology. *Nature Reviews Neuroscience, 2*, 209–215.

Harvey, P., & Sharma, T. (2002). *Understanding and treating cognition in schizophrenia: A clinician's handbook*. London: Martin Dunitz.

Posner, M., & Raichle, M. (1994/1997). *Images of mind*. New York: Freeman.

Sharma, T. (2003). *Brain imaging in schizophrenia: Insights and applications*. London: Remedica.

Sharma, T., & Harvey, P. (Eds.). (2000). *Cognition in schizophrenia: Impairments, importance, and treatment strategies*. New York: Oxford University Press.

SEMANTIC NETWORK

Linguistics. — A *semantic network* is a knowledge representation structure in the form of a graph with *nodes* ($\rightarrow$ REPRESENTATION). The nodes correspond to objects, concepts, or events ($\rightarrow$ CONCEPT, OBJECT). They are connected to each other by *arcs*, which specify the relationships between them. This type of graph is finite, oriented, labeled, usually connected, and cyclical.

The expression *semantic network* first appeared in 1966 in the thesis of the psychologist Ross Quillian. Quillian's idea was to use a formal model to represent the objective part of the meaning of words (→ MEANING AND SIGNIFICATION, SENSE). His plan was part of a project at the Massachusetts Institute of Technology to develop a computerized sentence-understanding system (→ LANGUAGE). The model was to provide the framework for developing a tool that could compare the senses of words and reason comparatively about their meanings (→ REASONING AND RATIONALITY). The adjective *semantic* in the computer-science context is somewhat misused relative to the linguistic meaning of the term, but although some linguists prefer to call these networks *associative* (→ SEMANTICS), the name *semantic network* seems to have become firmly entrenched in the literature.

The starting point and key element of the model is the *concept*. Each concept is described by a more general concept and a *discriminant property* (→ CATEGORIZATION). The discriminant property is composed of two nested elements: an *attribute* and a *value* attached to that attribute. For instance, the concept *salmon* is described as a fish (generic category) whose discriminant attribute is the color of its flesh (with pink as its value): *salmon = fish + color of flesh (= pink)*. The primary aim is to account for how subjects categorize concepts.

Quillian's ideas spread, and variations of semantic networks have proliferated, especially in artificial intelligence (see *artificial intelligence* below) as scientists attempt to represent knowledge. The aim is to put concepts into a larger structure in such a way that the meaning of a given concept emerges from the place it occupies in the network and the types of *relations* it has with neighboring concepts. Semantic networks thus combine the dual function of representing hierarchical *classes* and describing *properties* with attributes. Classes (superclasses, subclasses) denote relations of generalization and specialization, and each class groups together objects that share properties. The properties are attached to the classes and transmitted by *inheritance rules*, with a node inheriting the properties of the nodes located above it in the hierarchy (→ INHERITANCE). This type of inheritance is characteristic of the principle of economy that governs semantic networks, because it automatically assigns to an object the properties of more general objects located above it, no matter when the object is input into the network. Except for the relation *IS-A* common to all networks, the relations represented in a network vary across models and applications: *part-of*, *function* (*used-for*), and *consequence-of* are a few examples. Defining these relations is not a straightforward task, however. For instance, the relation *part-of* is not the same when we say that handlebars are part of a bicycle, carbon is part of carbon tetrachloride, blue is part of the American flag, and a juror is a part of a jury.

Semantic networks are supposed to be universal in that they represent conceptual units, but this poses the problem of the relationship between concepts and the particular lexical units of a given language (→ LEXICON). If there were a direct and univocal relationship between concepts and lexical units, then semantic networks would be strictly symmetrical across languages. This is far from true. For example, the French generic category *volaille* corresponds to the English *poultry*, but the generic category *chicken* has no perfect equivalent in French, because *poulet* excludes *coq*, *poule*, and *coquelet* (*cockerel, hen*, and *capon*) whereas *chicken* does not.

The user-friendliness of this knowledge-representation model most certainly accounts for its success and its extension to the representation of sentences, which led to the distinction between *conceptual semantic networks* and *propositional semantic networks* (→ PROPOSITIONAL FORMAT). The former networks, described above, represent permanent, long-lasting conceptual knowledge; the latter are used to represent instantiations of those concepts in a sentence by associating concepts (in the model) with the events that involve them. Among the various propositional semantic networks are John Sowa's *conceptual graphs*. A conceptual graph is a graphic representation of a proposition.

GABRIEL OTMAN

Artificial intelligence. — The idea of a semantic network goes back to Quillian's work from 1966 (see *linguistics* above). Although the expansion of semantic networks in the years that followed was somewhat haphazard, a famous article by William Woods in 1975 made it mandatory for network designers to accurately define the meaning of their representations. Some of the more substantial work that ensued includes studies on the KL-ONE language, developed by Ronald Brachman's team, and studies on the properties of Sowa's conceptual graphs, conducted by a highly active research community.

A semantic network is an oriented, labeled graph (or, more precisely, a multigraph, since two nodes in a graph can be connected by several *edges*). Each label, node, or edge has a meaning of its own that is independent of the rest of the network (which justifies the use of the word *semantic*). Of course, the latter criterion is very informal.

This criterion can be made stricter, however, by requiring that the symbols be mapped via a reference relation to an interpretation universe, as in a standard semantic logic (→ INTERPRETATION, LOGIC, SEMANTICS, SENSE/REFERENCE, SYMBOL). Many studies on networks start from this assumption, but in doing so, they relegate networks to the rank (no doubt interesting) of notational variations of logic. In fact, there does not have to be a reference relation, but if not, the nonformality of the meaning criterion must be regarded as an inevitable shortcoming.

Even if it cannot render the wealth of a semantic network, it is interesting to associate a network to its canonical translation in *first-order logic*. To do so, one selects a language in which the node labels correspond to unary predicates, and the edge labels, to binary predicates. A network is translated by the conjunction of the formulas associated with each of its edges, where the logic formula associated with label relation R between node A and node B is $(\forall x) (A(x) \supset (\exists y) (B(y) \land R(x, y)))$. If we suppose that relation R is the copula *be*, then the corresponding predicate is equality; the formula becomes logically equivalent to $(\forall x) (A(x) \supset B(x))$, which expresses the inclusion of A's extension in B's extension and makes A's individuals inherit B's properties ($\rightarrow$ CATEGORIZATION, INHERITANCE). The reverse process is to translate an arbitrary logic formula into a semantic network, but this is usually impossible. In particular, disjunctions, negations, and nested quantifiers are problematic. But it is precisely when only a subset of logic is used that one can devise networks with better algorithmic properties than ordinary inference systems. Processes like partitioning (Gary Hendrix), for example, can be used to translate modality ($\rightarrow$ MODALITY).

One can set aside logic altogether and design specific algorithms for networks by drawing more or less freely from the neurophysiological mechanisms of spreading activation among neurons ($\rightarrow$ ACTIVATION/INHIBITION, CONNECTIONISM, NEURAL NETWORK). This approach was initiated by Scott Fahlman (in 1977) and was taken up and extended recently by Lokendra Shastri and Venkat Ajjanagadde, for example. One can also take the opposite approach and extend the logic in such a way that its deductive system corresponds to inferences made by networks. The similarity between Fahlman's inhibition mechanisms and inference blocking in nonmonotonic logics is a good illustration of this approach. To a certain extent, object-oriented programming can be regarded as a generalization of the inheritance mechanism, whose importance has become apparent through work on semantic networks ($\rightarrow$ OBJECT).

More recently, description logics have supplied a satisfactory formal framework for inferences supported by a number of semantic networks, and this has made it possible to prove decidability results (for example, Bernhard Nebel) and complexity results (Francesco Donini and colleagues), which are critical in representing knowledge ($\rightarrow$ COMPLEXITY, REPRESENTATION).

DANIEL KAYSER

SELECTED BIBLIOGRAPHY

Donini, M., et al. (1991). Tractable concept languages. *IJCAI-89: Detroit, Michigan, USA: Proceedings of the Twelfth International Joint Conference on Artificial Intelligence, August 20–25, 1989* (pp. 458–463). San Mateo, CA: Morgan Kaufmann.

Fahlman, S. (1979). *A system for representing and using real-world knowledge*. Cambridge, MA: MIT Press.

Fensel, D., Wahlster, W., Lieberman, H., & Hendler, J. (Eds.). (2003). *Spinning the semantic web: Bringing the World Wide Web to its full potential*. Cambridge, MA: MIT Press.

Gazzaniga, M. (Ed.). (2000). *The new cognitive neurosciences* (Section VI, *Memory*) (2nd ed.). Cambridge, MA: MIT Press.

Kintsch, W. (1998). *Comprehension: A paradigm for cognition*. Cambridge, England; New York: Cambridge University Press.

Kosslyn, S., & Koenig, O. (1992/1995). *Wet mind: The new cognitive neuroscience*. New York: Free Press.

Kosslyn, S., & Rosenberg, R. (2001). *Psychology: The brain, the person, the world*. Boston: Allyn & Bacon.

Lehmann, F. (Ed.). (1992). *Semantic networks in artificial intelligence*. Oxford, England: Pergamon Press.

Shastri, L., & Ajjanadadde, V. (1993). From simple associations to systematic reasoning: A connectionist representation of rules, variables and dynamic bindings using temporal synchrony. *Behavioral and Brain Sciences, 16*, 417–494.

Sowa, J. (ed.). (1991). *Principles of semantic networks: Explorations in the representation of knowledge*. San Diego, CA: Morgan Kaufmann.

SEMANTICS

Linguistics. — Four approaches in cognitive research bear the name *semantics: logical semantics, linguistic semantics, psychological semantics*, and *cognitive semantics*.

1. Logical semantics has a long-standing tradition. It strives to judge the truth of expressions and the conditions under which language can state the truth; hence its other name, *truth-conditional semantics* (→ LANGUAGE, LOGIC, TRUTH). This branch of semantics underwent considerable modification with the formalization of logic, so it is therefore also rightly called *formal semantics*.

In this approach, meaning is defined as a relationship between a symbol and the object it denotes, in the world of what is, in a possible world, or in a counterfactual world (→ COUNTERFACTUAL, MEANING AND SIGNIFICATION, SYMBOL). It contributes to maintaining the division between syntax, semantics, and pragmatics proposed by Charles Morris and Rudolf Carnap (→ PRAGMATICS, SYNTAX). To describe natural languages, it applies principles, such as compositionality, that are used in the semantics of logic languages. Logical semantics has not produced an elaborate lexical semantics (→ LEXICON), but it offers a detailed understanding at the sentence level of many problems like quantification, indexicality, and scope. In *text semantics* (→ TEXT), the principal theoretical framework is still Hans Kamp's highly programmatic theory. His *discourse-representation structures* (DRS) are logical notations that permit clear statements of problems like indeterminate reference and anaphora (→ SENSE/REFERENCE).

Logical semantics benefited from the thrust of logical positivism. Its philosophical utility is great, for truth is one of the major themes of Western philosophy. However, its descriptive capabilities remain rather limited next to the complexity of the formalizations it employs. Despite its antipsychologism on principle (→ LOGICISM/PSYCHOLOGISM), formal semantics underwent a shift toward a more *mentalist* perspective between the mid-1970s and mid-1980s, principally by way of the computational theory of mind (→ COGNITIVISM, MIND). According to Jerry Fodor (in 1975), for example, cognitive processes culminate in the formal manipulation of symbols in a *language of thought* (→ LANGUAGE OF THOUGHT). Moreover, the famous book by Philip Johnson-Laird, *Mental Models* (1983), tried to reconcile psychology and some elementary features of mental-model theory (→ REASONING AND RATIONALITY).

2. Linguistic semantics originated in European linguistics and has been developing gradually since the turn of the twentieth century. It defines meaning as a linguistic relationship between signs, or more precisely, between signified concepts (→ SIGN). Signified concepts in turn have their psychological or even physical correlates, but the correlates do not define the concepts as such. The principal contemporary authors (for example, Bernard Pottier, Algirdas-Julien Greimas, Igor Mel'chuk, and Eugenio Coseriu) remain divided on crucial issues like the autonomy of semantics and the conceptual status of minimal units. Cognitive theories of conceptual primitives (for example, Roger Schank's theory) are rooted in this trend.

3. Psychological semantics, where meaning is defined as the relationship between signs and representations or mental operations (→ REPRESENTATION), dates back to the late nineteenth century. Today, we owe to this approach various theories of semantic networks (Ross Quillian) (→ SEMANTIC NETWORK), text understanding (Walter Kintsch), and models that require text comprehension. The most influential theory in linguistics, especially cognitive linguistics, is Eleanor Rosch's *typicality theory* (→ CATEGORIZATION). Some authors (such as Ray Jackendoff) have come to the conclusion that studying natural language semantics amounts to studying cognitive psychology.

4. A final approach is cognitive semantics, which may seem like an extension of psychological semantics. But cognitive semantics is not an experimental discipline. Its principal protagonists are linguists: George Lakoff and Ronald Langacker. Its point of view is basically mentalistic insofar as it relates all linguistic phenomena to mental operations. In France, Gustave Guillaume's *psychomechanics* is a good example of a cognitive linguistic approach proposed even before the term was coined.

Naturally, cognitive semantics runs into philosophical issues. It is currently leaning toward describing experience and consciousness (Jackendoff) (→ CONSCIOUSNESS, EXPERIENCE), which brings it closer to phenomenology and transcendental philosophy. For Mark Johnson, universal semantic structures condition our experience and the formation of selfhood (→ IDENTITY). He therefore concludes along with Jackendoff that the semantic structure *is* the conceptual structure (→ CONCEPT), or as Langacker put it, that meaning is identified with conceptualization (→ MEANING AND SIGNIFICATION). If one challenges logical theories of the concept—as every approach to cognitive semantics has done to a greater or lesser extent—then one must devise a theory of ideas that fits into a linguistic framework. This is the pathway proposed in particular by Langacker, in his statement that linguistic semantics must undertake the structural analysis and explicit description of abstract entities like thoughts and concepts. But if the nonautonomy of language in general, and sense in particular, is declared, does linguistics become a science of the mind? Langacker says he shares with Lakoff the vision of a nonobjectivistic linguistics that reflects the full wealth of our mental life.

Mentalistic theories of linguistic meaning, particularly those that claim allegiance to psychology, have been the target of a number of objections. One problem is their universalism. The core of cognitive semantics in this case draws from the philosophical tradition. The search for conceptual primitives, universals, and cognitive archetypes, for instance, is obviously part of this tradition. A second difficulty has to do with our poor understanding of mental states and processes, which limits their explanatory value. Finally, problems arise when one attempts to relate the mental to the linguistic. Two approaches have been taken. The "representationalistic" approach relates linguistic units to elements of thought, and properties of linguistic units are explained in terms of the properties of the elements of thought they represent. This poses the classic problems of word-concept correspondence and effability (relationship between the "number of thoughts" and the number of words or sentences). Another approach is to relate language and thought without necessarily relying on the notion of representation. It entails mapping linguistic data to thought operations, which one might call the "operationalistic" route. This approach has given rise to two distinct research trends. The first is procedural semantics; the second, cognitive semantics per se (Lakoff, Leonard Talmy), came later, and has overtly kept its distance from what is known as the *symbolic paradigm*, which is logical in inspiration. Cognitive semantics relates meaning to operations in mental spaces.

Note that the representationalistic and operationalistic views are not dualist in the same manner and do not use the same methodology to relate the two levels they distinguish. The former starts from a preconception of the mental level, generally logical, and then relates its units to linguistic units. Inversely, the latter starts from linguistic descriptions and uses them to delineate mental space, with language acting as "an open window onto cognition" (Jackendoff, Claude Vandeloise).

The different approaches to semantics are unequally developed and unequally recognized across the various disciplines. In computer science and artificial intelligence, formal semantics is naturally the best known and the most widely used. In cognitive research in general, psychological semantics is the prevailing reference. Linguistic semantics remains poorly recognized in these fields, other than in partial approaches or by a few authors here and there.

FRANÇOIS RASTIER

Neuroscience. — Sometimes, an effective way to stimulate research in a given field is to provocatively point out a certain state of the art, at the risk of being challenged. A case in point is the new thrust given to neuropsychology by Fodor's remark that neuropsychology—whose observations of double dissociations have allowed it to excel in demonstrating the modular organization of mental processes—was incapable of providing evidence of *modules* in the organization of central processes (→ MODULARITY, NEUROPSYCHOLOGY). Since the 1980s, a large number of patients have been described as having highly specific impairments in different realms of everyday knowledge. From such cases, the idea emerged that even a system as central as semantics, which encompasses all of an individual's knowledge, is organized into functional modules. Granted, these modules are less encapsulated than peripheral ones, but their existence makes it quite clear that the distributed hypothesis is not fully applicable to biological reality.

Accordingly, there are patients who suffer from partial losses of knowledge. And the number of cases of category-specific disorders increases each year: some patients have trouble naming living things, others fail on objects they can handle, and so on (→ CATEGORIZATION, DOMAIN SPECIFICITY). Another troublesome fact is that there are patients without a general language impairment (→ LANGUAGE) who cannot name an object they can see, yet they can express knowledge about it (*optical aphasia*). Even more interesting is that scientists have come up with entirely plausible theoretical explanations for every one of these neuropsychological cases, and new models have emerged as a result. Finally, in the vast majority of cases, lesions that give rise to specific semantic disorders are located in the left hemisphere, which is consistent with both brain activity research and studies on normal subjects where tachistoscopic visual-hemifield presentation is used.

ÉRIC SIÉROFF

SELECTED BIBLIOGRAPHY

Allwood, J., & Gärdenfors, P. (Eds.). (1999). *Cognitive semantics: Meaning and cognition*. Philadelphia: J. Benjamins.

Cruse, D. A. (2000). *Meaning in language: An introduction to semantics and pragmatics*. Oxford, England; New York: Oxford University Press.

Fensel, D., Wahlster, W., Lieberman, H., & Hendler, J. (Eds.). (2003). *Spinning the semantic web: Bringing the World Wide Web to its full potential*. Cambridge, MA: MIT Press.

Fodor, J. (1975). *The language of thought*. New York: Crowell.

Fodor, J. (1987). *Psychosemantics: The problem of meaning in the philosophy of mind*. Cambridge, MA: MIT Press.

Forde, E., & Humphreys, G. (Eds.). (2002). *Category specificity in brain and mind*. New York: Taylor and Francis.

Jackendoff, R. (1983). *Semantics and cognition*. Cambridge, MA: MIT Press.

Jackendoff, R. (2002). *Foundations of language: Brain, meaning, grammar, evolution*. Oxford, England; New York: Oxford University Press.

Jacob, P. (1997). *What minds can do: Intentionality in a non-intentional world*. New York: Cambridge University Press.

Johnson-Laird, P. (1983). *Mental models*. Cambridge, MA: Harvard University Press.

Johnson-Laird, P. (1995). Mental models, deductive reasoning, and the brain. In M. Gazzaniga (Ed.), *The cognitive neurosciences* (pp. 999–1008). Cambridge, MA: MIT Press.

Kintsch, W. (1998). *Comprehension: A paradigm for cognition*. Cambridge, England; New York: Cambridge University Press.

Lakoff, G. (1987). *Women, fire, and dangerous things: What categories reveal about the mind*. Chicago: University of Chicago Press.

Langacker, R. (1986). Introduction to cognitive grammar. *Cognitive Science, 10*, 1–40.

Langacker, R. (1987–1991). *Foundations of cognitive grammar* (Vols. 1–2). Palo Alto, CA: Stanford University Press.

Lehmann, F. (Ed.). (1992). *Semantic networks in artificial intelligence*. Oxford, England: Pergamon Press.

Lyons, J. (1995). *Linguistic semantics: An introduction*. Cambridge, England; New York: Cambridge University Press.

Martin, A., Ungerleider, L., & Haxby, J. (2000). Category specificity and the brain: The sensory/motor model of semantic representations of objects. In M. Gazzaniga (Ed.), *The new cognitive neurosciences* (2nd. ed., pp. 1023–1046). Cambridge, MA: MIT Press.

Rastier, F., Cavazza, M., & Abeillé, A. (2002). *Semantics for descriptions*. Stanford, CA: CSLI Publications.

SEMIOTICS

Linguistics. — References to semiotics in the cognition research are frequent, but they are generally oblique. We know that Charles Morris and Rudolf Carnap divided semiotics into syntax, semantics, and pragmatics (→ PRAGMATICS, SEMANTICS, SYNTAX). Noam Chomsky and many other linguists took up this tripartite division, although their debates rarely refer to the semiotics that overarches the three parts. Yet, semiotics is the very foundation of what is known as the *symbolic paradigm* in cognitive research (→ COGNITIVISM, SYMBOL). Moreover, with the recent upsurge of topics like multimodality and multimedia, semiotics has begun to attract more and more interest.

The science of signs was first called *semiotics* by John Locke. This name was reused by Charles Peirce, and then by Morris and Carnap. In the

French-speaking world, the linguist Ferdinand de Saussure called the discipline *sémiologie* (semiology), and later Louis Hjelmslev coined the word *sémiotique* (semiotic) to refer to sign systems. This terminology lasted until the 1960s (Roland Barthes, *Elements of Semiology* in 1964). With the foundation of the International Association of Semiotics in 1969, the term used in the English-speaking community was adopted worldwide and has now become the rule in the academic disciplines (except those relating to communication).

These terminological differences are also indicative of underlying epistemological differences. The most important one concerns the founding discipline of the science of signs: in the Peircian tradition, the foundation is philosophical logic ($\rightarrow$ LOGIC); in the Saussurian tradition, it is linguistics. The former looks in particular at formal languages (for example, Richard Montague's *Formal Philosophy*, which pursues Carnap's project in its own way) and strives to incorporate the fundamental categories of the study of natural languages into formal language theories. In this view, semiotics is concerned with classifying signs and formally defining relations among them ($\rightarrow$ SIGN). The latter tradition, on the contrary, takes language as the starting point ($\rightarrow$ LANGUAGE): Hjelmslev's *Prolegomena to a Theory of Language* (in 1943) presents a general semiotics designed to permit the description of any system of signs. This kind of semiotics retains on principle a Saussurian nonrealism, so that the problem of reference is no longer posed in its traditional terms, and a form of holism wherein systems exist before their elements and relations exist before their terms ($\rightarrow$ HOLISM, SENSE/REFERENCE).

At the present time there are four unequally represented approaches in semiotics, each one granting a different scope to its object of study. (1) The first approach confines its field of investigation to systems of nonlinguistic signs such as road signs, coats of arms, and uniforms. Its principal representatives are functionalist linguists like Georges Mounin and Louis Prieto. (2) The second approach defines language as the set of principles shared by natural languages and nonlinguistic sign systems (Hjelmslev, Algirdas-Julien Greimas). It tries to find semiotic relations and fundamental structures (like the semiotic square, which Greimas posits as the a priori form of all meaning; $\rightarrow$ MEANING AND SIGNIFICATION). (3) The third approach extends the concept of semiotics beyond systems of intentional signs, and it can be defined accordingly as the study of how the world and its signs become meaningful. In the tradition based on the Augustinian theory of natural signs, semiotics enables the study of indicators and cues: a cloud signifies rain in a different way than the word *rain* does. According to Umberto Eco, though, semiotics can uncover the unity of these different ways of signifying, provided the sign is defined very generally as something that takes the place of something else. This view of semiotics often leads to a kind of phenomenology (like Peirce's "phaneroscopy"). (4) Finally, some authors extend semiotics beyond the human world by granting a justifiable place to animal semiotics (or *zoosemiotics*). Bringing together the social sciences and the sciences of nature and life, these authors make use of notions like genetic code to promote a sort of pansemiotism, a renewed form of the philosophy of nature.

Each of these four approaches corresponds to an epistemological type. The first makes semiotics a descriptive discipline based on the comparative method, and as such, it remains among the social sciences. The second, more ambitious, assigns semiotics the task of serving as a norm to all human sciences (Hjelmslev). The third amounts to a philosophy of meaning. The fourth tends to eliminate the distinction between the sciences, and between science and philosophy.

These divergent ways of conceiving of general semiotics have not prevented specific semiotics from proliferating—on the contrary. *Discourse semiotics*, which in the 1970s set out to make up for the lack of a well-developed text linguistics, was divided into subdisciplines according to the type of discourse (legal, political, religious, etc.) (→ DISCOURSE, TEXT). Other approaches focus on sensory criteria relating to the expression modalities (visual semiotics, auditory semiotics, etc.; → PERCEPTION). Still others specialize in different cultural practices (semiotics of dance, cinema, advertising, cooking, etc.), while others look at particular systems (gestural semiotics) or arbitrarily defined segments of reality (semiotics of narrative, psychosemiotics, etc.).

The connection between specialized semiotics and the established academic disciplines is worth mentioning: Is the semiotics of music the same thing as musicology, that of images, the same as iconology? Now as far as general semiotics is concerned, two pathways for establishing the discipline can be envisaged: a federative one that would bring together the different semiotics to form an interdisciplinary field, and a unifying one that would consider specific semiotics to be subdisciplines of one and the same science. Only the second route has been explored so far. Its ambitions are undoubtedly tied to the philosophical origin of semiotics, but the other side of the coin is a lack of strong academic roots: semiotics still has not really taken a stand as an autonomous discipline.

FRANÇOIS RASTIER

SELECTED BIBLIOGRAPHY

Chandler, D. (2002). *Semiotics: The basics*. New York: Routledge.

Eco, U. (1975). *A theory of semiotics* (Trans.). Bloomington: Indiana University Press. (Original work published 1975.)

Eco, U. (1984). *Semiotics and the philosophy of language* (Trans.). Bloomington: Indiana University Press. (Original work published 1984.)

Greimas, A.-J. (1990). *The social sciences: A semiotic view* (P. Perron & F. Collins, Trans.). Minneapolis, MN: University of Minnesota Press. (Original work published 1976.)

Greimas, A.-J., & Courtès, J. (1982). *Semiotics and language: An analytical dictionary* (L. Crist, Trans.). Bloomington, IN: Indiana University Press. (Original work published 1979.)

Peirce, C. (1991). *Peirce on signs: Writings on semiotics.* Chapel Hill, NC: University of North Carolina Press.

Saussure, F. de. (1959). *Course in general linguistics* (C. Bally, A. Sechehaye, & A. Reidlinger, Eds.; and W. Baskin, Trans.). New York: McGraw-Hill. (Original work published 1916.)

SENSE

Linguistics. — Since Nicolas Beauzée in the eighteenth century, a distinction has been made in French semantics between *sens* (sense) and *signification* (meaning) (→ MEANING AND SIGNIFICATION, SEMANTICS), although usage varies and some authors interchange the two words. In English linguistics, the sense/meaning distinction is not clear cut either, especially since *meaning* refers to various forms of intentionality (→ INTENTIONALITY). In addition, *sense* is often used in English to speak of the conceptual meaning or core meaning of a word.

In lexical semantics, the *meaning* of a word can refer to its assumed invariable content, and *sense*, to its various acceptations or uses in context (→ CONTEXT AND SITUATION, LEXICON). Different levels of description bring out another distinction: one speaks of the meaning of a word, but the sense of a text (→ TEXT). This distinction reflects two different traditions: the logicogrammatical tradition (→ GRAMMAR, LOGIC) and the hermeneutical-rhetorical tradition.

The above distinctions are not made in cognitive semantics. The relationship between meaning and lexical sense is seen as the relationship between a *type* and a *token* (→ TYPE/TOKEN), or between a prototype and an exemplar of a category (→ CATEGORIZATION). Moreover, when the level under study is the text, the *principle of compositionality* is maintained in various forms, generally more lenient ones: the sense of a text becomes the "composition" or synergy of the meanings of its constituent propositions.

One might object to the idea that meaning is a type, being defined as such by linguists on the basis of its observed senses in discourse, which are tokens (→ DISCOURSE). In classical theories of meaning, and even in certain theories of lexical prototypes, a word has an unchanging or at least privileged meaning of its own. This intrinsic meaning is a stable concept (→ CONCEPT); it reflects a thing endowed with a permanent substance, an essence. It is with respect to this meaning that one defines variations in sense or acceptations, often viewed as accidents or mishaps of that essence—or, in more modern terms, as peripheral to the core meaning. The meaning of a word, then, is defined with respect to the reference paradigm, although this paradigm (whether direct or indirect) cannot account for the word's sense, nor can it explain why or how the reference varies across contexts, even if we assume that the meaning gets distorted in the process. If we relate the various lexical senses to the texts in which they occur, and then relate those texts to their genres and discourse types, it becomes clear that references are codified by the norms that govern them (→ NORMATIVITY). In fact, the hierarchy between sense and meaning could be reversed. If so, a word's sense would not be its meaning distorted by context. And its meaning would no longer be a type distorted in various ways in the set of tokens that constitute its senses, but rather a standardized sense, stripped of context. The type would then become a collection of accidents, a convention-based summary of the tokens deemed relevant to its definition.

FRANÇOIS RASTIER

SELECTED BIBLIOGRAPHY

Bartlett, B. (1975). *Beauzée's Grammaire générale: Theory and methodology.* The Hague, The Netherlands: Mouton.

Lyons, J. (1995). *Linguistic semantics.* Cambridge, England; New York: Cambridge University Press.

SENSE/REFERENCE

Philosophy. — The distinction between *sense* and *reference* (the latter sometimes translated *denotation*) was introduced by Gottlob Frege in response to the following problem. An identity relation like $a = b$ (e.g., *the evening star = the morning star*) is clearly informative, and it differs in that respect from the tautology $a = a$ (→ IDENTITY). Now, if the identity relation held only for the things referred to, then an identity statement would not be a source of new information, since a and b refer to the same thing; and if it held only for the names in it, then it would not help gain any knowledge. A distinction must therefore be made between two properties present not only in the constituents of an identity statement, but also in any sign (→ SIGN). One property is the sense of the sign, which supplies the way in which an object is given—its *mode of donation*; the other is its reference—that is, what it refers to or denotes (→ MEANING AND SIGNIFICATION, SENSE). In a true, nontautological identity, the two terms have the same reference but a different sense. According to Frege, every sign has both a sense and a reference. This holds in particular for proper names, whose sense is grasped by learning the name, and whose reference is a particular individual. It also holds for sentences (as particular cases of proper names), whose sense is what Frege calls a *thought*, and whose denotation is a *truth value*, truth or falsity (→ LOGIC). Frege extended the sense/reference opposition to indirect discourse, where the indirect denotation of words is their usual sense (→ DISCOURSE).

Frege's theory of sense triggered a large body of work aimed at addressing some of the issues he opened up. In their essays on demonstratives or on substance terms, influential theorists objected that proper names do not have senses but give direct access to their reference. In this theory, called the *direct reference theory* (David Kaplan), one thinks about the object denoted when using a proper name, without mediation by a particular description. Other neo-Fregean theories—where the denoted object can itself be a constituent of the sense—acknowledge the legitimacy of a *de re* mode of donation (or sense) (→ EXTERNALISM/INTERNALISM).

Frege's sense can be identified using one of two criteria, truth-conditional substitutability or epistemic substitutability (→ EPISTEMIC). The different weights given to one or the other of these criteria led philosophers like John Perry and Gareth Evans to propose rival theories to describe the sense/reference opposition.

Frege was careful to distinguish the sense of a sign from the *representation* it evokes: a sign's sense is objective and invariable; its representation is subjective and fluctuates across individuals (→ REPRESENTATION). This distinction is sometimes ignored, particularly in internalistic theories, where the concept of sense has been used to define the psychological content of mental states. Hilary Putnam's externalistic arguments led most philosophers to abandon this identification between sense and narrow psychological content.

JOËLLE PROUST

SELECTED BIBLIOGRAPHY

Frege, G. (1997). *The Frege reader* (M. Beaney, Ed.). Oxford, England: Blackwell.
Kaplan, D. (1989). Demonstratives. In J. Almog, J. Perry, & H. Wettstein (Eds.), *Themes from Kaplan*. Oxford, England: Oxford University Press.
Kripke, S. (1972). *Naming and necessity*. Oxford, England: Blackwell.

SIGN

Linguistics. — The major models of meaning or signification involve different types of *signs* (→ MEANING AND SIGNIFICATION). *Icons* are signs whose signifier represents the referent in an analogical way. The analogy is conventional and icons are always canonical. Natural languages do not have iconic signs (except for certain ideographic writing systems), but iconism is highly present in linguistics. In cognitive semantics, for example, iconic representations of linguistic meanings are abundant, and the choice of this graphic metalanguage is often based on the assumption that cognitive space is an abstract display of visual space (→ REPRESENTATION, SEMANTICS, SPACE). *Indexes* are signs whose meaning can be determined only relative to a real communication situation or one represented in a text (→ COMMUNICATION, CONTEXT AND SITUATION, TEXT). Natural languages do not have genuine indexes, but rather *indexical signs* like demonstratives, possessives, pronouns, and all signs used for deictic purposes.

Historically, the most important model of meaning is Aristotle's, known today under the name of *semiotic triangle:* its apexes form the word-concept-thing triad (→ CONCEPT). This model was taken up again and popularized in English-speaking countries by Charles Ogden and Ivor Richards (in 1923); it has remained practically unquestioned and is still predominant today in linguistics and philosophy of language. The semiotic triangle serves as a conceptual framework for cognitive research, where, according to Philip Johnson-Laird, for instance, the idea is to show how language is related to the world through mediation by the mind (→ LANGUAGE, MIND). In line with Ogden and Richards, the term *symbol* can be used to mean the type of sign in this triad, although this very ambiguous word is often employed to refer to the signifiers of a formal language (as in symbolic logic, for example) rather than to the signs of a natural language (→ LOGIC, SYMBOL). Maintaining the semiotic triangle keeps semantics dependent upon an ontology, the only explanatory framework capable of relating words to the world via the mediation of concepts. To this day, this *mentalistic* position governs all branches of cognitive semantics and allows them to rightfully use that name.

The other major paradigm in traditional semantics is the *indexical paradigm*. An index is a sign that conveys an inference (→ REASONING AND RATIONALITY). It was formerly used in rhetoric to articulate necessary or plausible proofs. In cognitive research, pragmatics reorganized the indexical paradigm (→ PRAGMATICS). Dan Sperber and Deirdre Wilson, for example, proposed an inferential model of communication (in opposition to the code model) according to which communicating is producing and interpreting indices (→ INTERPRETATION).

Signs must be understood with respect to the types of systems that organize them. For linguists, it is particularly important to make the distinction between linguistic signs and symbols, for many reasons. (1) The signifiers of linguistic signs are doubly articulated; symbols are not. (2) Linguistic signs can vary indefinitely, depending on the token (→ SENSE, TYPE/TOKEN), whereas symbols keep the same reference, even if unknown, within a given computation of meaning (→ SENSE/REFERENCE). (3) Symbols are not diachronous, whether within a computation or across computations; they have no history other than their original institution. (4) Linguistic signs are neither constants nor variables. (5) Symbols are strictly countable at the time they are instituted; there is an indefinite number of signs in a language. (6) The meanings of symbols are strictly composed by applying syntactic rules (→ SYNTAX), whereas linguistic signs do not obey the *principle of compositionality*, in such a way that the symbol-to-computation relation is akin to the element-to-set relation, whereas the sign-to-text relation is a local-to-global one. (7) Linguistic signs can be used metalinguistically, but symbols cannot (→ METACOGNITION); in other words, natural languages exhibit hermeneutic circularity, but formal languages do not. (8) Their interpretation framework differs, both for identifying their signifiers and for identifying the concepts they signify; in a computation, symbol interpretation is momentarily postponed, whereas signs must always be, and always are, interpreted.

The *symbolic paradigm* in cognitive research sees the logical symbol as a fundamental sign, in that mental representations are taken to be made up of logical symbols organized into propositions (→ COGNITIVISM, PROPOSITIONAL FORMAT).

In *cognitive semantics*, authors such as Ronald Langacker have reduced the semiotic triangle to two poles, the sign and the concept. In criticizing logical semantics, they abandoned the theory of direct denotation while retaining a weakened version of the principle of compositionality. Moreover, they now use icons rather than logic symbols to represent the concepts signified. Concepts nevertheless continue to be situated in another order of reality than signifiers, but, via a mentalistic conception of the space of states of affairs, concepts are related to cognitive domains in a mental space reminiscent of absolute space in transcendental philosophy (→ DOMAIN SPECIFICITY). Cognitive schemes have retained from their Kantian ancestors the figurative aspect of shapes in a space, but for the lack of a priori concepts of understanding, they have lost their mediating function.

The fact remains that the goal shared by all cognitive paradigms, by which they follow the same track as in general grammar prior to the creation of comparative linguistics (→ GRAMMAR), consists in moving up from language to thought, and from expression to concept.

FRANÇOIS RASTIER

SELECTED BIBLIOGRAPHY

Chandler, D. (2002). *Semiotics: The basics*. New York: Routledge.

Eco, U. (1975). *A theory of semiotics* (Trans.). Bloomington: Indiana University Press. (Original work published 1975.)

Eco, U. (1984). *Semiotics and the philosophy of language* (Trans.). Bloomington: Indiana University Press. (Original work published 1984.)

Peirce, C. (1991). *Peirce on signs: Writings on semiotics*. Chapel Hill, NC: University of North Carolina Press.

SOCIAL COGNITION

Psychology. — *Social cognition* is the field of knowledge and know-how related to persons (oneself and others); to interpersonal relations between individuals, identified by their personal and functional characteristics as they interact with each other, directly or indirectly (communication, mutual positioning, influence); to relations within a human group or among groups; and to social situations (→ COMMUNICATION, CONTEXT AND SITUATION, INTERACTION). This knowledge and know-how bears upon the emotions, affect (→ EMOTION), motives, and intentions that drive social agents, whether in a habitual way or in particular circumstances; it also bears upon the processes of adjustment, influence, avoidance, and dissimulation. By directing their attention, it enables subjects to determine which of the many observable but often subtle behaviors manifested by other persons are useful cues for interpreting the events that take place in the human environment (→ ATTENTION, INTERPRETATION). These events, whether accidental or relatively stable over time, are integrated and manifested at very different levels: fleeting facial expressions, messages, decisions, conduct reflecting a personality trait, ways of operating, general attitudes, social scenes, and so on. The events can be immediate, things that occurred in the near or distant past, or things that will or may occur in the future. Such events thus have a retroactive impact on the interpretation of the past or present, and a proactive impact on the anticipation of effects. Anticipation is a key component in the monitoring and regulation of behavior in that it plays a major role in controlling repetition, modification, and partial or total inhibition (→ ACTIVATION/INHIBITION, CONTROL).

These constituents of social cognition have a pragmatic component too (→ PRAGMATICS). In real-life situations, subjects must understand and/or act in view of attaining goals and of avoiding any undesirable effects if those goals prove incompatible with the goals of others (→ ACTION). Individuals may postpone, divert, trick, charm, or negotiate in their attempts to avoid or handle conflicts. Some of the other determinants of social information processing and social problem solving include judgments, inferences, deductions, categorizations, and evaluations, which very often rest on highly subjective and personalized grounds, even when they are artfully rationalized (→ CATEGORIZATION, INFORMATION, REASONING AND RATIONALITY). As Pierre Oléron and his collaborators showed, probability, uncertainty, and irreversibility must be taken fully into account. Emotional processes, which are highly visible in empathy and identification, are an integral part of understanding social situations. In addition, social cognition includes knowledge of the norms, conventions, and scenarios that help us understand and control social life at all levels (→ NORMATIVITY). Less used in the scientific discourse are terms like *social intelligence, psy-*

chological competence, and *interpersonal competence*, which span these different dimensions and refer to the goal-oriented knowledge underlying successful actions.

Social cognition is studied from four relatively independent perspectives: *cognitive social psychology, developmental psychology, intelligence testing*, and the *social psychology of cognitive development*.

1. Cognitive social psychology frames the person in his or her relationships with other persons, groups, and social structures, all seen as particular environmental stimuli processed by cognitive operations that discern properties and establish causal links (→ CAUSALITY AND MENTAL CAUSATION). The conceptual tools are usually the same as those used to account for cognition in general. Studies in this line (for example, Germaine de Montmollin's work) are based on causal attribution theory (Fritz Heider, Harold Kelley) and on the idea of "naive theories of personality," elaborated by individuals to serve as mediators for making sense of human events (Salomon Asch, Jerome Bruner, and Renato Tagiuri).

2. Developmental psychology looks at self-knowledge, knowledge of others, adaptation to interactions and social situations (such as communication, games and play, power relations), and knowledge of psychological phenomena (→ METACOGNITION). In the 1970s, the study of the development of social knowledge was marked by the concepts of decentration, perspective-taking, and role-taking. Social cognition was described as progressing toward the differentiation of points of view (self vs. others, apparent behavior vs. underlying intentions) and as involving the ability to take mutual interests into account in the short and longer terms (John Flavell, Robert Selman). At the same time, several authors began to defend the idea that children acquire early implicit social knowledge that they manifest in effective communication behaviors that are attuned to the addressee (Janine Beaudichon, Helen Borke, Tatiana Slama-Cazacu).

Another series of studies emerged in the 1980s and 1990s to examine young children's representations of the psychological states of persons and how those representations evolve with age (→ REPRESENTATION). According to Henry Wellman, such representations form a "naive theory of the human mind" by supplying the child with an organized, explanatory, and predictive framework for grasping human behavior (→ THEORY OF MIND). The underlying processes that build these representations are described in various models, including *modular models, post-Piagetian models*, and models based on *self-other matching* or *early intersubjectivity*. In modularist models, it is a question of the maturation and activation of specialized cognitive mechanisms, particularly mechanisms that detect intentionality (Simon Baron-Cohen, Alan Leslie) (→ DOMAIN SPECIFICITY, INTENTIONALITY, MODULARITY). In post-Piagetian models, which retain Jean Piaget's ideas on the coordination of perspectives, psychological knowledge is at first grounded in the child's experience of his or her own mental attitudes (→ EXPERIENCE), and then this knowledge is applied to other persons through differentiation and simulation (Paul Harris, Michael Tomasello, etc.). In models of self-to-others matching, it is an infant's experience of functional similarity, contingency, or reciprocity between his or her own behaviors and those of others (imitation, coordinated behavior) that enables early sharing of mental states and then gradual awareness of psychological relationships per se (Andrew Meltzoff, Sally Rogers, and Bruce Pennington) (→ CONSCIOUSNESS). Finally, according to models of early intersubjectivity, there exists a partly innate capacity to respond to others and to act directly upon others at the psychological level (emotions and motivations) through expressive behaviors. Such behaviors serve as the basis for understanding that there exist representations between people and the world (Peter Hobson, Colwyn Trevarthen).

3. For the purposes of measuring intelligence, most investigators from the psychometric tradition leave little room for the social component. One exception is Edward Thorndike, who defines three different types of intelligence: social, mechanical, and abstract (→ DIFFERENTIATION). Joy Guilford, who proposed a factorial breakdown of intellectual abilities, also found a factor pertaining to the behavior of others. Scales of social maturity such as Edgar Doll's in the United States or Marie-Claude Hurtig and René Zazzo's in France measure the adaptive component of social intelligence by situating subjects with respect to their age group on a series of everyday social behaviors. However, difficulty designing social-intelligence tests that meet the usual reliability standards of psychometrics has contributed to making these attempts very marginal.

Selman's work (Piagetian in inspiration) on the five *levels of social perspective-taking* that succeed each other in the course of childhood is noteworthy. His description can be applied in a broader way to account for the various interpersonal negotiation strategies that coexist and prevail in adults, in accordance with the circumstances and the personality of the social actors. The first three are negotiation by physical force, negotiation by recourse to power, and negotiation by persuasion; these levels are characterized by dominance/submission and by the use of techniques such as anger, bribery, seduction, and so on. The last two are negotiation by interpersonal collaboration, where empathy, communication, and consideration of different points of view dictate the outcome (the decision), and negotiation by integration-synthesis of different perspectives and of possible reasoning modes or outcomes. In a similar approach, Lawrence Kohlberg described the development of moral judgment.

4. Finally, the social psychology of cognitive development is interested in individuals as they acquire knowledge in social settings. The social context is regarded as a framework for selecting and processing information (*social marking*) based on collective representations, and as providing opportunities for comparing differing viewpoints through a process of sociocognitive conflict that triggers socially rooted destabilization and restablization (Willem Doise, Gabriel Mugny, etc.). In a variation on this view, the emphasis is placed on help-seeking and tutoring (Fajda Winnykamen). This approach has two origins: the study of social learning (Albert Bandura) (→ LEARNING) and the study of the internalization of skills acquired during social interactions, with expert adults playing an important role in that process (Lev Vygotsky).

A recurring problem in the social cognition research is the weakness of the correlations between observed levels of social understanding, assessed using fictitious social settings, and the quality of social behavior in adaptive real-world situations. Several explanations have been proposed: inadequacy of the experimental setups themselves, which are devoid of personal implications and are not conducive to the creation of real contexts where social skills can be actualized; oversimplification of the manner of attaining social goals in experimental tasks, which masks the specificities of the indirect and subjective routes taken to process intrapersonal and social variables; and failure to take into account the dynamic facet of the sequence of regulations by means of which adjustment is achieved through the substantial involvement of executive control processes. Comparative research in developmental psychopathology and neuropsychology is contributing to bringing out functional or structural dependencies or "independencies" between the different components: social cognition, social behavior, regulation mechanisms, and so forth (→ AUTISM, COGNITIVE PSYCHIATRY, NEUROPSYCHOLOGY).

JEANINE BEAUDICHON AND MARIE-HÉLÈNE PLUMET

SELECTED BIBLIOGRAPHY

Adolphs, R. (2003). Cognitive neuroscience of human social behavior. *Nature Reviews Neuroscience, 4*, 165–178.

Bandura, A. (1986). *Social foundations of thought and action: A social cognitive theory.* Englewood Cliffs, NJ: Prentice-Hall.

Bandura, A. (1997). *Self-efficacy: The exercise of control.* New York: Freeman.

Baron-Cohen, S., Tager-Flusberg, H., & Cohen, D. J. (Eds.). (1993). *Understanding other minds.* Oxford, England; New York: Oxford University Press.

Bartsch, K., & Wellman, H. (1995). *Children talk about the mind.* New York: Oxford University Press.

Beaudichon, J. (1982). *La communication sociale chez l'enfant* [Social communication in the child]. Paris: Presses Universitaires de France.

Beaudichon, J. (1998). *La communication: De la théorie à l'action* [Communication: From theory to action]. Paris: Armand Colin.

Bruner, J. (1990). *Acts of meaning*. Cambridge, MA: Harvard University Press.

Cacioppo, J., Bernston, G., Taylor, S., & Schacter, D. (Eds.). (2002). *Foundations in social neuroscience*. Cambridge, MA: MIT Press.

Doise, W., & Mugny, G. (1984). *The social development of the intellect* (A. St. James-Emler & N. Emler, Trans.). Oxford, England; New York: Pergamon Press. (Original work published 1981.)

Doise, W., & Mugny, G. (1997). *Psychologie sociale et développement cognitif* [Social psychology and cognitive development]. Paris: Armand Colin.

Flavell, J., & Miller, P. (1998). Social cognition. In W. Damon (Ed.), *Handbook of child psychology: Vol. 3. Social, emotional, and personality development* (5th ed., pp. 851–898). New York: Wiley.

Meltzoff, A., & Prinz, W. (Eds.). (2002). *The imitative mind: Development, evolution, and brain bases*. Cambridge, England; New York: Cambridge University Press.

Montmollin, G. de (1991). Cognition sociale [Social cognition]. In H. Bloch et al. (Eds.). *Grand dictionnaire de la psychologie* (pp. 137–139). Paris: Larousse.

Oléron, P. (Ed.). (1981). *Savoirs et savoir-faire psychologiques chez l'enfant* [Psychological knowledge and know-how in the child]. Brussels, Belgium: Mardaga.

Selman, R. L. (1981). The development of interpersonal competence. *Developmental Review, 1*, 401–422.

Shore, B. (with Bruner, J.). (1996). *Culture in mind: Cognition, culture, and the problem of meaning*. New York: Oxford University Press.

Vygotsky, L. (1962). *Thought and language* (Rev. ed.; A. Kozalin, Trans. and Ed.). Cambridge, MA: MIT Press. (Original work published 1934.)

Winnykamen, F. (1991). *Apprendre en imitant* [Learning through imitation]. Paris: Presses Universitaires de France.

Wyer, R., & Srull, T. (Eds.). (1994). *Handbook of social cognition*. Hillsdale, NJ: Erlbaum.

SPACE

Psychology. — Psychological space encompasses the spatial properties of objects (including the body) and the spatial relations between them (→ OBJECT). The cognitive psychology of space investigates the nature and origin of the spatial knowledge needed to achieve mastery of the environment.

Where? and *What?* are two crucial questions: Where is a given object (and how can it be reached)? And what is that object (and how can it be used)? This long-standing distinction, which separates *localization* (direction and distance) from *identification*, was validated in cognitive neuroscience (see *neuroscience* below) when it was shown that these two kinds of operations were performed by different neural circuits and could therefore be dissociated in brain-damaged patients (→ NEUROPSYCHOLOGY). The pathway called *dorsal* (occipitoparietal) does the locating and the pathway called *ventral* (occipitotemporal) does the identifying. The existence of these neural circuits has been confirmed using functional neuroimaging techniques (→ FUNCTIONAL NEUROIMAGING).

Spatial localization depends on what *reference system* is at stake. The *egocentric* system has the subject's own body as the origin (e.g., *to my right*), whereas the *exocentric* system locates with respect to external cues (e.g., *across from the window*). Egocentric references must be updated every time the person moves, whereas exocentric references are subject-independent. These two reference systems probably depend in turn on a *geocentric* frame of reference organized around the direction of gravity (Jacques Paillard).

Two types of processing are applied to spatial data. *Sensorimotor processing* handles the portions of the physical world that the organism encounters through its perceptual and motor systems (→ ACTION, PERCEPTION). Within this "sensorimotor dialogue" with the environment, to borrow Paillard's expression, extracorporeal space is framed in an egocentric way and is continuously updated as the subject and/or surrounding objects move. This is what happens, for example, when a object in motion is followed by the eyes and then grasped by the hands. *Semantic processing* (conceptual or representational) is based on the activation of mental representations stored in memory (→ CONCEPT, MEMORY, REPRESENTATION, SEMANTICS). It builds spatiocognitive maps, in image or propositional format, that summarize the relative locations of objects and the body, as well as the paths that link different points to each other (→ MENTAL IMAGERY, PROPOSITIONAL FORMAT). Insofar as it generates abstract knowledge that is independent of current sensorimotor actions, this type of processing is organized in an exocentric frame of reference.

The perceptual-motor systems that enable access to spatial properties in humans are vision, audition, touch, and somatovestibular proprioception. It was long believed, as Jean Piaget did, that these systems, which are separate at birth, become coordinated only through multisensory experience (→ EXPERIENCE). But today we know that newborns already exhibit cross-sensory coordination: they direct their gaze at a sound source and reach out in the direction of visible objects (→ INFANT COGNITION). A rudimentary degree of unity of the senses thus enables the early acquisition of coherent spatial knowledge. The acquisition process, which spans several years, originates in the motor activity that triggers changes in the sensory flow, permits the extraction of constants that specify locations and objects (James Gibson), and coordinates the subject's perceptual and motor spaces. Because of its discriminative capabilities and its vast perceptual field, vision is the most powerful perceptual modality in the spatial domain; it is also the dominant one. This means that if visual spatial data are inconsistent with auditory, tactile, or proprioceptive data, the visual input will override the rest and the subject may not even be aware of the incongruity between the senses.

In the debate about the origin of spatial knowledge, the opposition between nativism and empiricism is now outdated. It has been replaced by *interactionism*, wherein experience actualizes preexisting potentialities. The stages of development described by Piaget (the construction of topological geometry first, then projective and Euclidian geometries) have also been partially questioned (→ COGNITIVE DEVELOPMENT). It nevertheless remains true, as Piaget suggested, that development is characterized both by changes in the reference systems used and by the emergence of the ability to represent space from different points of view.

YVETTE HATWELL

Neuroscience. — In cognitive neuroscience, the concept of space has primarily been approached through the neuropsychological study of *hemineglect* (→ NEUROPSYCHOLOGY). Patients who suffer from this disorder have trouble processing (detecting, identifying, attending to) information situated in the half of space controlateral to the lesioned brain hemisphere (→ INFORMATION). The hemineglect syndrome, frequently observed in cases of right brain damage, can affect the visual, auditory, or tactile modalities—all used to apprehend space—without a concomitant elementary sensory or motor deficit. The lesions are usually in the parietal lobe, but subcortical or frontal damage may also cause the syndrome. The mechanisms in charge of representing and processing spatial information (→ REPRESENTATION) appear to be subtended by the inferoposterior parietal regions of the right hemisphere, certain parts of the thalamus, and also the frontal premotor cortex. Depending on the explanatory model, the hemineglect syndrome is ascribed to an attention deficit (Michael Posner) (→ ATTENTION), an imbalance of activation between the cerebral hemispheres (Marcel Kinsbourne), or a perturbation of the space representation frame itself (Edoardo Bisiach).

Cognitive neuroscience has shown that two separate neural circuits handle the two essential facets of the processing of objects in space: their localization and their identification (→ MENTAL IMAGERY, PERCEPTION). The "where" circuit is the *dorsal* pathway, which includes the regions situated along an occipital-parietal axis extending into the superior parietal lobe. This pathway is responsible for locating objects and analyzing the spatial attributes of perceived scenes. The "what" circuit is the *ventral* pathway, which is situated along an occipitotemporal axis extending into the inferior temporal gyrus. This pathway is specialized in shape processing and, more generally, in treating the figural characteristics of objects (identification operations). John Haxby's work in functional neuroimaging has validated this two-circuit description (→ FUNCTIONAL NEUROIMAGING).

OLIVIER HOUDÉ

Linguistics. — The various conceptions of space that emerge through language and discourse do not correspond to any preexisting model, since space in linguistic usage is heterogeneous, discontinuous, phenomenological, topological, and language-specific rather than three-dimensional, Eu-clidian, isotropic, and homogeneous (→ DISCOURSE, LANGUAGE). Space has a dual function: it is a referent of linguistic expressions, where it is structured according to the possibilities and constraints specific to their grammar (→ GRAMMAR), and it is a form for organizing other entities, which grants it a structuring role.

Different approaches to expressions of spatiality are indicative of the way not only language but also its links to culture, the body, and cognition are theorized. The study of verbal renditions of space has given rise to contradictory viewpoints on the status of language. For the proponents of *physical-biological determinism*, a subject's location and orientation are expressed in accordance with environmental constraints, and especially with the native properties of the human organism (for example, verticality is defined by the laws of gravity and by the evolution of *Homo erectus*, characterized by the upright stance); for the proponents of *relativism*, verbalizations of space originate instead in the way the body, human beings, and the world are categorized in a mythical-cultural system (→ CATEGORIZATION).

Verbalizations of space—from space as a referent structured by language to space as an organizing principle—can be approached from three angles: the linguistic devices available for talking about space, the organization of spatial descriptions in discourse and social interaction (→ INTERACTION), and the way space functions in metaphors.

Among the linguistic devices used to refer to space, *deixis* plays an essential role. Deictic expressions link contextual space to an interlocution, defined by the copresence of speakers, and the space containing the objects they are pointing out (→ CONTEXT AND SITUATION). Deictic markers are organized around what Karl Bühler called the "origo" of deixis, which is defined by the triad *I-here-now*. This triad is structured first and foremost by the language-dependent opposition between the terms that refer to *here* and those that refer to *elsewhere*, not only relative to the distance from the speaker but also to other dimensions such as the vertical position of places (*up* vs. *down*), the location within a specific territory (*on the forest side* vs. *on the seaside*, as in Dyirbal, spoken in Australia), and whether the object being situated is within sight (→ PERCEPTION), is reachable, or is given or new in the current discourse (as in Daga, spoken in New Guinea). The result is a set of complex interrelationships between local deixis and other dimensions such as topicality and figure-ground relations.

Outside the realm of "the here," the structured localization modes found in oppositions like *to the left* versus *to the right* and *in front of* versus *behind* are defined along two fundamental dimensions: *orientation* and *configuration*. The orientational dimension is organized by absolute references (such as the four directions, the stars, or salient parts of the landscape) or by relative references based either on the inherent properties of the concerned objects (for example, the asymmetry of the cabinet in *The pen fell in front of the cabinet*) or on contextual relationships (as in *The dart landed in front of the tree*, where the dart's location is not understood with respect to the tree but to the speaker or addressee). Such contextual relationships are in turn governed by different schemas (for example, the mirror or facing relation that opposes front and back in English, and the asymmetrical relation of alignment that opposes them in Haussa, Africa). The configurational dimension refers to the way objects and space are structured by the chosen localization mode. For example, the street is not configured in the same way in the German phrase *auf der Strasse* as it is in the (British) English phrase *in the street;* in the first case, the pavement is the dimension that determines the preposition, whereas in the second, it is the volumetric space that includes the building fronts along the street (American English usage—for example, *on Haight Street*—is analogous to the German). The configurational dimension thus brings to bear selection and idealization processes. These processes show that locating objects in space requires symbolic and cognitive operations to format, focalize, categorize, and organize data captured from the world.

Other forms of structuring are found in the cognitive and interactive strategies used to describe space. From the cognitive standpoint, spatial verbalizations (studied mainly in descriptions of houses and apartments) have their own specific modes of discourse planning, either revolving around a path along which elements are described in succession, or around the figurative aspects of a map, where the described elements laid out in a space grasped in its entirety (→ MENTAL IMAGERY). These two strategies rely on different space-organization schemas. From the interactive standpoint, spatial verbalizations (studied mainly in descriptions of itineraries) include negotiation of a point of view, a set of reference points, and a way of expressing spatial entities, all geared to the addressee. Ways of referring to known places (landmarks) and unknown places (to-be-located) are chosen only as a conversation unfolds. The choice involves more than the simple activation of a mental map; it is based on a series of confirmations, questions, evaluations, negotiations, and readjustments of a proposed description, during which each interlocutor's categorizations are brought to bear in order to find the relevant descriptors (for example, a description of how to get somewhere will not be worded in the same way if directed at a young vagrant and a traveling salesperson, and it will be apparent in the directions given whether the speaker lives in the neighborhood or learned about it from some other source). Descriptions of itineraries provide a good example of contextual variations in space-representation modes (→ REPRESENTATION).

A specific characteristic of spatial expressions is that they are not limited to referring to spatial entities. Spatial metaphors are employed in a variety of semantic domains, especially for expressing temporality, and they clearly illustrate how space shapes our thought (→ DOMAIN SPECIFICITY, SEMANTICS, TIME AND TENSE). *Text deixis*, achieved by expressions referring to place in a discourse, also relies heavily on spatial reference points: the page is depicted as a vertical space, speech as a linear space (→ ORAL, TEXT). More generally, localistic hypotheses assign space the role of fundamental structuring framework, not only for our experiences and knowledge, but also for language in general. This provides the rationale for adopting spatial categories for descriptions in linguistics. The *locative cases*, which express movements and spatial locations in some languages, are regarded as the prototypes of case values in general, by way of an iconic analogy between grammatical values and spatial values (for example, the figure of a trajectory—where an entity moves from a source location to a target location—is often employed to describe the fact of entering or leaving a situation or state, gaining or losing property, learning or forgetting something, and so forth).

These illustrations point out some of the possible ways that language and reference are spatialized. Different forms of spatialization are used effectively both by the cognitive schemas operant in our everyday experiences and by scientific models. They ensure the transition from representations of space, treated as a referent, to spaces of representation, treated as structuring forms, as places where knowledge is inscribed and distributed.

LORENZA MONDADA

SELECTED BIBLIOGRAPHY

Behrmann, M. (2000). Spatial reference frames and hemispatial neglect. In M. Gazzaniga (Ed.), *The new cognitive neurosciences* (2nd ed., pp. 651–666). Cambridge, MA: MIT Press.

Bisiach, E. (1997). The spatial features of unilateral neglect. In P. Thier & H. Karnath (Eds.), *Parietal lobe contributions to orientation in 3D space* (pp. 465–495). Berlin, Germany; New York: Springer.

Bloom, P., Peterson, M., Nadel, L., & Garrett, M. (Eds.). (1996). *Language and space.* Cambridge, MA: MIT Press.

Gibson, J. (1979). *The ecological approach to visual perception.* Boston: Houghton Mifflin.

Haxby, J., et al. (1991). Dissociation of object and spatial visual processing pathways in human extrastriate cortex. *Proceedings of the National Academy of Sciences USA, 88,* 1621–1625.

Kinsbourne, M. (1987). Mechanisms of unilateral neglect. In M. Jeannerod (Ed.), *Neurophysiological and neuropsychological aspects of spatial neglect.* North-Holland, New York: Elsevier.

Levinson, S. (2003). *Space in language and cognition: Explorations in cognitive diversity.* Cambridge, England; New York: Cambridge University Press.

Newcombe, N., & Huttenlocher, J. (2000). *Making space: The development of spatial representation and reasoning.* Cambridge, MA: MIT Press.

Paillard, J. (Ed.). (1991). *Brain and space,* Oxford, England; New York: Oxford University Press, 1991.

Piaget, J., & Inhelder, B. (1956). *The child's conception of space* (F. J. Langdon & J. L. Lunzer, Trans.). New York: Norton. (Original work published 1948.)

Posner, M., et al. (1987). How do the parietal lobes direct covert attention? *Neuropsychologia, 25,* 135–146.

Posner, M. , & Raichle, M. (1994/1997). *Images of mind.* New York: Freeman.

Robertson, I., & Halligan, P. (1999). *Spatial neglect: A clinical handbook for diagnosis and treatment.* Hove, England; New York: Psychology Press.

Vandeloise, C. (1986). *L'espace en français* [Description of space in French]. Paris: Seuil.

SUBDOXASTIC

Philosophy. — Contemporary cognitive psychologists frequently attribute to people representational states that do not seem to interact in the usual ways with other typical mental states such as beliefs and desires (→ BELIEF, DESIRE, REPRESENTATION). To take a notorious example, Chomskyian linguists often attribute to people "knowledge"of elaborate grammatical rules of which they are unaware and which do not combine with other beliefs they might possess at the same time (→ CONSCIOUSNESS, GRAMMAR). Chomsky himself might have been born "knowing" grammatical rule *R*, and as a linguist, he might believe that *if R then P* (where *P* is some particular claim about a language); but he might not be the least bit inclined to conclude *that P*—indeed, he may for some time have explicitly denied *both R and P*. Steven Stich calls such relatively isolated cognitive states *subdoxastic* (subbelief) states: they are contentful states that do not enter into standard inferential patterns with other relevant beliefs (→ REASONING AND RATIONALITY). They are, in Jerry Fodor's terms, *informationally encapsulated* (→ INFORMATION, MODULARITY). Since the precise degree of encapsulation varies in different cases (for example, in early vision, natural language syntax, semantics; → DOMAIN SPECIFICITY, LANGUAGE, PERCEPTION, SEMANTICS, SYNTAX), there is considerable controversy about whether they correspond to the states of Fodor's *modules*, to Chomsky's (1976) *cognized states*, or to what still others have called merely *tacit* or *unconscious knowledge.*

GEORGES REY

SELECTED BIBLIOGRAPHY

Chomsky, N. (1976). *Reflections on language.* London: Fontana/Collins.

Davies, M. (1989). Tacit knowledge and subdoxastic states. In A. George (Ed.), *Reflections on Chomsky* (pp. 131–152). Oxford, England: Blackwell.

Fodor, J. (1983). *The modularity of mind.* Cambridge, MA: MIT Press.

Fodor, J. (2000). *The mind doesn't work that way: The scope and limits of computational psychology.* Cambridge, MA: MIT Press.

Hauser, M., Chomsky, N., & Fitch, W. (2002). The faculty of language: What is it, who has it, and how did it evolve? *Science, 298,* 1569–1579.

Stich, S. (1978). Beliefs and subdoxastic states. *Philosophy of Science, 45,* 499–518.

SUPERVENIENCE

Philosophy. — Two of our most deep-rooted intuitions about mental phenomena seem to conflict: on one side, mental properties depend on physical properties, but on the other, mental properties cannot be reduced to physical properties (→ DUALISM/MONISM, PHYSICALISM, REDUCTIONISM). To reconcile these intuitions, philosophers of language proposed the concept of *supervenience*. This term goes back to the *Aristoteles Latinus*. It was used first in emergentist theories of evolution (→ EMERGENCE) and then in moral philosophy to express the idea that moral or evaluative properties such as goodwill or courage supervene on natural properties, without being reduced to them. Donald Davidson applied the concept to the relationship between the mental and the physical, to defend the idea that no two events can be identical in every physical aspect while differing in their mental aspects. The supervenience of a set of *A*-properties on a set of *B*-properties is both a relation of determination and a nonreductive relation (asymmetrical). But can it satisfy both of these conditions?

In fact, the term *supervenience* is used to refer to several different concepts (Jaegwon Kim). In *weak supervenience*, *A* supervenes weakly on *B* if and only if two things that have the same *B*-properties necessarily have the same *A*-properties. But this relation is too weak. It precludes envisaging a possible world where two physically identical objects are not mentally identical, but it authorizes the existence of a possible world that is physically identical to ours yet radically different mentally. A remedy is to introduce *strong supervenience:* if something has property *A*, it also has property *B* such that, necessarily, anything that has *B* has *A*. But this relation seems to imply the coextension of *A* and *B*, and hence, reduction. *Global supervenience* has also been proposed: *A* supervenes globally on *B* if two *B*-indiscernible worlds are also *A*-indiscernible. This relation is compatible with the existence of a world that deviates from ours in minor physical details, but is radically different mentally. The relationships between these supervenience concepts can be studied to distinguish degrees of physicalist and reductionist commitment in the various doctrines. It is generally agreed nonetheless that the supervenience of the mental on the physical is a minimal requirement for naturalism (→ NATURALIZATION), although the concept serves to specify only the ontological implications of a doctrine and says nothing about the nature of the mentalistic and physicalistic explanations that might be proffered.

PASCAL ENGEL

SELECTED BIBLIOGRAPHY

Davidson, D. (1980). *Essays on actions and events* (2nd ed.). Oxford, England: Clarendon Press.
Kim, J. (1993). *Supervenience and mind*. Cambridge, England: Cambridge Universirty Press.

SYMBOL

Philosophy. — *Symbols* are objects that possess a semantic interpretation (→ INTERPRETATION, SEMANTICS). A symbol always refers to what it represents by virtue of a rule: the physical aspect of the sign must be distinguished from its *normative* aspect, that is, from the rule that governs its use (→ NORMATIVITY, REPRESENTATION, SIGN). The rule is what allows for the distinction between the accessory part of a symbol and its essential part. Two physically different symbols that stand for the same thing and express the same rule—say, the Arabic and Roman numerals 1 and I, both of which stand for the number *one*—are equivalent both in *sense* and in *reference* (→ SENSE/REFERENCE).

A *symbolic system* is a closed set of signs. A *formal* symbolic system has two additional properties, which qualify it as a *calculus:* (1) all elements in the system can be reduced by decomposition to a finite list of elementary constituents, and (2) rules exist for determining what symbol associations produce new "well-formed" expressions (→ LOGIC, SYNTAX).

In "classical" artificial intelligence (see *artificial intelligence* below), as in psychology and cognitivist philosophy of mind (→ COGNITIVISM, LANGUAGE OF THOUGHT, MIND), it is argued that thinking amounts to manipulating symbols, notably in a calculus. It is by virtue of their physical form that symbols can interact causally (→ CAUSALITY AND MENTAL CAUSATION); but it is by virtue of their normative properties that the system that manipulates them can generate true formulas (→ TRUTH).

JOËLLE PROUST

Artificial intelligence. — In ancient Greece, the word *symbol* was used to refer to a sign of recognition of a long-standing friendship, acknowledgment of a debt of hospitality, or recognition of a contract (→ SIGN). From this usage, the term has retained its everyday meaning: a flag and a fleur-de-lis are symbols in that they embody, in material objects, other realities (here, national unity and French monarchal legitimacy). More generally, a symbol is any object or sign that refers to something other than itself by virtue of a relation of analogy.

In computer science, where executable operations are performed on sequences of zeros and ones, a symbol is necessarily represented by such a string. This being the case, the relationship between these bit strings and what they stand for is highly context- and usage-dependent.

The relationship between a sign and its sense can be set by simple convention, without being legitimatized by any kind of formal analogy; the symbolization in this case is highly tenuous (→ SENSE). A string of characters (which is always reducible to a bit string since each character is reducible to such a string) can also evoke a word, a proposition, or a sentence in ordinary language, in which case the sense follows from shared usage and will be recognized by an entire social community (→ LANGUAGE, PROPOSITIONAL FORMAT). Finally, it may be that a string inserted in a set of formal manipulations behaves in an equivalent manner to its referent in the environment (→ SENSE/REFERENCE). In this case, there is a formal analogical relation between the symbol and what it designates. This type of relation is particularly well-suited to mathematical objects, since it specifies their properties without recourse to intuition. Since David Hilbert in the early twentieth century, a branch of mathematics has been working on such a formalization.

In artificial intelligence, the ideas one hopes to refer to by means of symbols—for example, the notions of table, doctor, or man—can hardly ever be expressed by means of a mere set of syntactic relations (→ SYNTAX). One must therefore search for mechanisms that go beyond the formal manipulations listed in mathematical logic (→ LOGIC) in an attempt to come closer, if possible, to the evocative power of words. This is a current topic of study in research on knowledge representation (→ REPRESENTATION).

Among the methods used to process information (→ INFORMATION), techniques called *symbolic* are commonly distinguished from *numerical* techniques, which include formal neural networks and, more generally, connectionist approaches (→ CONNECTIONISM, LEARNING, NEURAL NETWORK). Does this mean that symbols are opposed to numbers (→ NUMBER)? At the strictly formal level, nothing allows us to make this statement, since a number is just a particular symbol endowed with particular properties. However, to the extent that symbols have the power to evoke, their meaning relies partly on a mental function (→ MEANING AND SIGNIFICATION, MIND), whereas numbers result from a supposedly objective measure.

JEAN-GABRIEL GANASCIA

SELECTED BIBLIOGRAPHY

Pinker, S., & Mehler, J. (Eds.). (1988). *Connections and symbols*. Cambridge, MA: MIT Press.
Pylyshyn, Z. (1984). *Computation and cognition: Toward a foundation for cognitive science*. Cambridge, MA: MIT Press.

SYNTAX

Philosophy. — *Syntax* is the study of word combinations in sentences and of derivation relations between propositions (→ LANGUAGE). *Completeness* (in the broad sense) warrants the equivalence between syntax and semantics (→ SEMANTICS), to the extent that any formula in a coherent formal system (propositional logic or predicate logic; → LOGIC) has a model, that is, an interpretation (→ INTERPRETATION, MODEL). On the other hand, Kurt Gödel demonstrated the incompleteness of formal arithmetic: its syntactic and semantic properties are no longer equivalent.

The idea of defining a universal syntax, which we owe to Rudolf Carnap, consists in searching for the formal a priori conditions of all scientific discourse (whether logical or descriptive) and of the relationship between language and experience (→ EXPERIENCE). Under the influence of Alfred Tarski, this project was transformed into the search for a universal semantics.

According to Noam Chomsky, syntax is a recursive mechanism for producing a virtually unlimited number of sentences. The fact that thought is organized in a systematic manner, and that it is also endowed with productivity, led Jerry Fodor to contend that thought, too, has a syntactic structure (→ LANGUAGE OF THOUGHT).

JOËLLE PROUST

Linguistics. — While grammar proposes an inventory of all regularities in a language, syntax (as it is traditionally defined) studies rules for combining words to make sentences (→ GRAMMAR, LANGUAGE). Syntax differs from *morphology*, which pertains to the way meaningful units are combined to form words, and from *discourse analysis*, which looks at relationships between sentences (→ DISCOURSE, MORPHOLOGY). In a structuralist or distributional perspective, syntax is the study of how *morphemes* (smallest meaningful units; → MEANING AND SIGNIFICATION) are combined to make phrases and how phrases are combined to make sentences. If syntax is concerned with rules for combining attached morphemes (for example, prefixes, suffixes), it covers morphology (in which case it is called *morphosyntax*). There are different types of syntactic phenomena, including *categories* and *subcategories*, *phrase constituents*, types of *constructions*, and *anaphoric relations*.

1. The study of linguistic categories brings out the link between *lexicon* and syntax (→ CATEGORIZATION, LEXICON). The distinction is generally made between *grammatical categories* (closed classes) and *lexical categories* (open classes): from a synchronic point of view, one can easily create a verb (*to fax*), a noun (*a networker*), or an adjective (*evaluatable*), but one cannot create a preposition, pronoun, or article; from a diachronic point of view, a word can be shifted from a lexical category to a grammatical category (for example, when the grammaticalization process that creates an auxiliary from a full verb), but never the reverse. The traditional or philosophical approach classifies words into parts of speech. The *structuralist* approach defines syntactic categories as classes of morphemes with the same distribution, that is, capable of occurring

in the same syntactic contexts (for example, common nouns can occur between an article and an adjective) (→ CONTEXT AND SITUATION). In this approach, *my, your*, and *his* are not possessive adjectives but articles, because they occur in the same contexts as *the* and *a*. Subcategories (such as transitive or intransitive) further specify the acceptable contexts for a given word. More recent theories break down syntactic categories into sets of features. The presence of common features explains why a coordinating conjunction can be used to compound a noun and an adjective (*Jack is the representative of his district and proud to be so*) or a noun phrase and a clause (*The little girl said her name and that her nickname was Bibi*). Theories grouped under the heading *categorial grammars* do not have rules to describe phrases but use complex categories to describe the set of all possible combinations of lexical units.

2. The structural school, which became "generative" with Noam Chomsky, defines grammatical groups as phrases, that is, category sequences classified according to their possible and impossible contexts. A noun phrase, for example, can occur at the beginning of a sentence or follow a preposition. Since a phrase can itself include another phrase, the outcome is an embedding of immediate constituents, easily depicted in a tree-like format. Take the sentence *The door of my room is open.* The noun phrase *the door of my room* is an immediate constituent of the sentence; it has the prepositional phrase *of my room* as its own immediate constituent, which in turn has the noun phrase *my room* as an immediate constituent. In this approach, dependency relations are rendered by the respective positions of the phrases in the syntactic tree structure, and traditional grammatical functions (subject, object, etc.) need not be brought to bear (→ FUNCTION). According to other traditions such as *dependency grammars* (Lucien Tesnière), grammatical functions are important and must be defined as relations between words, not between phrases. In this case, graphs (and not trees) are preferred for denoting cases of multiple dependencies, as in *Jean persuades Marie to come*, where *Marie* is both the object of *persuades* and the subject of *to come*.

3. The study of different syntactic constructions was renovated by *generative transformational grammar*, which proposes a formal definition of systematic relations between active and passive sentences, declarative and interrogative sentences, and so on. In this approach, semantic kinships between an active and passive sentence are explained in terms of their shared deep syntactic structure (canonical). Formal rules (*Move the object to the subject position*, etc.) are applied to derive all observed surface structures (→ SEMANTICS). The various transformations were first enumerated and then grouped on the basis of purely formal criteria. For example, relative clauses, interrogative sentences, and cleft sentences fall into the same group because they share essential

syntactic properties, in spite of their different meanings and uses. In Chomsky's most recent grammar, the set of transformation rules was replaced by a small number of more general, more abstract principles (for example, application of the two rules *A passive verb cannot govern a direct object* and *A sentence with a conjugated verb must have a subject* explains why the object becomes the subject in the passive voice). In *unification grammars*, the syntactic properties associated with words are reorganized in such a way that transformations are not needed, and one can work directly on surface structures.

4. An important phenomenon handled by generative-like syntaxes is anaphoric relations within sentences, which generally go beyond the simple question of pronouns. In elliptic sentences like *Paul likes oranges and Marie bananas*, the omission of the second verb can be regarded as the trace of an anaphora whose antecedent is the first verb. The inclusion of anaphoric relations in syntax prevents it from being treated as a purely formal system, since it must manipulate referential cues. The idea that syntactic rules are heterogeneous in nature can explain the concept of *degree of grammaticality*. The extent to which a sentence deviates from grammaticality depends on what syntactic rules it breaks: violating agreement rules (*He come tomorrow*), for instance, will not be considered as bad as violating embedding rules (*I know the girl to whom the man who wrote is dead*). In this view, syntax is a more complex set of modules than Chomsky's initial generative system.

A critical question regarding syntax concerns its *autonomy*. Syntax is often given the task of establishing the link between sound and meaning (→ PERCEPTION). The autonomous syntax view—propounded by the generativists and attacked by Ronald Langacker and other advocates of an integrated cognitive linguistics—does not refute the existence of interactions with morphology (as in agreement phenomena) or with phonology (as in liaison constraints), but it contends that one can study well-formedness rules irrespective of their meaning or phonetic realization.

Clearly, syntax needs semantic information, as in cases of ambiguous adjective attachment, for example. In *A blond judo teacher*, the adjective *blond* has semantic constraints that prevent it from being selected as a modifier of *judo*. But syntactic properties are generally independent of semantic properties, so the way words are assigned to grammatical categories cannot be predicted from their form or their meaning alone. One cannot say, for instance, that verbs denote actions and adjectives denote properties: there are stative verbs (*be, remain*) and nouns that denote an action (*destruction, breakage*) or a property (*whiteness, frailty*). But grammatical functions cannot be reduced to semantic properties either (the subject of a sentence is not necessarily the doer of the action) (→ THEMATIC RELATION).

In the view that syntax is autonomous with respect to phonology or morphology (Arnold Zwicky), syntactic rules pertain to abstract properties that may have a given phonological or morphological realization, but they do not bear directly on those realizations. A language can force speakers to employ the nominative case, but it cannot make them begin with a consonant or end with *-us*. Another example is the prenoun positioning of certain adjectives in French (for example, *un gros homme* versus *un homme gros*), which is merely a stylistic preference, not a syntactic rule. Moreover, studying syntactic properties separately has contributed to updating the typology of languages: according to Joseph Greenberg's classification, there are only three major types, SOV, SVO, and VSO (S = subject, O = object, V = verb), since there is no canonical order where the object precedes the subject.

Finally, concerning syntax and formal semantics, following Emil Post logicians began to define formal systems as having a syntax (well-formedness principles governing the propositions of the language) and a semantics (rules for interpreting independent well-formed propositions) (→ INTERPRETATION, LOGIC). In this sense, artificial languages like computer programming languages have a syntax (for example, an *if* must be followed by a *then*). This view of syntax was applied by Chomsky, through his generative grammar, to natural languages. The task of syntax is to describe all grammatical strings (that is, all strings recognized by speakers as belonging to their native language), and no others. One can henceforth conceive of syntactic analysis as an algorithm that starts from any combination of words in the language, determines whether or not it is well-formed, and assigns it as many syntactic descriptions as there are ways of obtaining it from the rules of the system. A sentence that is assigned more than one parsing is said to be syntactically ambiguous, as in *I can see the wife of the man sitting in the yard*, where the relative clause *[who is] sitting in the yard* can be attached to the noun *wife* or to the noun *man*. Computations of this type are the true basis of automatic syntactic analysis programs.

ANNE ABEILLÉ

SELECTED BIBLIOGRAPHY

Baltin, M., & Collins, C. (Eds.) (2001). *Handbook of contemporary syntactic theory*. Malden, MA: Blackwell.

Carnap, R. (1937). *Logical syntax of language*. London: Routledge and Kegan Paul.

Carnie, A. (2002). *Syntax: A generative introduction*. Malden, MA: Blackwell.

Chomsky, N. (1969). *Aspects of the theory of syntax*. Cambridge, MA: Harvard University Press.

Chomsky, N. (1995). *The minimalist program*. Cambridge, MA: MIT Press.

Fodor, J. (1975). *The language of thought*. New York: Crowell.

Greenberg, J. (Ed.). (1966). *Universals of language*. Cambridge, MA: MIT Press.

Radford, A. (1997). *Syntax: A minimalist introduction*. Cambridge, England; New York: Cambridge University Press.

Tesnière, L. (1959). *Éléments de syntaxe structurale* [Elements of structural syntax]. Paris: Klincksieck.

T

TEXT

Psychology. — Text comprehension and text production can legitimately be approached jointly because performance on these two activities is highly correlated (with a shared variance of more than 40 percent). Furthermore, from the standpoint of cognitive psychology, both can be modeled as a system of interrelated components (conceptual, textual, syntactic, lexical, perceptual-motor, and motor; → ACTION, CONCEPT, LEXICON, PERCEPTION, SYNTAX), each of which is thought to implement processes specific to a given type of representation (→ REPRESENTATION). In the study of both comprehension and production, the psychologist's task is first to define these components and determine their architecture (i.e., organization and processing mode), and then to look into how they function (in serial or in parallel, top-down or bottom-up information flow, etc.; → INFORMATION) and what constraints they must satisfy (limited processing capacity; → ATTENTION, CONTROL, MEMORY).

For Walter Kintsch and Teun van Dijk, and for Charles Perfetti as well, comprehension during listening and reading (→ LANGUAGE, READING) is achieved via word-by-word and sentence-by-sentence processing (and, as the case may be, paragraph-by-paragraph processing) aimed at constructing an integrated mental representation for interpreting literal information in accordance with the listener's or reader's prior knowledge (→ INTERPRETATION). This interpretation is oriented by the goal set for the discourse or text at hand (→ DISCOURSE). It is built from explicit lexical information organized into sentences, which are arranged in turn to form texts with different structures and constraints (narratives, scientific articles, user's manuals, etc.). The words and their arrangement activate concepts and concept relations in memory (the concepts and concept relations together forming a schema for a given domain). As Morton Ann Gernsbacher showed, some of these concepts and relations are irrelevant and have to be inhibited (→ ACTIVATION/INHIBITION). The relevant ones are activated and become the building blocks of original mental structures, or *mental models*, as Philip Johnson-Laird called them (→ REASONING AND RATIONALITY). This construction process is achieved by means of *inferences* that activate information that is not explicitly stated. The inferences may be *anaphoric*—in which case they serve to determine whether certain words in the succession of sentences refer to the same or different entities—or they may be *causal*—in which case they connect events or states by linking causes to effects (→ CAUSALITY AND MENTAL CAUSATION). Inferred information is combined with stated information to form an organized sequence of chunks that is gradually incorporated into the overall representation. This structuring process takes place under severe capacity constraints that may hinder understanding when the processing load is too great. Specific *markers* (such as connectives and punctuation marks) can be used to trigger processes like parsing, integration, inference making, and/or inhibition. Knowledge of these markers helps the reader or listener implement the right processes at the right times, and this can at least partly reduce the risk of cognitive overload.

In line with John Hayes and Linda Flower's view, text production begins with the elaboration of a more or less complete, overall mental representation. This representation is then submitted to the sentence-generation process, which takes place in accordance with the goal set by the author of the message. These two processes are contingent upon the author's conceptual knowledge, linguistic knowledge (lexicon, syntax), rhetorical knowledge (text structures), mastery of the oral (studied in particular by Willem Levelt) or written production modality, and knowledge of the addressee (→ COMMUNICATION, ORAL, SOCIAL COGNITION). Here again, the different operations are constrained by limitations in the speaker's or writer's processing capacity. The same individual will attain different performance levels depending on the production situation (more or less conducive to direct interactions; → INTERACTION) and on his or her knowledge of the domain (→ DOMAIN SPECIFICITY), mastery of text structures, and relationship to the addressee.

MICHEL FAYOL

SELECTED BIBLIOGRAPHY

Barthes, R. (1977). *Image, music, text* (S. Heath, Trans). New York: Hill & Wang.

Costermans, J., & Fayol, M. (Eds.). (1997). *Processing interclausal relationships in the production and comprehension of texts*. Hillsdale, NJ: Erlbaum.

Gernsbacher, M. A (1994). *Handbook of psycholinguistics*. San Diego, CA: Academic Press.

Johnson-Laird, P. (1983). *Mental models*. Cambridge, MA: Harvard University Press.

Kintsch, W. (1998). *Comprehension: A paradigm for cognition*. Cambridge, England; New York: Cambridge University Press.

Le Ny, J.-F., & Kintsch, W. (Eds.). (1982). *Language and comprehension*. Amsterdam; New York: North-Holland.

Levelt, W. (1989). *Speaking: From intention to articulation*. Cambridge, MA: MIT Press.

Perfetti, C., Britt, M. A., & Georgi, M. (1995). *Text-based learning and reasoning*. Hillsdale, NJ: Erlbaum.

Perfetti, C., Rieben, L., & Fayol, M. (1997). *Learning to spell: Research, theory, and practice across languages*. Hillsdale, NJ: Erlbaum.

Rastier, F. (1997). *Meaning and textuality* (F. Collins & P. Perron, Trans.). Toronto, Ontario; Buffalo, NY: University of Toronto Press.

THEMATIC RELATION

Linguistics. — The term *thematic relation* refers to the connection between a verbal *predicate* and each of its *arguments* (or *actants*, in Lucien Tesnière's terminology). Each actant assumes a specific role in the predication. Apart from the particular usage of the term *actant* in Algirdas-Julien Greimas's semiotics (→ SEMIOTICS), Tesnière's theory (presented in his book on structural syntax), whose principal assumptions will be presented here, laid the foundation for several lines of research in linguistics and cognitive science.

Tesniere's syntactic dependency theory is based on a general principle of syntactic structure (→ SYNTAX) applicable to phrases whose head belongs to one of the four major parts of speech: verb, noun, adjective, and adverb. The head of a phrase is the *governor*, to which one or more subordinates is attached, either directly or after a *translation* (change of category) (→ CATEGORIZATION). The link between the governor and the governee is both structural and semantic (→ SEMANTICS): the structural link goes from the governee to the governor; the semantic link goes in the opposite direction. Thus, a noun head can have determiners and adjectival phrases as its subordinates, but also prepositional phrases derived by translation from noun phrases, relative clauses or noun phrases, and infinitive or participle phrases derived by translation from a verb phrase.

The subordinates of a verb phrase are subdivided into actants (including the grammatical subject) and *circonstants*. Actants are attached to the verb by one of the following relations: subject (first argument), direct object (second argument), or indirect object (third argument), or, in languages with case marking, by a case with an actant function (→ FUNCTION). The maximum number of arguments a verb can take on is its *valency*, but some argument slots may not be filled.

However, the hypothesized concordance between structural link and semantic incidence put Tesnière in a problematic situation in several cases. The three types of actants are semantically likened to the primary functions of the nominative, accusative, and dative cases in Latin. Because of this, the subordinates introduced in Latin by a genitive or ablative marker have an a priori circumstantial function. For instance, in French, subordinates introduced by *à* (at, to) are third arguments insofar as their semantic function is like that of a dative, and subordinates introduced by *de* (of) are never actants because they are usually seen as ablatives. Take the French sentences *Jean achète une voiture à Paul* (literally, *Jean buys a car at Paul*) and *Alfred change de veste* (literally, *Alfred changes of jacket*). The constituents *à Paul* and *de veste*, manifestly governed by the verb, are seen as circonstants. Inversely, certain circonstants in French can occur without a preposition, as in *Il travaille la nuit et dort le jour* (literally, *He works the night and sleeps the day*).

Nonetheless, when integrated by Igor Mel'chuk into his meaning-text model at the two levels of syntax, deep and surface, Tesnière's theory opened up three main lines of research (→ MEANING AND SIGNIFICATION). The first deals with the distinction between actants and circonstants. This approach was taken up in Germany, where in 1969 Gerhard Helbig and Wolfgang Schenkel published a sketch of the first short dictionary of German verb valency. Valency theory was then applied to Latin by Heinz Happ, at the same time as it was utilized for French by Winfried Busse, who with Jean-Paul Dubost soon published a very comprehensive valency lexicon of French verbs at the macro- and microstructural levels (→ LEXICON). In all of this work, the distinction between actants and circonstants is generally made using deletion and moving tests, but because of the intermediate category of optional actants (e.g., *I hear someone/something/*), thematic relations must also be interpreted semantically (→ INTERPRETATION). The basic difference from Tesnière's theory is that all local directive subordinates (places of origin, passage, and destination) occupy a specific, intermediate position between actants and circonstants.

The second, most prevalent line of research focuses on the semantic characterization of verb arguments. There seem to be two tendencies, one more linguistic and the other more computational and/or cognitive. Linguists have proposed various case grammars (→ GRAMMAR). Some investigators (Jerome Gruber, John Anderson, and Ray Jackendoff) defend the localistic hypothesis, according to which local thematic relations are conceptually primary. In 1981 thematic roles were integrated into Noam Chomsky's generative grammar as a module of their own (→ MODULARITY), also known under the name *argument structure* (Joan Grimshaw). In the typology of languages, many researchers strive to classify the case-marking systems of languages on the basis of thematic role (Gilbert Lazard and Gisa Rauh). One of the fruits of this research is Hansjakob Seiler's participation theory. The idea of a participant is useful for comparing languages with and without case marking while incorporating the morphological, syntactic, semantic, and speaker-related properties of thematic relations (→ MORPHOLOGY).

In artificial intelligence (AI) and in cognitive science, thematic relations appear either directly in the labels given to the arcs of semantic or conceptual networks (→ SEMANTIC NETWORK) (e.g., agent, object, recipient, origin, etc.) or indirectly in the breakdown of complex predications into primary relations (e.g., change, cause, act), as in theories like Roger Schank's conceptual dependency theory and Jackendoff's lexicoconceptual representation theory (which is localistic in inspiration) (→ CONCEPT, REPRESENTATION). In cognitive semantics, a method of the former type is Walter Kintsch and Jean-François Le Ny's text processing by predicate analysis (→ PROPOSITIONAL FORMAT, TEXT); some methods of the latter type are Charles Fillmore's semantics of scenes and frames, Leonard Talmy's theory of the interplay of antagonistic forces in representations of events and actions (→ ACTION), and Jean-Pierre Desclés's inventory of cognitive archetypes. David Dowty's prototype semantics is also used to approach thematic relations, for many predicative frames are hybrid variants of the prototypical agent and patient roles.

The third line of research looks at the interdependency between the properties of thematic relations and the properties of aspect in predication (→ ASPECT). This interdependency, which is studied within a functional-linguistic framework by Simon Dik, and from a cognitive perspective by Jacques François and Guy Denhière, has been demonstrated by many studies in descriptive and general linguistics—for example, for Malay-Indonesia languages (Alain Lemarechal) and Hindi (Annie Montaut).

The concept of thematic relation has thus proven useful not only in descriptive linguistics and language typology, but also in theoretical and computational linguistics, psycholinguistics applied to text processing, and artificial intelligence. Its success outside of linguistics per se can be explained by its use of the logical concepts *function* and *argument* (→ LOGIC). For example, Dik's recent model of functional grammar merges various elements from research based on Tesnière's work: in a formal predicate logic enriched by the introduction of operators at different levels, Dik distinguishes *core predication*—where the arguments are linked to the (usually) verbal predicate by thematic relations—from *extended predication*, which takes the "satellites" of different semantic types into account.

JACQUES FRANÇOIS

SELECTED BIBLIOGRAPHY

Anderson, J. (1971). *The grammar of case: Towards a localistic theory*. Cambridge, England: Cambridge University Press.

Lazard, G. (1998). *Actancy* (Trans.). Berlin, Germany; New York: Mouton de Guyter. (Original work pubished 1994.)

Tesnière, L. *Éléments de syntaxe structurale* [Elements of structural syntax]. Paris: Klincksieck, 1959.

Wilkins, W. (Ed.). (1988). *Thematic relations*. San Diego, CA: Academic Press.

THEORY OF MIND

Psychology. — Coined by David Premack and Guy Woodruff in their original article "Does the Chimpanzee Have a Theory of Mind?," the expression *theory of mind* refers to the ability to explain and predict one's own actions and those of other intelligent agents (that is, agents that, unlike physical objects, are the causes of their own actions) (→ ACTION, ANIMAL COGNITION, MIND). The question raised is whether this ability is specifically human, as the title of the above article suggests. A more recent issue concerns the possible lack of a theory of mind in certain humans, as suggested by Simon Baron-Cohen, Alan Leslie, and Uta Frith in their famous article "Does the Autistic Child Have a Theory of Mind?" (→ AUTISM).

For these authors, understanding behaviors implies being able to infer that behaviors are induced by mental states, which in turn implies having a theory of mind (→ CAUSALITY AND MENTAL CAUSATION)—"theory" because it supports predictions for testing hypotheses about inobservables, theory of mind because the inferred inobservables are mental states. Only in this strict sense could the expression *theory of mind* be defined. In fact, this definition has become but one theoretical position among others and is now contributing to the heated debate about what "methodology" enables us to foresee and predict behaviors.

Two major research trends take opposing positions on this issue. In the first, which remains faithful to Premack and Woodruff's definition, the methodology we use to understand and predict behavior is subtended by a naive psychological theory about the structure and functioning of the mind; this theory activates a set of rules for manipulating symbols based on inference making (→ REASONING AND RATIONALITY, SYMBOL). We make use of this naive psychological theory in our social interactions (→ COMMUNICATION, INTERACTION, SOCIAL COGNITION), just as we apply the principles of naive physics to our everyday interactions with objects. In other words, psychological knowledge is not a special kind of knowledge; it too functions on the basis of a naive epistemology (→ EPISTEMOLOGY). The proponents of this kind of methodology are called *theory-theorists*. They are divided into two factions, depending on their view of the origins of the methodology: *modularist nativists* and *interactionists* of various types (→ MODULARITY).

The second trend postulates the implementation of a *simulationist* type of methodology to explain how we are able to understand and predict intentional behaviors (→ INTENTIONALITY). A simulation-based methodology utilizes motivational and emotional resources (→ EMOTION), along with the individual's practical reasoning skills. As such, it is both a heuristic that requires only a minimal amount of brain activity and a means of gaining access to the range of mental states through simulation of the mental states of others. Here again, the origin of this capacity divides the authors into groups on the basis of whether the mental states inferred and predicted to explain intentional behaviors are *perceptual* (for example, attention, as an indicator of interest), *volitional* (desire), or *epistemic* (knowing that, believing that, thinking that, etc.) (→ ATTENTION, DESIRE, EPISTEMIC, PERCEPTION).

The field of research aimed at explaining this ability—still called *mind reading* by authors hoping to avoid the polysemous expression *theory of mind*—lies at the intersection of several disciplines in cognitive science: philosophy of mind, primatology, linguistics, psychology, and developmental psychopathology.

In developmental psychology (→ COGNITIVE DEVELOPMENT), the expression *theory of mind* often takes on a still broader meaning and refers to the child's understanding of the mind as a representational device (John Flavell, Joseph Perner) (→ METACOGNITION, REPRESENTATION). This view provides the rationale for speaking not of a single theory of mind but of several theories of mind, each corresponding to a different facet or step in the comprehension process, considered as innate and modular—which does not mean that process doesn't have to develop—or as acquired individually or by acculturation (and thus elaborated).

In this approach, three types of tasks are used to find out about children's theories of mind and account for their access to *metarepresentation*, that is, to an understanding of representation as a product of mental activity and not as a mere copy of reality. In visual perspective-taking tasks, access to metarepresentation shows up as the child's ability to grasp the idea that one and the same object can be represented in different ways in subjects who have different percepts. In appearance/reality distinction tasks, access to metarepresentation is attested by the ability to recognize that one's own beliefs can be false because they are the result of a perceptual illusion (→ BELIEF). Finally, belief-attribution tasks test the capacity to resolve conflicts between epistemic propositional content (true vs. false) and epistemic propositional attitudes (*I believe that, I think that, I know that*, etc.) (→ PROPOSITIONAL ATTITUDE). False-belief attribution presupposes reasoning based on the fact that individuals act in accordance with the state of their representations and not in accordance with the state of the world (*I may believe that something is true when it is in fact false*). Convergent findings ground the idea that children begin to master metarepresentation between the ages of 4 and 5 years, probably within a task-dependent developmental hierarchy.

JACQUELINE NADEL AND ANNE-MARIE MELOT

SELECTED BIBLIOGRAPHY

Astington, J. (1993). *The child's discovery of the mind*. Cambridge, MA: Harvard University Press.

Astington, J., Harris, P., & Olson, D. (Eds.). (1988). *Developing theories of mind*. Cambridge, England; New York: Cambridge University Press.

Baron-Cohen, S., Leslie, A., & Frith, U. (1985). Does the autistic child have a "theory of mind"? *Cognition, 21*, 37–46.

Bartsh, K., & Wellman, H. (1995). *Children talk about the mind.* New York: Oxford University Press.

Gallagher, H., & Frith, C. (2003). Functional imaging of theory of mind. *Trends in Cognitive Sciences, 7*, 77–83.

Gopnik, A., Meltzoff, A., & Kuhl, P. (1999). *The scientist in the crib: Minds, brains, and how children learn.* New York: William Morrow.

Meltzoff, A., & Gopnik, A. (1997). *Words, thoughts, and theories.* Cambridge, MA: MIT Press.

Mitchell, P. (1996). *Introduction to theory of mind: Children, autism and apes.* New York; London: Arnold.

Mitchell, P., & Riggs, K. (Eds.). (2000). *Children's reasoning and the mind.* Hove, England: Psychology Press.

Perner, J. (1991). *Understanding the representational mind.* Cambridge, MA: MIT Press.

Premack, D., & Woodruff, G. (1978). Does the chimpanzee have a theory of mind? *Behavioral and Brain Sciences, 1*, 513–526.

Wellman, H. (1990). *The child's theory of mind.* Cambridge, MA: MIT Press.

Wimmer, H., & Perner, J. (1983). Beliefs about beliefs: Representation and constraining function of wrong beliefs in young children's understanding of deception. *Cognition, 13*, 103–128.

TIME AND TENSE

Psychology. — There is not a single domain of knowledge that is unrelated to time. Yet all attempts to define it have been in vain, so varied are its facets. A testimony to the complexity of time is the diversity of ways it has been approached in psychology. To mention only a few, we find studies on the concepts of past, present, and future; studies on memory for events and the temporal organization of memories; ontogenetic research on the development of temporal concepts like duration and succession; and analyses of reasoning processes whenever space or speed is involved (following the pioneering work by Jean Piaget) (→ COGNITIVE DEVELOPMENT, MEMORY, SPACE). One question, though, has always headed the list of important issues in the psychology of time: the relationship between *objective time* and *subjective time*. Humans have devised increasingly accurate systems for measuring time, but the subjective assessment of duration still raises many questions. Time is not directly perceivable—indeed, none of our five senses is capable of perceiving it (→ PERCEPTION).

Right from the very beginning of scientific psychology, many psychophysics studies were conducted to describe the laws governing the relationship between physical time and perceived time (→ PSYCHOPHYSICS). The effects of various factors were examined, including the nontemporal parameters of stimuli, events that compose or delineate time intervals, subjects' states of alertness and motivation, and so on. After drawing up a synthesis of data collected over a period of fifty or so years, Paul Fraisse argued that time estimation in fact depends on the number of changes perceived. This view has continued to have an unfailing influence, even after the new surge of research on psychological time, with cognitive psychology granting a predominant role to information-processing mechanisms.

Today, there are several theoretical trends that differ by the answer given to a critical question: Is time (parameter *t*) treated as a piece of information per se, that is grasped, encoded, and stored by specific internal mechanisms (→ INFORMATION)? The proponents of internal timer-based models rely on a number of findings, including the fact that human adults are not the only ones to process time. Conditioning studies have revealed that animals are fully able to accurately estimate the duration of their own actions, or the time elapsed between two of their actions (→ ACTION, ANIMAL COGNITION, LEARNING). In addition, human newborns have been shown to very finely discriminate the rhythm and duration of stimuli in their surroundings, particularly the sounds of their language (→ INFANT COGNITION, LANGUAGE). Adults in their daily lives often estimate the duration of their own actions and of external events, without recourse to sophisticated measurement instruments.

The advocates of the opposing position, who refute models of a temporal processor, argue that such models cannot account for the diverse facets of temporal processing in humans (Richard Block). Following Fraisse's line of thinking, they defend the idea that subjective duration depends on how much nontemporal information is processed during the interval whose duration is being estimated. According to Robert Ornstein, the more complex this information is and the more there is of it, the greater the storage size and the longer the subjective duration.

An important step will be taken in validating internal timer models if new functional neuroimaging techniques are able not only to identify its biological substrates, but also to show that they differ from those subtending attention and memory processes (→ ATTENTION, FUNCTIONAL NEUROIMAGING). Even so, this will not answer some of the many other perplexing questions about time that continue to puzzle human beings. As Étienne Klein said, time is not an isolate of thought; it cannot be stripped down.

VIVIANE POUTHAS

Linguistics. — Like some languages (German and Russian) but unlike others (the Romance languages), English has two separate words, *time* and *tense*, to refer respectively to the temporal semantic relation and the morphological phenomenon that marks time in verb conjugations (→ MORPHOLOGY, SEMANTICS), although these two linguistic categories are related in a privileged, albeit complex way. Time as a semantic relation is not the same as cosmic time, of interest in physics, nor is it experienced time, a concern of psychology and phenomenology (see *psychology* above). In linguistics, not only do utterances represent time (as they do space and objects; → OBJECT, SPACE), but temporality is an essential dimension of linguistic representation (→ REPRESENTATION): everything that is said is necessarily situated in time. Utterances sometimes considered to be atemporal (like analytic truths) are simply presented as true all the time.

Linguistic time (tense) is fundamentally deictic: the process (state or event) is situated before (past), at the same time as (present), or after (future) the time of the utterance. The problem then becomes explaining why a language like French offers five tenses (not counting two-auxiliary forms) solely for expressing the past. In an attempt to answer this type of question, grammarians and linguists have gradually added some new distinctions: tense, the time frame that situates the process, is opposed to *aspect*, the time that is internal to the process (→ ASPECT); and *absolute time* (the relationship between the process and the utterance time) is opposed to *relative time* (relative to another moment specified by the context; → CONTEXT AND SITUATION). For example: *He knew* (absolute time: past) *that he would come* (relative time: later); *He found out* (absolute time: past) *that she had walked across the lawn* (relative time: earlier).

The next thing to determine is the nature and properties of the moment relative to which a process or event is situated. Hans Reichenbach's tense theory is generally used as a framework or starting point for analyzing such phenomena. In addition to *event time* (denoted E) and *speech time* (S) (an opposition that can only be used to describe three absolute temporal relations), Reichenbach defined *reference time* (R), which, when combined with E and S, accounts for relative time. For example: *Her work was finished* ($R = E < S$), *Her work has been finished for two hours* ($E < R = S$), and *Her work had been finished for two hours* ($E < R < S$). The complement [*for* + duration] measures the distance between E and R; it is thus incompatible with the preterite (**Her work was finished for two hours;* the asterisk indicates an ungrammatical sequence).

Recent developments of this model include the study of the mechanisms used to identify the reference time in a narration (the progression of narrative time), and the change from *points* to *intervals* for representing the three times (E, R, and S). Hans Kamp and Christian Rohrer attempted to explain chronological relationships between events in narrative text in terms of the reference time (→ TEXT). Typically, the simple past or preterite introduces a past event that constitutes the text's reference point; each new statement in the preterite moves the point of reference forward by one step (*succession effect*), whereas the imperfect presents a past state that encompasses the current point of reference, introduced by the last sentence in the preterite (*simultaneity effect*). However, many counterexamples that bring to bear pragmatic and encyclopedic knowledge have been forwarded to show that verb tense does not always work in the typical way (→ PRAGMATICS). For instance, in the sequence *The policemen arrested Luc; he was driving too fast*, the imperfect cannot express exact simultaneity with respect to the reference point introduced by the first sentence. In this case, it marks immediate precedence.

The use of intervals instead of Reichenbach's points led to new developments (in the models proposed by Wolfgang Klein and Laurent Gosselin) that cast serious doubt on linguistic analyses of tense. (1) The *reference interval* (called *topic time* by Klein) corresponds to that part of the event taken into account in the utterance (and thus, that which is declared if the sentence is declarative). (2) The relationship between the reference interval and the *event interval* defines the grammatical aspect (→ GRAMMAR). For example, the preterite (perfective) makes the two intervals exactly coincide, whereas in the imperfect (imperfective), the reference interval is included in the event interval (of which neither the beginning nor the end is included): [*for* + duration] thus measures the distance between the beginning of the event and the beginning of the reference interval, as in *He had been walking for two hours*. (3) Absolute time no longer follows from the relationship between the event and the utterance time, but between the reference interval and the speech interval: in *When I looked through the door, the baby was sleeping*, the imperfect expresses the past in that it situates the reference interval as prior to the utterance, but nothing indicates that the event is currently over (simply because the reference interval is included in the event interval). (4) Likewise, relative time is determined by the relationship between two reference intervals (belonging to two different statements) and not directly between the events themselves. For example, in *Marie thought he would come*, nothing prevents the two events from being partially concomitant. (5) An adverbial of time that is a syntactic part of the verb phrase locates the event interval (→ SYNTAX), whereas a detached adverbial pertains to the reference interval (as in *At eight o'clock, he was sleeping*).

In semantic analysis (→ SEMANTICS), calculating temporal relations from syntactic and lexical markers in the text poses the problem of how to treat the contextual polysemy of markers and the holistic linguistic meaning (that is, the impact of the text's overall meaning on the meaning of its parts) (→ HOLISM, LEXICON, MEANING AND SIGNIFICATION). The same tense can indicate various temporal relations (in addition to aspectual and modal ones; → MODALITY), depending on the context in which it occurs, which itself is defined by markers that are often polysemous as well. To arrive at satisfactory representations of time, then, one must take a holistic approach to figuring out the temporal meaning of sentences, one that considers the interactions among the various polysemous markers in the text.

LAURENT GOSSELIN

SELECTED BIBLIOGRAPHY

Aschersleben, G., Bachmann, T., & Musseler, J. (Eds.). (1999). *Cognitive contributions to the perception of spatial and temporal events*. Amsterdam; New York: Elsevier.

Block, R. A. (1990). *Cognitive models of psychological time*. Hillsdale, NJ: Erlbaum.

Buzsáki, G., Llinas, R., Singer, W., Berthoz, A., & Christen, Y. (1994). *Temporal coding in the brain*. Berlin, Germany; New York: Springer-Verlag.

Bybee, J., Perkins, R., & Pagliuca, W. (1994). *The evolution of grammar: Tense, aspect, and modality in the languages of the world*. Chicago: University of Chicago Press.

Comrie, B. (1985). *Tense*. Cambridge, England; New York: Cambridge University Press.

Dickey, M. (2001). *The processing of tense: Psycholinguistic studies on the interpretation of tense and temporal relations*. Dordrecht, The Netherlands; Boston: Kluwer.

Fraisse, P. (1963). *The psychology of time* (J. Leith, Trans). New York: Harper & Row; London: Eyre and Spottiswoode. (Original work published 1957.)

Gosselin, L. (1996). *Sémantique de la temporalité en français: Un modèle calculatoire et cognitif du temps et de l'aspect* [The semantics of temporality in French: A computational and cognitive model of tense and aspect]. Louvain-la-Neuve, Belgium: Duculot.

Kamp, H., & Rohrer, C. (1983). Tense in texts. In R. Bauerle, C. Schwarze, & A. von Stechow (Eds.), *Meaning, use and interpretation of language*. Berlin, Germany: De Gruyter.

Klein, W. (1994). *Time in language*. London; New York: Routledge.

Ornstein, R. E. (1969). *On the experience of time*. Hardmondsworth, England: Penguin Books.

Piaget, J. (1969). *The child's conception of time* (A. J. Pomeras, Trans.). New York: Basic Books. (Original work published 1946.)

Reichenbach, H. G. (1947). *Elements of symbolic logic*. New York: Dover.

TRUTH

Philosophy. — Although certain philosophers have taken the concept of truth to be unanalyzable (Gottlob Frege), several types of theories have been set forth. "Substantial" theories define the meaning of the word *true* and describe the nature of potential bearers of the predicate "true." "Modest" theories are confined to specifying the usage conditions of the word, or the extension of the predicate, but not its meaning.

Correspondence theory posits that a proposition (sentence, belief) is true if and only if there exists a fact that corresponds to it and makes it true (Aristotle, Bernard Bolzano, Bertrand Russell) (→ BELIEF, LANGUAGE). A true proposition is supposed to describe the corresponding fact by expressing its structure. In *coherence theory*, truth does not depend upon a relationship between language and reality, but upon a coherence relation between sentences (Keith Lehrer). *Verificationist theory* identifies truth with verifiability: saying that a proposition is true is saying that there is a method for verifying it (Charles Peirce, Michael Dummett). In the *pragmatic theory* of truth, truths are beliefs that are useful in helping us act (William James) (→ ACTION, PRAGMATICS).

Deflationary theories of truth contend that one cannot devise any kind of substantial theory of truth by identifying a particular property of true sentences. Different versions exist. Having noted that the truth value of proposition p is always the same as the truth value of the proposition p *is true*, Frank Ramsey proposed *redundancy theory*: saying that a sentence is true consists simply in repeating what it asserts. Peter Strawson suggested that the predicates "true" and "false" serve to mark agreement or disagreement and should therefore be analyzed as performative utterances. Dummett proposed that the truth of a sentence be interpreted in terms of assertability. Alfred Tarski's *semantic theory* of truth (→ SEMANTICS) defines the concept of "truc in L" (where L is a formal language) as an equivalence between any true sentence and its translation: X is true if and only if p, where X stands for the sentence p. The two expressions X and p are equivalent. This equivalence schema supplies a partial characterization of truth in L (more exactly, the adequacy condition of any definition of "true in L"). Donald Davidson proposed applying this same concept to natural languages: the sentence *Snow is white* is true in English if and only if snow is white. He showed how a theory of meaning could be derived from this kind of theory of truth.

JOËLLE PROUST

SELECTED BIBLIOGRAPHY

Dummett, M. (1978). *Truth and other enigmas*. Oxford, England: Clarendon Press.
Engel, P. (1991). *The norm of truth: An introduction to the philosophy of logic* (M. Kochan & P. Engel, Trans.). Toronto, Ontario; Buffalo, NY: University of Toronto Press.
Horwich, P. (1990). *Truth*. Oxford, England; Cambridge, MA: Blackwell.

TURING MACHINE

Artificial intelligence. — A *Turing machine* is a model (→ MODEL) of computing imagined by the mathematician Alan Turing. It is an extension of the concept of *automaton* (see below): input symbols are recorded on a "tape" and transitions between states cause the "reading head" to move on the tape and, whenever necessary, change the symbols marked on it (→ SYMBOL). It would be pointless to actually build such a device, since the model cannot be used to perform practical computations. Nevertheless, the theoretical possibility of building one has played an important role in demonstrating the computability of many classes of problems.

The mathematical object studied in automaton theory is an abstraction of the physical idea of an automaton. It is described by a discrete set of states containing an initial state and a set of final states, along with a law that governs how the automaton will evolve when given a discrete flow of symbols. The law is represented by a state table that, for each state and for each symbol, gives either the unique next state (deterministic case) or the set of possible next states (nondeterministic case), which may potentially be a probabilistic set (*stochastic automaton*).

DANIEL KAYSER

SELECTED BIBLIOGRAPHY

Copeland, J. (2003). Turing, Alan. In L. Nadel (Ed.), *The encyclopedia of cognitive science* (Vol. 4, pp. 427–430). London: Nature Publishing Group, Macmillan.

Davis, M. (2000). *The universal computer: The road from Leibniz to Turing*. New York: Norton.

Hodges, A. (1983). *Alan Turing: The enigma*. New York: Simon and Schuster.

Millican, P., & Clark, A. (Eds.). (1996). *The legacy of Alan Turing*. Oxford, England: Clarendon Press; New York: Oxford University Press.

Turing, A. M. (1992). *Collected works of A. M. Turing: Mechanical intelligence* (D. C. Ince, Ed.). Amsterdam; New York: North-Holland.

TYPE/TOKEN

Philosophy. — Since the American philosopher and logician Charles Peirce, an occurrence of a sign has been called a *token* and the sign itself has been called a *type* (→ SIGN). In the sentence *The cat is on the mat*, which contains six words, the word *the* occurs twice, in first and fifth positions. The two *the*'s are two numerically distinct tokens of the same word type. The whole sentence can also be considered as a type or a token: every time someone utters the sentence *The cat is on the mat*, the utterance is a new token of this sentence type (see *linguistics* below).

The type/token distinction, a critical one in semantics (→ SEMANTICS), was imported into the philosophy of mind (like many other distinctions or concepts borrowed from the philosophy of language) (→ LANGUAGE, MIND). Accordingly, one often distinguishes between types and tokens of mental states. This distinction is the foundation of a well-known version of materialism, *token physicalism* (→ PHYSICALISM). In token physicalism, it is contended that the identity between mental states and physical states of the brain can be established only at the token level: every token of a mental state is a token of a brain state, but one cannot reduce a mental-state type to a brain-state type (→ REDUCTIONISM).

FRANÇOIS RECANATI

Linguistics. — Linguistic types and tokens do not have the same status, since types pertain to language (competence) and tokens pertain to discourse (performance) (→ COMPETENCE/PERFORMANCE, DISCOURSE, LANGUAGE). The distinction between type and token can be studied at three levels of linguistic description.

At the word level, this distinction separates a canonical expression from its graphic or phonic variants, on the one hand, and its conventional meaning from its contextual variations, on the other (→ CONTEXT AND SITUATION, MEANING AND SIGNIFICATION); to account for the relationship between meaning as a type and particular acceptations in context, cognitive semantics borrowed from psychology the concept of *prototype* (→ CATEGORIZATION, SEMANTICS). At the sentence level, the type/token opposition separates the sentence as a type, capable of being interpreted literally, from the utterance, which can have derived interpretations (for example, the interpretation

Close the window for the sentence *It's cold in here*) (→ INTERPRETATION); this distinction hinges on pragmatic considerations (→ PRAGMATICS). Finally, at the text level, text genres are types, and particular texts are tokens (→ TEXT). Note, however, that cognitive linguistics has not yet really studied the problem of genres. Comprehension frames, which are analyzed in cognitive psychology, are only indirectly related to this problem.

FRANÇOIS RASTIER

SELECTED BIBLIOGRAPHY

Hutton, C. (1990). *Abstraction and instance: The type-token relation in linguistic theory.* Oxford, England; New York: Pergamon Press.

Jackson, F., Pargetter, R., & Prior, E. (1982). Functionalism and type-type identity theories. *Philosophical Studies, 42*, 209–225.

Peirce, C. (1992). *The essential Peirce: Selected philosophical writings, 1893–1913* (N. Houser & C. Kloesel, Eds.). Bloomington, IN: Indiana University Press.

V

VALIDATION

Philosophy. — *Validation* is a type of method used for justifying the statements of a science (→ EPISTEMOLOGY). Validation in the formal sciences can be distinguished from validation in the empirical sciences. In the formal sciences, *demonstration* is the validity criterion: a proposition capable of being validated is a proposition capable of being demonstrated, that is, derivable in an axiomatic system (→ LOGIC). In the empirical sciences, a proposition to be validated must be *deducible* from a general law (with initial conditions); in addition, it must be *testable* by means of an experimental test that does not presuppose its own truth (→ EXPERIENCE, TRUTH). This type of validation is called *hypotheticodeductive* (→ REASONING AND RATIONALITY). A proposition can be confirmed or rejected on this basis. But as Karl Popper showed, it cannot, strictly speaking, be verified because a true consequence can follow from false premises. A proposition that cannot be validated in any manner has no informative content, even if in some cases it can be granted a heuristic value.

JOËLLE PROUST

Artificial intelligence. — Like any other software system, a *knowledge-based system*, or KBS (→ KNOWLEDGE BASE) must be validated in order to guarantee that it correctly solves the problems for which it was designed (→ PROBLEM SOLVING). A characteristic of knowledge-based systems is that the knowledge they process is specific to a given *domain of application* (→ DOMAIN SPECIFICITY). This knowledge is represented in the knowledge base and is separate from the procedures that use it. Thus, validating a KBS basically amounts to validating its knowledge base. A complete validation requires ensuring the perfect fit between the knowledge represented in the KBS and the real knowledge of an expert in the domain. Achieving such a validation is in fact impossible, because all formalizations of reality are by nature reductive.

There are two main approaches to KBS validation: *testing*, and *verification of properties* of the knowledge base. Testing entails comparing the output of the KBS with the results obtained by a domain expert on all problems in the test set. In cases of disagreement between the expert and the KBS, the problem that arises is how to single out the cause of the discrepancy in the knowledge base. To do this, one can make use of the KBS's explanatory capabilities (→ EXPLANATION), for instance, by presenting the expert with a history of the sequence of rules that led to the KBS output. An important problem in attaining a high-quality validation by testing is being able to guarantee that the test problem set is representative. This is possible if a list of the problems that constitute the basic expertise in the domain under study has been compiled, as is often the case in medicine, for example, where files on treated patients supply a collection of particular problems describing that field of expertise. The results of a validation by testing are difficult to evaluate, given that the criterion for KBS success is relative. In particular, the success rate should be compared with the percentage of test cases upon which different domain experts agree.

Automatic verification of certain properties of a knowledge base is another side of KBS validation. The general idea is to see how the formal properties of the knowledge representation (in the formalism chosen for encoding the data) might reflect certain abnormalities or on the contrary certain qualities of the knowledge in the KBS (→ REPRESENTATION). Once these properties are defined, one can look into how they can be verified automatically and then design the verification algorithms. For example, if the knowledge base is a set of rules, one might be interested in detecting flaws like the presence of redundant or conflicting rules. More general properties of the knowledge base, such as *consistency* and completeness, can also be formally defined. Intuitively, a knowledge base is consistent if, for all correct input, none of the results inferred from the data in the knowledge base is contradictory. This problem has been studied and formalized for knowledge bases expressed in logical-rule format (→ LOGIC). Correct input is formalized as sets of facts that satisfy certain integrity constraints representing the semantic constraints of the domain (→ CONSTRAINT, SEMANTICS). Different automatic tools for verifying knowledge base consistency have been developed in conjunction with particular formal knowledge-representation systems.

Compiling a knowledge base can be seen as an incremental modeling process (→ MODEL) that supplies a series of increasingly accurate models, starting from an analysis model and finishing with an operational model (the final knowledge base). Once defined, the successive models must be validated, and the consistency of the processes that transform the models must be guaranteed.

MARIE-CHRISTINE ROUSSET

SELECTED BIBLIOGRAPHY

Granger, G. (1983). *Formal thought and the sciences of man* (Trans.). Dordrecht, The Netherlands; Boston: Reidel. (Original work published 1960.)

Popper, K. (1959). *The logic of scientific discovery* (Trans.). London: Hutchinson; New York: Harper & Row. (Original work published 1935.)

Vermesan, A., & Coenen, F. (Eds.). (1999). *Validation and verification of knowledge based systems: Theory, tools and practice.* Boston: Kluwer.

W

WILL

Philosophy. — The concept of will generally refers to a psychological phenomenon that is often difficult to distinguish from desire and intention; it is conceived of as a mental event (a volition) within an agent, and is a determinant of his or her actions (→ ACTION, DESIRE, THEORY OF MIND). In this sense, it can either be seen from a *dualist* angle, as a mental cause that is separate from the physical effects it produces (→ CAUSALITY AND MENTAL CAUSATION, DUALISM/MONISM), or from a *materialist* angle, as being identical to a brain event that causes a series of physical events (→ PHYSICALISM). But if a will is an inner mental event (physical or nonphysical), does it follow that the action begins when that event occurs, in such a way that to do *A*, an agent need only have the will to do *A?* Trying to do *A* is not doing *A*. To get around this aporia, some philosophers, such as Elizabeth Anscombe, argue that the terms *willful* and *intentional* when qualifying an action do not refer to any particular mental event, but to a complex set of psychological attitudes (in particular, desires and beliefs; → BELIEF) and behaviors. However, this conception runs up against a problem: in practical reasoning and in intentional actions (→ REASONING AND RATIONALITY), there indeed seem to be distinct psychological events, identifiable with intentions or volitions, that cause actions.

PASCAL ENGEL

SELECTED BIBLIOGRAPHY

Anscombe, G. E. M. (1957). *Intention*. Ithaca, NY: Cornell University Press; Oxford, England: Blackwell.
O'Shaughnessy, B. (1980). *The will: A dual aspect theory*. Cambridge, England; New York: Cambridge University Press.

WRITING

Psychology. — Writing is a complex activity involving cognitive processes like spelling and text production, which are studied in psycholinguistics, and motor processes (→ ACTION, LANGUAGE). Only writing as a movement is defined here.

Viewed as a motor task, writing involves producing sequences of graphic symbols (letters, numbers) that correspond to predefined spatial forms (production of *morphokineses*, to use the terminology of Jacques Paillard) while following a set of conventional rules, such as progressing from left to right in our alphabetic system (production of *topokineses*, again according to Paillard) (→ SPACE, SYMBOL). For normal-sized writing, the morphokinetic component is ensured by distal motricity (fingers, wrist) and requires a proactive type of movement control (anticipatory) specific to automated movements (→ AUTOMATISM, CONTROL). Wrist movements produce lateral oscillations along a nearly rectilinear x' axis; finger movements generate front-back oscillations on a y' axis more or less parallel to the axis of the hand. One can understand why certain peripheral models (John Hollerbach) consider writing to result from the coordinated coupling of two orthogonal oscillation systems, one responsible for the pen's horizontal movements in the graphic space, and the other, for its vertical movements. Letter writing is known to be governed by certain invariant principles (Paolo Viviani, Carlo Terzuolo) such as *spatial homothety* and *temporal homothety*, which stipulate that the size and duration ratios of the strokes in a letter (a stroke being defined as the part of the trajectory that falls between two speed minima) are maintained across variations in the letter's size and execution time, respectively (→ TIME AND TENSE). Local covariation of space and time, called the *isogony principle*, has also been demonstrated. This principle stipulates that angular speed remains constant across variations in the trajectory's curve radius. Greater stability in the spatial aspects of writing than in its temporal aspects has often been reported, so it is hypothesized that the spatial encoding of letters is a central process. Some authors consider *allographs* (specific spatial representations of a grapheme, such as lowercase and uppercase; → REPRESENTATION) to be a good candidate for the unit that gets stored centrally (Hans-Leo Teulings, Arnold Thomassen). Much less studied, the topokinetic component of writing relies on proximal motricity (elbow, shoulder). It is responsible for translation movements along the horizontal axis, and is controlled by movement feedback (mostly visual). Many arguments, especially neuropsychological ones (→ NEUROPSYCHOLOGY), have been set forth to support the independence of the morpho- and topokinetic components of writing (Andrew Ellis).

Given that writing is a slow-speed, serial activity (two or three letters per second), central models of writing (Gerard van Galen, Lambert Schomaker) have proposed hierarchical *modular architectures* (with independent production steps, for example, letter format programming, followed by size and speed parameterization) that function almost entirely in parallel (→ COMPUTATIONAL ANALYSIS, MODULARITY). This framework is used to study the effects of different linguistic and nonlinguistic variables, both word-related and letter-related (frequency, regularity, length, position, etc.), on written production (reaction time, movement time, size, speed, acceleration, etc.). Finally, a large number of *computational approaches* to writing have been described in the literature. Some of the issues studied are kinetic and/or kinematic control of movements in the task space (Anatol Feldman, Tamar Flash, Pietro Morasso), in the joint space (Stephen Grossberg, Rund Meulenbroek, David Rosenbaum), or relating to antagonistic muscle units (Réjean Plamondon). A yet unanswered question concerns how the different activities taking place at these various levels are coordinated.

ANNE VINTER

Neuroscience. — Until sometime in the 1980s, neuropsychologists believed that a writing disorder (*agraphia*) following brain damage could not exist on its own (→ NEUROPSYCHOLOGY). They contended that writing could be affected only in association with other deficits such as speech impairments (→ LANGUAGE, ORAL). Certain authors argued that writing demands a considerable amount of attention (→ ACTION, ATTENTION) and should therefore be more readily perturbed in brain-damaged patients with a confusional disorder. This "fragility" also shows up in the fact that agraphia is frequently observed at the onset of dementia (as in Alzheimer's disease; → AGING). Since the 1980s, many cases of isolated agraphia without other deficits have been described. They are currently classified into several different syndromes. *Central agraphia* includes impairment of the lexical processes responsible for irregular or ambiguous word writing (*lexical agraphia;* → LEXICON) or of the phonological conversion processes in charge of writing dictated nonsense words via a phoneme-to-grapheme conversion mechanism (*phonological agraphia*). *Deficient memory for graphemes* caused by alterations in the graphemic buffer have also been noted (→ MEMORY). *Peripheral agraphia* mainly affects graphic execution. While strictly spatial disorders like hemineglect rarely cause writing disabilities (→ SPACE), an essentially spatial type of agraphia is found in the classical Gerstmann syndrome. *Praxic difficulties* in producing the strokes that make up letters also exist, but the question of whether this type of impairment should be seen as a separate disorder is still under discussion. The brain lesions that provoke agraphia are almost always situated in the temporoparietal region of the left hemisphere.

Éric Siéroff

SELECTED BIBLIOGRAPHY

Caramazza, A. (Ed.). (1991). *Issues in reading, writing and speaking: A neuropsychological perspective*. Dordrecht, The Netherlands; Boston: Kluwer.

Ellis, A. (1984). *Reading, writing and dyslexia: A cognitive analysis*. Hove, England: Erlbaum.

Schomaker, L., & Van Galen, G. (1996). Computer models of handwriting. In A. Dijkstra & K. de Smedt (Eds.), *Computational psycholinguistic: AI and connectionist models of language processing*. London: Taylor and Francis.

Thomassen, A., & Van Galen, G. (1992). Handwriting as a motor task: Experimentation, modelling and simulation. In J. Summers (Ed.), *Approaches to the study of motor control and learning*. Amsterdam, The Netherlands: Elsevier.

Watt, W. (Ed.). (1994). *Writing systems and cognition: Perspectives from psychology, physiology, linguistics, and semiotics*. Dordrecht, The Netherlands; Boston: Kluwer.

List of Entries

Index